Review of
Radiologic Physics

William F. Sensakovic, PhD, DABR, MRSE (MRSC™)
Telerad Physics Teaching, LLC
Chair, Division of Medical
  Physics
Senior Associate Consultant
Associate Professor
Mayo Clinic Arizona

Walter Huda, PhD
Retired
Stewkley, Bucks,
  United Kingdom

Illustrations by
R. Brad Abrahams, DO, DABR
Interventional and Diagnostic Radiologist
Wayne Radiologists, PA
Goldsboro, North Carolina

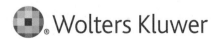 Wolters Kluwer

Philadelphia • Baltimore • New York • London
Buenos Aires • Hong Kong • Sydney • Tokyo

Acquisitions Editor: Nicole Dernoski
Development Editor: Eric McDermott
Editorial Coordinator: Thirupura Sundari
Marketing Manager: Kirsten Watrud
Production Project Manager: Matt West
Manager, Graphic Arts & Design: Steve Druding
Manufacturing Coordinator: Lisa Bowling
Prepress Vendor: TNQ Technologies

5th edition

9 8 7 6 5 4 3 2 1

Printed in Singapore

Library of Congress Cataloging-in-Publication Data

ISBN-13: 978-1-975199-04-3

Cataloging in Publication data available on request from publisher.

---

shop.lww.com

MKO723

To Jennifer, Bohdan, and Evelina who are the joy in my life. To my parents, Joy and Bill, sister, Holly, niece, Aspen, and father-in-law, Larry, who are always so supportive.

– William Sensakovic

To my parents, Stefan and Paraskevia Huda, for their resolute support and encouragement.

– Walter Huda

Ordinary language is totally unsuited for expressing what physics really asserts, since the words of everyday life are not sufficiently abstract. Only mathematics and mathematical logic can say as little as the physicist means to say.

– Bertrand Russell

Preface

This book is focused on imaging using x-rays (i.e., radiography, mammography, fluoroscopy, and CT), as well as nuclear medicine, ultrasound, and MR. The emphasis continues to be on clinically relevant radiologic physics, which relates to information that radiologists and radiologic technologists need to know to perform their clinical duties. Older texts emphasized learning physics facts and equations that enabled residents to pass an examination, but which was generally forgotten once a successful pass result had been obtained. By contrast, the current focus on clinical physics is to provide information that will remain relevant during a radiologist's and radiologic technologist's professional lifetime.

The format of the book is focused on relaying important information in a compact way. The text is bulleted to make information more digestible and less daunting. This is a design choice and means that extensive explanations of why or how are generally not given. The hope is that by keeping information digestible and emphasizing practice questions the book helps the student to make connections between topics and makes it a better companion to lecture and hands-on instruction where focus can be placed on explanations of why and how.

Only essential information is included that will help radiology residents and radiologic technologists understand how images are created, how to alter image quality, as well as the corresponding risks of the radiation used to make these images. Selection of material has been guided by whether the material is necessary to understand three issues: (a) the essentials (but not details) as to how any image is created; (b) aspects that impact on the image quality, and how these aspects can be controlled and optimized; (c) the factors that impact on imaging risks and other imaging costs, and how these characteristics can be minimized without adversely affecting diagnostic information.

Teaching radiologic physics to radiologists may be compared to teaching someone to drive a car, where the minute mechanical details of how internal combustion engines "work" can be safely ignored. Many of the details of radiologic physics are simply irrelevant to the practice of radiology and can therefore be ignored. Examples of irrelevant details include emission of Auger electrons during x-ray interactions, emission of internal conversion electrons during gamma decay, and production of neutrinos and antineutrinos in beta decay. Knowledge of such details is irrelevant to the practice of radiology by radiologists and has therefore been minimized or omitted. Similarly, topics such as shielding design for radiology facilities and understanding how to convert incident radiation into patient organ doses belong to the practice of medical physics, and have been excluded.

Physics is an inherently quantitative discipline that is intimately tied to mathematical equations. However, the mathematical aspects of radiologic physics are neither important nor helpful to imaging practitioners. With few exceptions, mathematical equations are useful only as a compact way to remember relationships that are important (e.g., between dose and tube current). Derivation of equations and knowledge of equations that do not directly relate image quality or dose are not clinically useful for the technologist or resident. Accordingly, equations have generally been removed from the main text, but some have been included for completeness as a separate section at the end of the book.

Although imaging practitioners do not typically need to have a detailed knowledge of quantitative imaging data, they do need to understand why certain numbers are important as well as their approximate magnitude. When the number of photons in nuclear medicine images average no more than about 100 per pixel, the random noise results in interpixel fluctuations of 10% or so and the resultant images will always be mottled unless a way is found to increase the number of photons that create the image. Where medical imaging parameters impact on achievable imaging performance, these have been included, and radiologists and radiologic technologists are expected to have "some idea" of their magnitude. Radiation workers need to know that saying the dose for a chest radiograph is 1 Gy is as ridiculous as saying that the size of a human femur is 25 ft!

Imaging practitioners need to understand why selectable protocol parameters such as tube voltage (kV) and relative output (mAs) are important and what they impact. Reducing the x-ray tube voltage will reduce the x-ray beam penetrating power, increase patient doses when performed using automatic exposure control, and increase subject contrast. Furthermore, the increase in contrast with decreasing tube voltage will be modest for soft-tissue lesions, but large in angiographic studies that use iodinated contrast material. Increasing the x-ray tube current and the corresponding tube output in radiography primarily influences the radiation intensity incident on the image receptor. Quadrupling the mAs will quadruple the radiation at the image receptor, which halves image mottle but does not affect image contrast or spatial resolution performance.

Contents

Introduction

I. RADIOLOGIC PHYSICS

Radiology is the most technology-dependent specialty in medicine, encompassing radiography, fluoroscopy, mammography, computed tomography, magnetic resonance, nuclear medicine, and ultrasound. Radiologic physics provides an understanding of the factors that improve or degrade image quality. It also provides information about the baseline risk of an examination and how that risk changes as factors change. All imaging modalities have a "cost" associated with their use. In MR, the cost might be increased patient heating or decreased patient throughput. For modalities that employ ionizing radiation, one of the "costs" is the radiation dose to the patient and staff working with these systems. Consider a CT examination where radiologists and technologists in a protocol committee need to understand how to specify the type/amount of radiation emerging from a CT scanner, select an appropriate amount for a patient undergoing a defined imaging task, and be able to understand the amount and significance of the radiation received by the patient.

Radiologists and technologists need to understand how to specify the CT output, which can be understood in terms of x-ray beam quantity and quality. The quantity of the x-ray tube output is specified as a volume CT dose index ($CTDI_{vol}$), but details of how $CTDI_{vol}$ is measured are of no importance to imaging practitioners (i.e., radiologists and technologists) and are therefore generally omitted in this book. The quality of the x-ray beam is the penetrating power expressed as an aluminum half-value layer, but the details of how this is measured or calculated are again of no interest to practitioners. What is required is an understanding that increasing the x-ray tube output (i.e., mAs) linearly increases $CTDI_{vol}$, and increasing tube voltage (i.e., kV) increases x-ray beam quality as well as output, and that the latter is supralinear.

Understanding CT x-ray beam quantities and qualities is the prerequisite to ensuring that the appropriate values are selected for use in x-ray beam examinations. Imaging practitioners need to understand the importance of x-ray beam quality because this determines patient penetration, as well as the corresponding CT image contrast. Low tube voltages are essential for angiography and imaging infants, whereas high beam qualities are important to minimize beam hardening artifacts in head CT, and for imaging large patients. The choice of $CTDI_{vol}$ influences image mottle, and imaging practitioners need to know that a routine adult head CT should use a $CTDI_{vol}$ of ~60 mGy. However, use of advanced (iterative) image reconstruction techniques may permit this value to be reduced without adversely impacting on diagnostic performance.

Practitioners are generally provided with information relating to the total amount of radiation used to perform a specific examination. In CT examinations, the dose-length product (DLP) is a measure of the total amount of radiation used to perform the examination and can be used to estimate patient doses and (any) corresponding radiation risks. An adult head

CT scan would likely use a DLP of about 1,000 mGy-cm. The patient effective dose for this type of routine head CT scan will be about 2 mSv, which is less than Americans receive from natural background each year, and a few percent of the current US regulatory annual dose limit for occupational workers. For a 25-year-old adult, the carcinogenic risk from this head CT scan would be less than 0.1%, compared to the 40% background risk of an American contracting cancer in their lifetime. Imaging practitioners must understand risk to identify worthwhile examinations (i.e., benefit > risk), and to convey this information to patients, staff, and referring physicians.

II. REVIEW BOOK STRUCTURE

The text assumes a background of instruction in radiologic physics and is not intended to replace the standard radiologic physics texts. As with previous editions, readers need to understand that this review book does not explain any topic in full detail. Focus is on making physics digestible and understandable but does not get into lengthy explanations of why or how. These kinds of explanations are left to the other instruction that readers undergo in their training. Radiation quantities are generally provided using SI units. An exposure of 1 R can be taken to be equal to an air kerma of 8.76 mGy. In the text, an air kerma of 10 mGy is typically approximated as an exposure of 1 R.

The first third of the book is entitled Foundations and needs to be mastered before residents can progress to the specifics of any imaging modality. The second part of the book is entitled X-ray Imaging Modalities and deals with all the ways in which x-rays can be used to generate images. The final third of the book deals with the Advanced Modalities that have only been developed in the latter part of the 20th century. Each chapter is divided into a few major sections, and each section is divided into a few subsections.

Each chapter is followed by questions designed to provide a self-test of the reader's knowledge and comprehension. The author would expect that any physics teacher would understand why a particular question was being asked, as well as being able to immediately identify the correct answer. In line with the move to teach clinically relevant radiologic physics, the focus of most questions in this book is qualitative, where residents are expected to know that increasing tube voltage will reduce image contrast, and vice versa. The review book also contains two practice examinations with questions that range over all the topics covered in this book.

Because equations have been mostly taken out of the main text, a separate section at the end includes full formulae for completeness. At the end of the book is a glossary of key terms commonly used in radiologic physics. The bibliography has been updated and provides an overview of books aimed at radiology residents as well as radiology technologists. The Appendices contain a summary of SI units, radiologic units, and photometric quantities, as well as a selection of websites relevant to medical imaging.

Foundations

CHAPTER 1

Foundations of Radiological Physics

I. FOUNDATIONAL CONCEPTS

A. Forces and Energy

- **Forces** cause bodies to deviate (push or pull).
  - Electrostatic force causes **protons** (+) and **electrons** (−) to attract each other.
- **Energy** is the ability to do work or cause change, and is measured in **joule (J) or electron volts (eV).**
  - In radiology, heating is typically in J while particle energy is in eV.
- **One electron volt (1 eV)** is the kinetic energy gained by an electron when it is accelerated across an electric potential of 1 volt (V).
  - Several **eV** are required to eject outer shell electrons from atoms.
- An electron gains 1,000 eV (**1 keV**) when accelerated across an electric potential of 1,000 V.
  - Several keV, or tens of keV, are generally required to eject the innermost (K-shell) electrons from atoms.
  - Several MeV (several thousand keV) is required to eject **nuclear particles** (e.g., alpha particles).

B. Electricity and Power

- **Electrons** are negatively charged (−), **protons** are positively charged (+), and **neutrons** have no net charge.
  - A voltage is created between two points by making one area a bit more positive or negative than another area (potential difference).
  - One volt (1 V) is needed to give one electron 1 eV of energy.
- Applying a **voltage** to an electrical circuit causes electrons to move.
  - The **positive region** of an electrical circuit is called the **anode,** and the **negative region** is called the **cathode.**
- Electrons are repelled from the cathode and attracted to the anode.
- **Electric current**, measured in ampere (A), is the flow of electrons through a circuit.
- **Power** is the rate of using energy and is measured in joules per second.
- When the voltage is 1 V and the current is 1 A, electrical power is 1 W.
  - Power of **1 W dissipates 1 joule of energy every second.**
- **X-ray generators** typically use **10 kW to 100 kW** of electrical power.
  - For reference, a typical TV uses tens of watts and a toaster less than 1 kW.
- Energy utilization in making x-rays, however, is relatively low because exposure times are kept short.
  - Energy is Power × Time.
  - **100 ms** is a typical **exposure time** for an abdominal x-ray examination.
  - **Energy is Power × Time; thus, 15 kW × 10 ms = 150 J.**

TABLE 1.1	Atomic and Mass Numbers of Atoms Commonly Found in Human Tissues		
Nucleus	**Protons (Atomic Number [Z])**	**Neutrons**	**Nucleons (Mass Number [A])**
Hydrogen	1	0	1
Carbon	6	6	12
Nitrogen	7	7	14
Oxygen	8	8	16
Calcium	20	20	40

C. Matter

- **Matter** is made up of atoms that contain **protons, neutrons, and electrons.**
- **Protons** have a **positive charge** and are found in the nucleus of atoms.
- The **atomic number (Z)** is the number of protons in the nucleus of an atom and is unique for each element.
- **Neutrons** are electrically **neutral** and are also found in the nucleus.
- The **mass number** (A) is the total number of protons and neutrons in the nucleus (Table 1.1).
- **Electrons** have a **negative charge**, are smaller than protons, and are found in shells around the nucleus.
  - The innermost shell is called the **K-shell (n = 1)**, the next shell the **L-shell (n = 2)**, and so on.
  - The maximum number of electrons in a shell is $2n^2$ and thus 2 electrons for the K-shell.
- The energy required to completely remove (i.e., ionize) an electron from an atom is called the **electron binding energy.**
- Binding energies are unique for each electron shell of each element.
- K-shell binding energies increase with atomic number (Z), as listed in Table 1.2.
- The **outermost electrons** in all atoms have **binding energies of several eV.**
- **Electron density** refers to the number of electrons per cubic centimeter (e/cm^3).
  - Interactions between radiation and matter increase with electron density.
- **As physical density increases, so does electron density**.
  - Electron densities are depicted in Table 1.3.

D. Electromagnetic Radiation

- **Electromagnetic radiation** is both a wave and particle.
- Electromagnetic radiation travels in a straight line at the **speed of light (c).**
- Electromagnetic waves are characterized by a **wavelength, frequency**, and **velocity.**
  - As a wave, it is oscillating electric and magnetic fields.

TABLE 1.2	K-Edge Energies of Atoms Encountered in Radiological Physics		
Element	**Atomic Number (Z)**	**K-Shell Binding Energy (keV)**	**K-Shell Binding Energy Relative to O (i.e., Tissue)**
Oxygen (O)	8	0.5	1
Calcium (Ca)	20	4.0	8
Iodine (I)	53	33	66
Barium (Ba)	56	37	72
Lead (Pb)	82	88	180

COMPLETE: Table 1.3 Add % diff relative to water.

TABLE 1.3	Typical Electron Densities of Human Tissues		
Material	**Effective Atomic Number (Z)**	**Nominal Density (g/cm³)**	**Percent Difference Relative to Water (%)**
Lung	7.5	0.3	−70
Fat	6.5	0.9	−10
Water	7.5	1.0	-
Soft tissue	7.5	1.04	+4
Bone	12	1.7	+70

- **Wavelength (λ)** is the distance between successive crests of waves, measured in meters (m).
- **Frequency (f)** is the number of wave oscillations per unit of time, measured in cycles per second.
  - One cycle per second is 1 hertz [Hz].
- The **wave velocity (v)** is the product of the wavelength and frequency, and measured in meter per second.
  - **High frequencies** have **short wavelengths**, and **low frequencies** have **long wavelengths**.
- **Visible light** and **x-rays** are a form of **electromagnetic radiation**.
- Electromagnetic radiation is **quantized**, meaning that it exists as discrete particles called **photons**.
  - **Photon energy (E)** is directly **proportional to frequency**.
- **Radio waves used in magnetic resonance imaging have low frequencies** (low photon energies), and **x-ray waves have high frequencies** (high photon energies).
- High-energy photons are called **x-rays** when produced by **electrons** but are called **gamma rays** when produced in a **nuclear process**.

E. **Ionization**
  - Energy transferred from energetic particles to atomic electrons can raise electrons to higher energy shells (**excitations**).
  - **Ionization** occurs when an electron is ejected from a neutral atom, leaving behind a **positive ion**.
  - Ionizing radiation is electromagnetic radiation with sufficient energy to eject atomic electrons.
    - **Radio waves, microwaves**, and **visible light cannot ionize atoms**.
  - **Ultraviolet light, x-rays**, and **gamma rays** are examples of **ionizing radiations**.
  - Particles can ionize electrons only if their **energy is greater than the electron binding energy**.
    - A 50 keV electron cannot eject a tungsten K-shell electron (K-shell binding energy is 70 keV), whereas a 100 keV electron can.
  - A **vacancy** in the K-shell will be filled by an electron from a higher shell, resulting in the emission of **characteristic x-rays or Auger electrons**.
    - **Auger electrons** are more likely in atoms with Z < 30 (like tissue).
    - **Characteristic x-rays** are more likely in atoms with Z > 30 (like tungsten).
  - Characteristic x-ray energy is the binding energy of the filling electron minus the binding energy of the vacancy.
    - **Iodine (K-shell binding 33 keV) characteristic x-rays** have energies **slightly less than 33 keV.**
  - Tissue characteristic x-rays are infrequent, and their low energies are absorbed locally, so we usually do not discuss them clinically.

▌II.▐ X-RAY PRODUCTION

A. Generators

- Voltages are increased from a few hundred volts (wall outlet) to tens of thousands of volts using a **transformer.**
- In modern systems, the **maximum (peak) voltage kV$_p$** is essentially the same as the effective voltage (**kV**).
  - Ripple in the voltage is less than 3%.
- Electrons flow from tube cathode to anode creating an electrical current.
  - X-ray tube currents are measures in **milliamperes (mA).**
- Exposure time is the duration of the tube current.
  - Exposure times are measured in **milliseconds (ms)** or seconds (s).
- Power dissipated in the x-ray tube in watts (W) equals the product of tube voltage (V) in volt and current (I) in amp.

$$100 \text{ kV} \times 1{,}000 \text{ mA} = 100 \text{ kW.}$$

- Generator power ratings are power that can be sustained for 0.1 s.

B. X-Ray Tubes

- Figure 1.1 shows the essential components of an x-ray tube.
- X-ray tubes are **evacuated containers** containing a **negative filament (cathode)** and a **positive target (anode).**
  - **Targets** in most x-ray tubes are **tungsten (W).**
- The x-ray tube filament is heated to a high temperature, which then emits electrons (thermionic emission).
- A **high voltage (kV)** from the generator is applied between the filament (cathode) and the target (anode).
- **Tube current (mA) is the flow of electrons** from the negative filament to the positive target.
- Each electron feeling a 100 kV voltage gains 100 keV of energy.
- **X-rays** are produced when the energetic electrons interact with the nuclei of atoms in the tungsten target.
- Only 1% of the energy deposited in a target is converted into x-rays, with the remainder **99% converted into heat.**

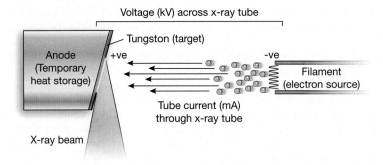

FIG 1.1 Essential components of the x-ray tube include a filament (electron source) and a target embedded in the anode. A voltage (kV) is applied across the x-ray tube with the filament negative, and a current (mA) flows from the filament to the target that is embedded in a positive anode. Applying a voltage of 100 kV results in electrons that each gain 100-keV energy after acceleration across the x-ray tube. Most of this energy is converted to heat, which is conducted from the target to the anode where it is temporarily stored before being dissipated.

- The **target is embedded in an anode** material that temporarily **stores the heat** produced in the target.
- The **focal spot** is the portion of the target producing x-rays.

C. Bremsstrahlung

- **Bremsstrahlung** x-rays are produced when energetic electrons interact with electric fields from the nucleus.
  - Bremsstrahlung means braking radiation in German.
- Energetic electrons are **decelerated by the nuclear electric field** and change their direction of travel.
- The energy lost when the energetic electron decelerates appears as an x-ray photon.
- **Bremsstrahlung** produces a **range of x-ray energies (spectrum)** up to a maximum energy.
- The **maximum bremsstrahlung** photon energy is numerically equal to the x-ray tube voltage.
  - A **voltage** of **100 kV** can produce **bremsstrahlung photons** with **energies** up to **100 keV** but no higher.
- Bremsstrahlung x-ray production increases as **voltage (kV)** and the **atomic number (Z) of the target increase.**
- **Most x-rays** produced are via **bremsstrahlung** processes.

D. Characteristic X-Ray Production

- Characteristic K-shell x-rays are produced when target **K-shell electrons** in the target are ejected by the incident electrons from the filament.
- To eject a K-shell electron, the incident electron must have an energy greater than the binding energy.
- Characteristic x-rays occur only at **discrete energy levels**, unlike the continuous energy spectrum of bremsstrahlung.
- The characteristic energies are determined by the material of the target.
- For tungsten, K-shell characteristic x-rays are produced when the applied voltage exceeds 70 kV.
  - A voltage of >70 kV will produce electrons with kinetic energy >70 keV, sufficient to eject K-shell electrons (binding energy 70 keV).
- **K-shell characteristic** x-ray **energies** are always **slightly lower** than the **K-shell binding energy.**
- **L-shell characteristic x-rays** always accompany K-shell x-rays, but these have very low energies and are absorbed by the x-ray tube glass envelope.

E. Spectra

- X-ray beams in diagnostic radiology contain a wide range of photon energies.
- A **spectrum** is a graph of x-ray tube output that shows the number of x-ray photons at each energy.
- For most radiological imaging, the average photon energy is much lower than the maximum photon energy.
  - The average energy is typically around one-third to half the maximum energy.
- In **angiography**, the spectrum obtained at **70 kV** will likely have an **average photon energy** of **35 keV.**
- **Abdominal radiography** performed at **80 kV** will likely have an **average photon energy** close to **40 keV.**
- A computed tomographic (**CT**) spectrum obtained at **120 kV** will likely have an **average photon** energy of about **60 keV.**
- The spectrum from x-ray tubes includes both bremsstrahlung and characteristic photons.
- Tungsten K-shell characteristic x-rays can contribute up to 10% of x-rays produced in radiography, fluoroscopy, and CT imaging.

- In mammography, x-ray tube targets may be **molybdenum (Z = 42). Molybdenum (K-shell binding energy 20 keV)** has characteristic x-rays with an average of about 18 keV.
- In mammography with **Mo targets, characteristic x-rays are a major contributor** to the spectra used clinically.

III. X-RAY AND GAMMA RAY INTERACTIONS

A. Absorption and Scattering

- Three possible fates of x-rays incident on matter are **scattering, absorption**, and **penetration (transmission).**
- **Coherent scatter** occurs when a low-energy x-ray photon is scattered from an atom without any energy loss (**delivers no dose**) (Fig. 1.2A).
  - **Coherent interactions** accounts for **less than 5%** of all photon interactions and is of minor concern in diagnostic radiology.
- X-rays are primarily **scattered** via **Compton interactions** (Fig. 1.2B).
  - The x-ray **transfers** a fraction of its **energy** to an **electron (Compton electron)** and the rest stays with the **scattered photon.**
- X-rays are absorbed via the **photoelectric (PE) effect** (Fig. 1.2C).
- In **PE** interactions, the x-ray **photon** is totally **absorbed** and transfers all **energy** to the ejected **electron (photoelectron).**
- Compton and PE interactions typically ionize atoms.
- Energetic **photoelectrons and Compton electrons** lose energy by interacting (colliding) with the electrons in adjacent atoms, **producing additional ionizations.**
  - **Each energetic electron** (i.e., Compton or PE) produces **hundreds to thousands of additional ionizations.**
- X-ray photons that pass through matter unaffected are said to penetrate an object (i.e., they are transmitted).
  - **Very few x-rays (<1%) penetrate** through an average-sized patient.
- The fate of x-ray energy incident on a patient is summarized in Figure 1.3.

B. Photoelectric Interactions

- The **PE** effect occurs between tightly bound (**inner shell**) electrons and incident x-ray photons.
- In a PE interaction, the x-ray photon is **totally absorbed** by an inner shell electron, which is subsequently ejected from the atom (photoelectron).
- Outer shell electrons fill the inner shell electron vacancies, with the excess energy emitted as characteristic x-rays or Auger electrons.

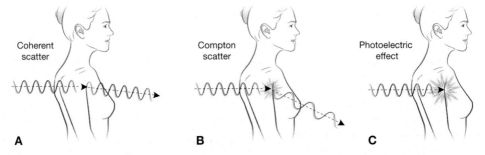

FIG 1.2 Coherent interactions produce a tiny amount of scatter and deposit no energy (A). Compton interactions deposit some energy and produce scatter (B). Photoelectric interactions absorb the incident photons and deposit energy at the site of interaction (C).

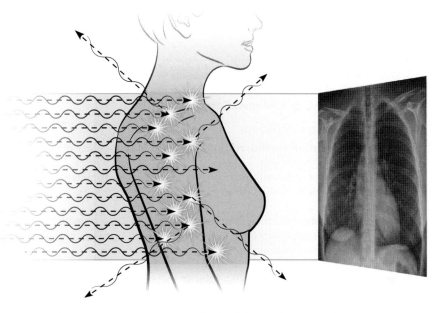

FIG 1.3 In most radiographic examinations, two-thirds of the incident x-ray photon energy is absorbed in patients, one-third is scattered out of the patient, with less than 1% transmitted to the image receptor to create the radiographic image.

- The probability of photoelectric interaction decreases rapidly as the photon energy (E) further increases above the K-edge.
  - **Above the K-edge**, PE interactions are proportional to $1/E^3$.
- The higher the electron binding energy, the greater the probability of a PE interaction.
- The **probability of photoelectric absorption increases with atomic number** and is proportional to Z^3.
- The **PE** effect is important when **beam energy is low** and/or **atomic number (Z) is high.**
- PE interactions account for the brightness seen in bone in extremity radiography, iodine in angiography, and barium in gastrointestinal imaging.
- **PE interactions** are more important in **mammography** because spectra primarily consist of low-energy x-ray photons.
- Photon-counting detectors in nuclear medicine depend on PE interactions in the high-Z detector.

C. Compton Interactions

- In **Compton scatter**, incident photons interact with outer shell electrons.
- A Compton interaction results in a **scattered photon** that has **less energy** than the incident photon and generally travels in a different direction.
- **Scattered photons may travel in any direction (i.e., isotropic)** including 180° to the direction of the incident photon (backscattered).
- The probability of a Compton interaction is proportional to the number of electrons available in the medium (i.e., **electron density**).
- The probability of Compton interactions is **inversely proportional** to the **photon energy (1/E).**
- For **soft tissue**, the probability of **PE vs Compton is equal at 25 keV.**

- PE and Compton probabilities are equal at 40 keV for bone.
- Compton interactions account for **most scattered radiation** encountered.
- In most x-ray examinations, about **a third** of the **total energy** incident on a patient is **scattered.**
- **Scattered photons** may reach the image receptor and **degrade image quality.**
- **Scatter** always **reduces lesion contrast,** which degrades lesion visibility.
  - **Scatter** does **not affect** either spatial **resolution** or **image mottle (noise).**
- **Scattered** radiation **from** the **patient** is the primary source of **operator radiation exposures** in **fluoroscopy-guided procedures.**

D. Linear Attenuation Coefficient

- The **linear attenuation coefficient (μ)** is the fraction of incident photons that interact while traveling in matter (Fig. 1.4).
- Linear attenuation coefficients are expressed in **inverse centimeters (cm^{-1}).**
- The **attenuation coefficient** accounts for all x-ray interactions, including **coherent, PE,** and **Compton.**
- The **linear attenuation coefficient increases** with increasing **density** of the material.
- Linear **attenuation** coefficients generally **increase** with increasing **atomic number.**
- In diagnostic radiology, **attenuation decreases** with increasing photon **energy.**
  - An exception is at a **K-edge,** where a sudden increase in photon attenuation occurs.
- When the value of μ is small, the numerical value of **μ represents the fractional loss of photons.**
- A μ of 0.1 cm^{-1} means that 10% of the incident photons are lost (i.e., absorbed or scattered) in 1 cm.
  - A **μ of 0.1** also means the remaining **90% of x-ray photons are transmitted.**
- **Transmission** of the primary beam through an average patient is only about **1% for skull radiography.**
  - Transmission of x-rays is **higher for chest x-rays** and **lower in abdominal radiography.**

E. K-Edge

- For the PE effect to occur with a K-shell electron, the incident x-ray energy must exceed the **binding energy** of the K-shell electron.
  - Photon absorption increases markedly when photon energy increases from "just below" to "just above" the binding energy of the K-shell electrons (K-edge).
- The binding energy of the K-shell electrons in **iodine is 33 keV**, and a sharp increase in the interaction of photons occurs at this energy (K-edge).

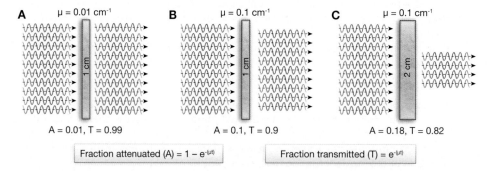

FIG 1.4 Linear attenuation coefficient for a monochromatic (single-energy) x-ray beam. **A:** Attenuation coefficient of 0.01 cm^{-1} means that roughly 1% of incident photons are lost in 1 cm. **B:** Attenuation coefficient of 0.1 cm^{-1} means that roughly 10% of incident photons are lost in 1 cm. **C:** Attenuation coefficient of 0.1 cm^{-1} means that roughly 10% of incident photons are lost in the first centimeter and roughly 10% of what is left is attenuated in the second centimeter.

- When the x-ray energy is **below 33 keV**, there is **much less attenuation by iodine**.
- When the x-ray energy is **just above 33 keV**, x-ray **absorption by iodine will be maximized**.
  - At x-ray energies **much higher** than 33 keV, x-ray **absorption by iodine** is **markedly reduced**.
- Maximizing absorption of x-rays by iodine in angiography requires an average energy of about 35 keV, achieved using tube voltages of about **70 kV**.
- In mammography, the beam passes through a **molybdenum** filter where x-rays above the K-edge (20 keV) are absorbed, whereas those below are transmitted.
  - Very low–energy x-rays are absorbed by higher shell Mo electrons.
- **Molybdenum (K-edge 20 keV), Rhodium (K-edge 23 keV),** and **Sliver (K-edge 25 keV)** are used as **x-ray filters** in **mammography**.
  - Mo, Rh, and Ag filters all **transmit** x-ray **energies** that are **just** *below* their respective **K-shell binding energies**.

▮ **IV.** X-RAY QUANTITY AND QUALITY

A. Beam Quantity

- **Kerma** is the energy given from photons to charged particles per unit mass of the irradiated material.
  - Kerma stands for the <u>K</u>inetic <u>E</u>nergy <u>R</u>eleased per unit <u>M</u>ass.
- The unit of kerma is joules per kilogram (J/kg), where 1 J/kg is 1 Gray (Gy).
  - 1 Gy is 1,000 mGy, and 1 mGy is 1,000 μGy.
- **Air kerma (K_{air})** delivered in a known amount of time is proportional to **beam intensity** (i.e., energy per second per mm^2).
- Kerma obeys the **inverse square law**, decreasing with the square of the distance from a source.
  - Doubling distance quarters kerma.
- The **entrance K_{air}** is a measure of the x-ray radiation intensity incident on the patient.
  - Entrance K_{air} in adult radiography is normally **a few mGy**.
- K_{air} at the **image receptor** is a measure of the x-ray radiation intensity that is used to generate the image.
  - In radiography, K_{air} at the **image receptor** is normally a **few micrograys (μGy).**
- Radiation intensities at the **image receptor** are **reduced** because of **attenuation** by the patient, increased **distance** from x-ray tubes, and **grid losses**.

B. HVLs and Beam Quality

- A **half value layer (HVL)** is the thickness of designated material that attenuates an x-ray beam by 50%.
- Material **atomic number** is the most important determinant of half value layer, as depicted by the data in Table 1.4.
- Increasing average photon energy will increase the HVL.
- In **mammography** (30 kV), the **HVL for soft tissues is ~1 cm.**

TABLE 1.4	Nominal Half Value Layers (HVL) for X-Ray Spectra Generated at 80 kV	
Material	**Atomic Number (Z)**	**Approximate Thickness to Attenuate 50% of Incident X-Ray Beam (mm)**
Soft tissue	7.5	30
Aluminum	13	3
Copper	29	0.3
Lead	82	<0.1

- In **abdominal radiography** (80 kV), the **HVL for soft tissues is ~3.0 cm.**
  - An anteroposterior abdomen (24 cm soft tissue) corresponds to eight half values, which transmits about 0.4% ($1/2^8$) of the incident beam.
- In **computed tomography** performed at 120 kV, the **HVL for soft tissue increases to ~ 4 cm.**
- **Beam quality** refers to the x-ray **beam penetration** and relates to average beam energy.
- Quality of an x-ray beam is measured as the **HVL in aluminum (mm Al).**
- Increasing average photon energy increases beam quality (i.e., penetrating power).
  - As the **average energy increases, more Al is required** to **attenuate** the x-ray beam by **50%.**
- In **mammography,** beam qualities are generally very low, with **HVLs** of about **0.5 mm Al.**
- For **radiography** performed at 80 kV, x-ray beam **HVLs** are about **3 mm Al.**
- **Filtering out low-energy photons** from a beam will also increase the HVL.

C. Tube Current and Exposure Time

- The **x-ray beam intensity** is generally taken to be **proportional** to the number of x-ray **photons per mm^2** in a given amount of time and is quantified by K_{air}.
- X-ray beam intensity is directly proportional to the x-ray **tube current (mA).**
  - Doubling the tube current will double the number of x-rays produced.
- X-ray beam intensity is directly proportional to the **exposure time (s).**
  - Doubling the exposure time will double the number of x-rays produced.
- The product of the tube current (mA) and exposure time (s) is known as the **mAs.**
- The x-ray beam intensity is directly proportional to the **mAs.**
  - Doubling the current at constant exposure time has the same effect as doubling the exposure time at constant tube current.
- Adjusting the **mAs** affects x-ray beam intensity (quantity) but does not change the **energy spectrum (quality).**
- When more x-rays are required, this is achieved by increasing the mAs.
- Increasing the mAs is best achieved by increasing the mA whenever this is possible.
  - **Longer exposure times** may result in **motion blur.**
- Figure 1.5 shows that doubling the mAs will double the number of x-ray photons (K_{air}) but not affect the beam energies.

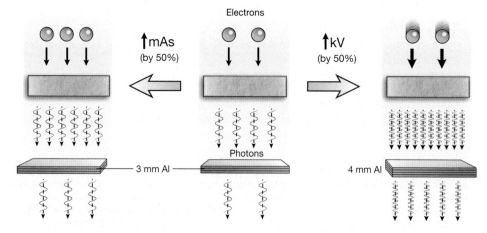

FIG 1.5 Increasing the mAs by 50% (left) increases the number of photons by 50% but does not change the x-ray beam penetrating power, so 3 mm Al still attenuates half the x-ray beam. Increasing the radiographic kV by 50% (right) increases the number of photons by well over 100% and increases the x-ray beam penetrating power so that 4 mm Al is now required to attenuate half the x-ray beam.

TABLE 1.5	Factors That Influence X-Ray Quantity and Quality	
Increase in:	**Results in X-Ray:**	
	Quantity	Quality
Tube voltage (kV)	Increase (as kV^2)	Increase
mAs	Increase (as mAs)	No change
Distance	Decrease (as $1/d^2$)	No change
Filtration	Decrease (exponential)	Increase

D. Tube Voltage

- When the tube **voltage increases**, (many) **more x-rays** are produced, and these x-rays are also **more penetrating**.
  - Changing **tube voltage** impacts both x-ray **beam quantity and quality**.
- In radiography, x-ray **beam intensity** is approximately proportional to the **square of the tube voltage ($K_{air} \propto kV^2$)** as depicted in Figure 1.5.
- In **computed tomography**, x-ray beam intensity obeys a **power law relationship** ($K_{air} \sim kV^{2.6}$).
- In **mammography**, there is **no simple relationship** between kV and the corresponding K_{air} output from the x-ray tube.
- **Increasing tube voltage** also **increases the average and maximum x-ray photon energy**.
- Changes in **tube voltage** affect **patient penetration, scatter**, and **absorption**.
- In radiographic imaging, **increasing the kV by 15%** requires **decreasing the mAs 50%** to maintain K_{air} at the **image receptor (15/50 rule)**.
- Radiographic **tube voltages** are normally adjusted to change **patient penetration**.
  - Changes in **photon energy** (i.e., kV) will also impact on the resultant **image contrast** and **dynamic range**.
- Whenever the **kV** is **adjusted**, there is always a **corresponding adjustment of the mAs** to ensure **appropriate K_{air}** at the image receptor.

E. Filtration and Beam Hardening

- X-ray beams emerging from the x-ray tube may contain **relatively low-energy photons**.
  - **Low-energy photons dose** the **patient** but add nothing to the image.
- **Filters** are added at the x-ray tube to **preferentially absorb low-energy photons in the beam**.

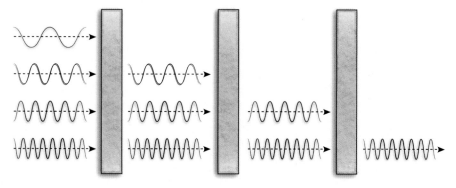

FIG 1.6 Schematic illustration of x-ray beam hardening for a polychromatic (i.e., spectrum) x-ray beam where attenuators preferentially absorb lower-energy photons. Lower-energy photons have higher attenuation coefficients than higher-energy photons.

- **Filters** are typically made from a **few millimeters of Aluminum** or a few tenths of a millimeter of copper.
- Mammography uses special filter materials such as rhodium, molybdenum, and silver.
- **Filtration** always **reduces** the x-ray tube output (**quantity**) but **increases** the beam penetration because the average beam energy increases (**quality**).
  - Use of **heavy filtration** will likely require use of **(expensive) x-ray tubes** with a **high x-ray output (K$_{air}$)**.
- Table 1.5 shows how quantity and quality are affected by the technique.
- **Beam hardening** refers to effect of a material (e.g., filter or patient) on a **x-ray beam** containing a range of x-ray photon energies.
- Beam hardening is the **preferential loss of lower-energy photons** by any material (e.g., filter or patient).
  - **Computed tomography** uses **very high filtration** to **reduce beam hardening artifacts.**
- As low-energy photons are absorbed, the mean photon energy increases, and the resultant x-ray beam becomes more penetrating (Fig. 1.6).
- **Filtered beams** with higher mean photon energies are **harder x-ray beams.**
- The **second HVL** will always be **greater** than the **first HVL** for a typical x-ray beam.
  - **Beam hardening** does *not* **occur with monochromatic x-ray** beams because all photons have the same energy.

Chapter 1 (Basics) Questions

1.1 How does kVp compare to kV in modern systems?
A. kVp is half of kV.
B. kVp is about the same as kV.
C. kVp is double kV.

1.2 X-rays are most likely generated in the x-ray tube _____.
A. filament
B. target
C. anode
D. window

1.3 Which target is most likely to produce the highest number of bremsstrahlung photons?
A. Molybdenum (Z = 42)
B. Tungsten (Z = 74)
C. "The same"

1.4 Which x-ray photon energy *cannot* be made at an x-ray tube voltage of 80 kV?
A. 20 keV
B. 50 keV
C. 80 keV
D. 100 keV

1.5 Characteristic x-rays have an energy that is _____ the target K-shell binding energy.
A. higher than
B. equal to
C. less than

1.6 Which type of examination is most likely to result in the production of tungsten K-shell characteristic x-rays?
A. Screening mammogram
B. Infant abdominal x-ray
C. Extremity radiograph
D. Adult chest x-ray

1.7 A dedicated chest x-ray unit operated at 120 kV would most likely have an average x-ray photon energy of:
A. 30 keV
B. 60 keV
C. 90 keV
D. 120 keV

1.8 What is the change in kerma if the mAs is doubled?
A. Quartered
B. Halved
C. No change
D. Doubled

1.9 What is the name for x-rays produced following a photoelectric interaction?
A. Characteristic x-rays
B. Compton scatter
C. Coherent scatter
D. Bremsstrahlung photons

1.10 What photon energies are most likely to undergo a K-shell photoelectric interaction with an iodine atom (K-edge 33 keV)?
A. 20 keV
B. 30 keV
C. 35 keV
D. 70 keV

1.11 Compton scatter proportion is largest in _____.
A. ultrasound
B. extremity radiography
C. infant radiography
D. body CT

1.12 What interactions combine to form the linear attenuation coefficient?
A. Compton
B. Coherent
C. Photoelectric
D. A, B, and C

1.13 What is the fraction of photons transmitted through 2 cm of material when the tissue linear attenuation coefficient is 0.1 cm^{-1}?
A. 0.1
B. 0.2
C. 0.8
D. 0.9

1.14 Which of the following materials has the highest K-edge energy?
A. Copper (Z = 29)
B. Molybdenum (Z = 42)
C. Rhodium (Z = 45)
D. Silver (Z = 47)

1.15 What is the typical K$_{air}$ incident on the image receptor for a body radiograph?
A. 0.03 μGy
B. 0.3 μGy
C. 3 μGy
D. 30 μGy

1.16 What is the HVL for an adult abdominal radiograph?
A. 0.3 mm Al
B. 1 mm Al
C. 3 mm Al
D. 10 mm Al

1.17 How much does the x-ray tube output increase when the x-ray tube current and exposure time are both doubled?
A. 2×
B. 4×
C. 8×
D. 16×

1.18 What is the increase in average x-ray photon energy when the tube current (mAs) doubles?
A. 0%
B. 25%
C. 50%
D. 100%

1.19 In radiography, increasing the x-ray tube voltage by 10% will result in what increase in x-ray tube output (K_{air})?
A. <10%
B. 10%
C. >10%

1.20 What interaction is responsible for the majority of x-rays emitted from a tube?
A. Photoelectric
B. Bremsstrahlung
C. Compton
D. Coherent

Answers and Explanations

1.1 **C** (kVp is about the same as kV). In early radiography, the peak and average voltages were very different (large voltage ripple); now, the kV is roughly the same for the entire exposure time, so these two values are roughly the same.

1.2 **B** (target). X-rays are produced when energetic electrons are decelerated in tungsten targets that are embedded in x-ray tube anodes.

1.3 **B** (Tungsten). Bremsstrahlung production is directly proportional the atomic number of the target, so tungsten (Z = 74) produces more than molybdenum (Z = 42).

1.4 **D** (100 keV). A voltage of 80 kV produces 80 keV electrons, which may *all* be converted into a bremsstrahlung photon with an energy of 80 keV (i.e., 100 keV photons are impossible).

1.5 **C** (less than). K-shell characteristic x-ray energies are always (slightly) lower than the target K-shell binding energy.

1.6 **D** (Adult chest x-ray). To make tungsten characteristic x-rays requires tube voltages exceeding 70 kV, and only adult chest x-rays would achieve this (e.g., 120 kV), with tube voltages for mammograms, infants, and extremities below 70 kV.

1.7 **B** (60 keV). For heavily filtered x-ray beams used in chest radiography, the average energy will be close to half the maximum energy of 120 keV.

1.8 **D** (Doubled). Doubling the mAs will double the number of electrons hitting the target. This will double the number of photons emitted. This will in turn double the energy given to electrons per unit mass in the irradiated material (i.e., kerma).

1.9 **A** (Characteristic x-rays). Photoelectric interactions occur by knocking out K-shell electrons; this can result in the production of (low energy) characteristic x-rays.

1.10 **C** (35 keV). 20 and 30 keV photons do not have sufficient energy to eject the iodine K-shell electron; maximum x-ray absorption is just above the k-edge, and at 70 keV, there will be 8 times fewer interactions than at 35 keV (PE varies as $1/E^3$).

1.11 **D** (body CT). Average photon energies is highest in CT, so most interactions will be Compton scatter.

1.12 **D** (A, B, and C). The linear attenuation coefficient includes all interactions (i.e., Compton, coherent, and photoelectric interactions).

1.13 **C** (0.8). 1 cm of tissue absorbs about 0.1, so 2 cm of tissue absorbs approximately twice as much (i.e., 0.2), which means that (approximately) 0.8 would be transmitted.

1.14 **D** (Silver). The exact atomic K-edge energies are 9 keV (Cu), 20 keV (Mo), 23 keV (Rh), and 25 keV (Ag). The last three numbers are very important in mammography, as these are common filter materials.

1.15 **C** (3 µGy). The radiation at the image receptor is any radiograph is most likely 3 µGy, which would be reported in the DICOM header as an exposure index of 300.

1.16 **C** (3 mm). At 80 kV (typical in adult abdominal radiography), the filtration of an x-ray tube would likely be 3 mm Al, which coincidentally results in an x-ray beam that has a half value layer (penetrating power) of 3 mm Al.

1.17 **B** (4×). Doubling the current (mA) and exposure time (s) will quadruple the mAs and therefore increase x-ray tube output by a factor of 4.

1.18 A   (0%). Changing the x-ray tube technique only affects the number of x-rays that are produced but does not modify the x-ray beam energy.

1.19 **C**   (> 10%). X-ray tube output in radiography is normally taken to be proportional to kV^2, so the increase in x-ray tube output (quantity) will be higher than the 10% increase in x-ray tube voltage.

1.20 B   (Bremsstrahlung). The beam is composed of characteristic and bremsstrahlung photons. The vast majority of the beam is photons from bremsstrahlung interactions.

X-Ray Imaging

▊ I. SCATTERED X-RAYS

A. Scatter

- **Scattered radiation** is always present in x-ray and gamma-ray imaging.
- **Compton interactions** are the dominant source of **scatter.**
  - **Coherent scatter** is a **minor** contributor to total scatter (<5%).
- The **ratio of scatter x-rays to primary x-rays** exiting a patient can be as high as **5:1** (e.g., abdominal radiography).
- **Scatter** is undesirable in diagnostic radiology because it **reduces contrast.**
  - When **substantial scatter** is present, resultant **images are "foggy"** like looking in the mirror after a hot shower.
- When a **lesion transmits half** the x-rays of adjacent tissues, the **contrast is 0.5 or 50%** (100 for tissues vs 50 for lesion).
  - A **scatter-to-primary ratio** of **1:1** adds 100 scatter photons everywhere, **reducing con-trast** to **0.25 or 25%** (200 for tissues vs 150 for lesion).
- **Scatter** does **not affect spatial resolution** or **mottle.**
- Abdominal radiography would be **"impossible"** without the **removal** of most of the **scattered x-rays.**
- **Scatter** radiation is **minimized** in most of radiographic imaging using **grids** (Fig. 2.1) and in nuclear medicine using collimators.
- Scatter is the **primary source of dose** for the **interventional radiologist.**

B. Scatter Factors

- **Scatter increases** markedly with **increasing field of view or FOV** (i.e., area of x-ray beam).
- **Collimation** reduces the total patient volume irradiated and **reduces scatter.**
  - Collimation benefits radiologists by improving contrast (less scatter) and also benefits patients because less radiation is incident and absorbed.
- For **small x-ray beam areas**, most of the **scatter** will **miss** the **image receptor.**
  - When small x-ray areas are used, such as 40 mm wide detectors in computed tomog-raphy (CT), scatter is of less importance.
- **Scatter** generally **increases** with **increased patient thickness.**
- When patient **thickness exceeds about 12 cm**, scatter removal is **essential.**
- **Scatter** is of much **less concern** for high Z materials such as calcium in **bone.**
  - In **extremity radiography**, most interactions with bone are **photoelectric effects** and there are fewer scatter photons.
- At **low voltages** (e.g., 25 keV for soft tissue), there is generally **more photoelectric absorption** and less Compton scatter (Fig. 2.2).
  - There is **less scatter in mammography** due to the low voltages used.

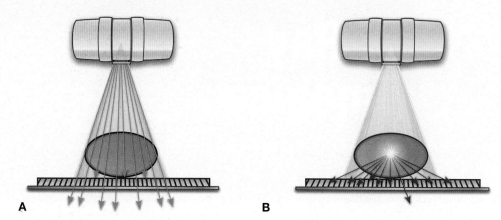

A   B

FIG 2.1 **A:** Approximately 70% of the primary x-rays (green) pass through a typical 10:1 grid ratio scatter removal grid. **B:** For the same grid, about 90% of the scattered x-rays (red) are absorbed by the grid. Increasing the grid ratio will reduce both primary and scatter photons transmitted through the grid, and vice versa.

- Table 2.1 summarizes the **voltages** used in **radiographic examinations**, and the resultant **scatter characteristics.**
- When radiographs are obtained using grids it is essential to obtain sufficient radiation intensity (i.e., K_{air}) at the image receptor to have acceptable noise in the image.
  - A K_{air} of about **3 μGy** results in a **satisfactory image for body radiography.**
- At **high voltages or filtrations**, the x-ray beam **penetration increases**, and less radiation is required to obtain the required receptor K_{air} (3 μGy).
  - This can result in **lower patient dose** if the mAs is also reduced but **more scatter** due to higher average beam energy (Fig. 2.3).

C. Scatter Removal

- **Antiscatter grids** are used to remove scatter in x-ray modalities (Fig. 2.1).
- Antiscatter **grids** are made up of many narrow **parallel bars** of **lead** or other highly attenuating material.
- X-rays pass **between** the **strips**, which are filled with low attenuation material such as **aluminum** or **graphite** to keep the strips correctly aligned.
- The **grid ratio** is the ratio of the strip height (H) along the x-ray beam direction to the gap (D) between the lead strips, where the grid ratio is H/D.

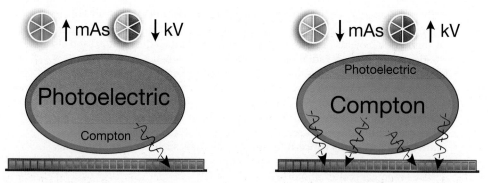

FIG 2.2 Use of low tube voltages (i.e., low photon energies) in x-ray imaging results in mainly photoelectric interactions (left), whereas increasing the tube voltage (i.e., higher photon energies) results in mainly Compton interactions (right). Using a high kV (i.e., more penetration) requires markedly lower tube currents to achieve any given intensity (K_{air}) at the image receptor.

TABLE 2.1	Tube Voltages, and the Amount of Scatter, in Radiographic Imaging		
Body Region	**Tube Voltage (kV)**	**Scatter in Image**	**Grid Required**
Distal extremity	55	+ (Very low)	No
Skull	80	+++ (Moderate)	Yes
Chest	125	++++ (High)	Yes
Abdomen	80	++++++ (Very High)	Yes

- Common radiographic **grid ratios** in radiography and fluoroscopy are ~**10,** with ~**45 lines per centimeter** (line density).
- **Grids** are generally **focused** and have diverging strips that must be used at the specified distance.
- **Grids** are placed between the **patient** and the **image receptor.**
  - Grids are **not seen on images** due to **image processing** and grid movement (**reciprocation**) that blur them out of existence.
  - The device that moves the grid is called a **Bucky,** named after its inventor.
- **Virtual grids** use scatter modeling to remove scatter after acquisition.
  - Virtual grids are **best when proper orientation of a physical grid is difficult or impossible.**
  - Virtual grids are **better than no grid but often less effective than physical grids.**

D. **Grid Characteristics**
  - **Primary transmission** is the percentage of (useful) primary radiation that passes through the grid.
  - Grids are expected to **transmit** about **70%** of the **primary** x-rays and absorb the remaining 30%.
  - Grids are expected to **absorb 90%** of (useless) **scattered photons** and transmit the remaining 10% (Fig. 2.1).
    - **Increasing** the grid **ratio reduces** both the **primary** and **scatter transmission** through the grid (Table 2.2).
  - The **Bucky factor** is the ratio of radiation incident on the grid to the transmitted radiation.
    - **Bucky factor** is the **increase** in **patient dose** due to the use of a grid.
  - In abdominal radiography (**Bucky factor ~ 5**), adding a grid requires an increase in technique (mAs) and patient dose by a factor of about 5.
    - Without a grid in abdominal radiography, however, image contrast is so low that the radiograph would be considered "**nondiagnostic.**"
  - The **contrast improvement factor** is the ratio of contrast with a grid to contrast without a grid.
  - **Contrast improvement factors** are **substantial** and can easily be a factor of **two or higher.**
  - Use of **higher grid ratios** improves image contrast but also **increases patient dose.**
  - **Artifacts** such as **grid cutoff** may be caused by **improper alignment** and the **wrong** focal spot to detector **distance** for focused grids.
    - **Portable radiography** uses parallel (not focused) grids with lower grid ratio to avoid grid artifacts.

E. **Geometric Magnification**
  - **Geometric magnification** occurs when there is an **air gap** between the **patient** and the corresponding **image receptor.**

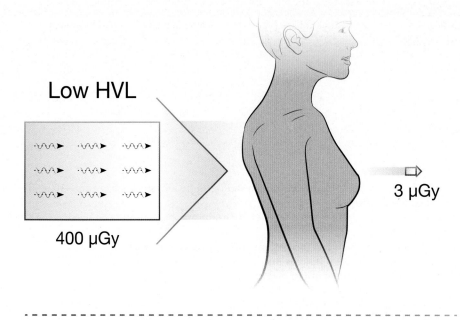

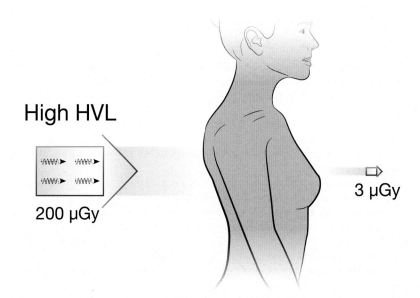

FIG 2.3 Effect of half-value layer (HVL) on dose. Top: A low HVL beam (e.g., low kV with high mAs) is less penetrating, so more radiation is needed to get an acceptable amount to the receptor. This results in increased patient dose. Bottom: A high HVL beam (e.g., high kV with low mAs) is more penetrating, so less radiation is needed to gen an acceptable amount to the image receptor. This results in decreased patient dose but worse image contrast.

- **Primary photons** will **reach** the **image receptor** but result in **geometrical magnification.**
  - **Magnification factor** is the source-to-detector distance divided by the source-to-object distance.
- **Scattered photons** are **less likely** to **reach** the **image receptor** when there is an **air gap.**
  - **Magnification mammography** removes the grid due to reduced scatter from the air gap.

TABLE 2.2	**Effect of Grid Ratio on Grid Transmission, Image Contrast, and Patient Dose**	
Grid Ratio	Low	High
Primary transmission	High	Low
Scatter transmission	High	Low
Image contrast	Low	High
Patient dose	Low	High

- A major drawback of **geometric magnification** imaging is the **increased focal spot blurring.**
- Use of **air gaps (magnification)** generally requires **using smaller focal spots** to minimize focal spot blurring.
- **Magnification imaging** is sometimes used in **mammography** and **neuroradiology.**
  - **Magnification** can be helpful for **improving lesion visibility** of a microcalcification cluster or a small blood vessel.

II. DIGITAL DETECTORS

A. Scintillators

- **Scintillators** are materials that emit light when exposed to radiation (Fig. 2.4).
- Absorption of a 35 keV x-ray photon generally produces about a thousand light photons.
- **Flat panel detectors** may use scintillators coupled to a two-dimensional (2D) array of light detectors (**photodiodes**) and charge storage (**thin film transistors**).
  - **Cesium iodide (CsI)** scintillator is commonly used in image intensifiers, CT, radiography, digital fluoroscopy, and mammography detectors.
- Scintillators are used in all **positron emission tomography (PET) and nuclear medicine (NM) detectors, well counters, and thyroid probes** as well.

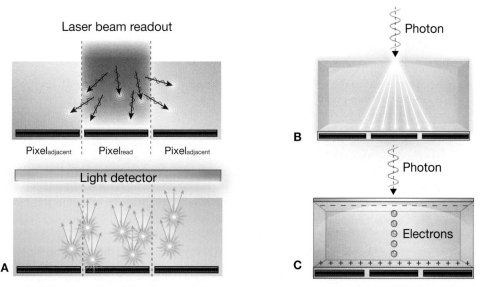

FIG 2.4 A: Photostimulable phosphor showing the laser beam incident on a pixel (upper) that results in light being scattered into adjacent pixels, which will result in light being released from adjacent pixels, and therefore increase blur. **B:** Scintillators absorb x-ray photons, and the resultant light will spread out on the way to the light detectors, resulting in blur that depends on the scintillator thickness; **C:** Photoconductor showing minimal spread of the charge (electrons) produced when x-rays are absorbed, and which is therefore expected to result in excellent resolution.

- Scintillators are **excellent x-ray absorbers** because of their **high density, high Z, and the K-shell binding energies.**
  - **CsI K-edge energies** are an excellent match to the **average x-ray energies** in radiography (e.g., **40 keV** at 80 kV).
- Scintillators are **indirect detectors** because the x-rays are absorbed to produce light, which is subsequently converted to charge in the light detector.
- **Scintillators** introduce image **blur** because of diffusion (**spreading**) of the **light** produced by absorbed x-rays (Fig. 2.4).
  - Radiographic **scintillator crystals** may be manufactured in **columns** to **minimize** light diffusion and reduce image **blur.**
- Table 2.3 shows how varying the **scintillator thickness** will impact on x-ray absorption, patient dose, and image blur.

B. Photoconductors

- **Photoconductors** absorb x-rays, which are converted into **charge** (electrons), as depicted in Figure 2.4.
  - A voltage across the photoconductor **collects** the **charge.**
- The **electronic signal** (i.e., charge collected) in a pixel is directly proportional to the amount of x-ray **energy deposited** in the region.
  - Photoconductors are **direct detectors** because the liberated charge is collected and measured without converting to something else (e.g., light).
- Photoconductors such as **amorphous selenium (a-Se)** have a low Z and very low K-edge binding energy (**13 keV**) which makes them **poor x-ray detectors** at 80 kV and higher.
- a-Se is an **excellent absorber** of *low-energy* x-rays and is widely used in **mammography** (**20 keV**).
  - **Photoconductors** are also found in radiography and fluoroscopy.
- Charge does *not* spread out during the collection process, resulting in less blur than in scintillators.
  - **Photoconductors** generally have **sharper** images **than scintillators.**

C. Photostimulable Phosphors

- **Photostimulable phosphor** plates are made of barium fluorohalides (e.g., BaFBr).
  - Photostimulable phosphors were the first digital detectors to replace screen-film, and the process was historically known as **computed radiography.**
- X-ray photons are absorbed in the phosphor with some of the **absorbed energy** "**stored,**" which thereby creates a **latent image.**
- After exposure, plates are read out using **red lasers** to **release** the "**stored**" energy that is **emitted** as **blue-green** light (Fig. 2.4).
  - The amount of **released blue-green light** from each pixel represents the amount of x-ray **photons reaching** this **pixel.**
- The detected light pattern, typically consisting of **5 million pixels (2,000 × 2,500)**, is digitized and stored in a computer.
- **White light** is used to **erase** photostimulable phosphor plates, which can then be **reused.**
- **Thick phosphors** are **impractical** because readout **light scatters** into **adjacent pixels** releasing light that increases image blur (Fig. 2.4).

TABLE 2.3	Effect of Scintillator Thickness on X-Ray Absorption Efficiency, Patient Dose, and Image Blur		
Detector Thickness	**X-Ray Absorption Efficiency**	**Patient Dose**[a]	**Image Blur**
Thick	High	Low	High
Thin	Low	High	Low

[a]Fixed number of *detected* photons.

- **Photostimulable phosphors** images are **not** as **sharp** as those obtained using scintillators or photoconductors.
- **Thin photostimulable phosphors, like thin scintillators,** absorb fewer photons and thus **increase patient dose.**

D. Gas Detectors

- Gas detectors are **not typically used for imaging** but are used in radiation measurement detectors.
- A **voltage** across the detector (chamber) measures the **electrons liberated** by Compton and photoelectric interactions.
  - High voltages make ionization chambers, and very high voltages make Geiger-Mueller counters.
- The **signal** produced by absorption of x-rays is the **total electron charge liberated** in the gas, which is collected by the positive anode.
- Imaging gas detectors would likely use **high–atomic number gases.**
- **Gas detectors** are generally operated at **high pressure** to improve their ability to absorb x-rays.
- **Gas detectors are used clinically as dose calibrators and survey meters (ionization chambers and Geiger-Mueller counters).**

E. Digital Detector Characteristics

- Digital detectors are either **integrating detectors** or **photon counters.**
- **Integrating detectors** record the total amount of energy absorbed by an area (almost all x-ray detectors are ionization chambers).
- **Photon counters** record the number of photons that hit an area (all NM and PET as well as cutting-edge CT).
  - Photon counters have a **better image quality**, but engineering limitations have hindered wide adoption at **high count rates** until recently (e.g., in CT).
- All digital detectors have a **linear response.**
  - Doubling the x-ray intensity will double the signal detected in any digital x-ray detector.
- The **(linear) response** of all digital x-ray detectors is markedly different from the **sigmoidal response** of **film and image intensifiers.**
- **Digital detectors** can tolerate x-ray intensities **100 times lower,** and **100 times higher,** than those required for analog (i.e., wide latitude or dynamic range).
- The **dynamic range** of digital radiographic systems is **>10,000:1.**
  - **Dynamic range** for **screen-film** is about **40:1.**
- **Too little radiation** will result in a **mottled (noisy)** image, but **contrast and spatial resolution are generally not affected.**
  - When the digital detector signal is low, **electronic noise** becomes important and may degrade image quality.
- When **too much radiation** is used with a digital detector, image quality is rarely affected, but patients do receive unnecessary dose.

III. DIGITAL IMAGING

A. Digital Data

- A **patient** may have many **studies** and each study may have many **series** and each series will be one or more **instances** (i.e., **Images**).
- **Analog signals** can be **digitized** using an **analog to digital converter** and stored in a computer.
- To **display digital data** requires a **digital to analog converter.**
- **Computers store data** in **bits**, each one of which can take on values of either 0 or 1.
  - A byte is a collection of 8 bits.
- **Small medical images are hundreds of kilobytes (kB)** (1 kB is 1,024 bytes).

- **Large medical images** are tens of **megabytes** (MB) (1 MB is 1,024 kB) of data.
- Series may be hundreds of megabytes or **gigabytes** (GB) (1 GB is 1,024 MB).
- **Radiology departments** have very large storage requirements, normally measured in **terabytes (TB)** (1 TB is 1,024 GB).
- Large images and image series can take a long time to transfer from storage to the workstation and require a fast Ethernet.
  - Gigabit Ethernet transfers up to 1 gigabit per second across a network.

B. Digital Image Data

- **Pixels** are individual **picture elements** in a 2D image or voxels (**volume elements**) in three dimensions.
- The number of pixels in a given dimension is called **matrix size.**
- The total number of **pixels** in an **image** is the product of the number of pixels assigned to the horizontal and vertical dimensions.
- If there are **1,000 (1 k)** pixels in both the horizontal and vertical dimensions, then the image contains **1 megapixel (MP)—1 k × 1 k pixels.**
- The information content of images is the **product of the number of pixels and the bit depth.**
  - A pixel with 1 byte bit depth (i.e., 8 bits of storage) can show up to 256 shades of gray (2^8).
- Most **medical images have a bit depth of 2 bytes** (>65,000 shades of gray) but do not use all the possible values.
- An image with a 1 k × 1 k matrix and 2-byte bit depth requires 2 MB of memory.
- Table 2.4 lists matrix sizes and data content for radiological images.

C. Workstations

- A **soft-copy display** refers to presenting images on flat panel monitors.
  - A monitor where the horizontal dimension is longer is called a **landscape** display, whereas a longer vertical dimension is a **portrait** display.
- Standard diagnostic workstations have 3 MP, with a matrix size roughly 2,048 × 1,600.
- **3 MP** pixel monitors are typically used for nonmammography workstations and **5 MP** for mammography workstations.
  - **Large MP monitors** allow most or all of a large matrix image to be shown at native resolution **without zooming and panning,** thus making **reading faster.**
- Test patterns to evaluate monitor performance have been developed by the **Society of Motion Picture and Television Engineers (SMPTE).**
- The SMPTE pattern includes intensities ranging from 0% to 100% in 10% increments.

TABLE 2.4	Radiological Digital Image Matrix Sizes and Data Content		
Modality	Typical Matrix Size[a]	Byte per Pixel	Nominal Image Size (MB)
Nuclear medicine	128 × 128	1	1/64
Magnetic resonance imaging	256 × 256	2	1/8
Computed tomography	512 × 512	2	1/2
Digital ultrasound	512 × 512	1	1/4
TV digital photospot/ Digital subtraction angiography	1,024 × 1,024	2	2
Digital radiography	2,560 × 2,048	2	10
Mammography and tomosynthesis	4,096 × 6,144	2	50

[a]Matrix sizes may vary for some modalities like magnetic resonance imaging. A typical value is shown.

- Display is adequate when all intensity steps are seen and a **5% square in a 0% background** (dark) and **95% square in a 100% background** (white) can be **visualized.**

D. Artificial Intelligence

- **Artificial intelligence (AI)** attempts to create programs capable of performing tasks typically requiring human intelligence.
- **Machine learning** is an AI technique where a machine may learn to perform tasks directly from data without explicit task programming from human expertise.
  - In **supervised learning**, the machine is given a set of data with the correct answers (labels) from which to learn.
  - In **unsupervised learning**, the machine is given data but does not have access to the correct answers (labels).
- **Neural networks** are a type of machine learning where many regression models (nodes) are connected to each other and arranged into layers to create an output (the final layer).
- **Deep learning** is machine learning using **neural networks with many layers,** which allow the machine to model the data more precisely at the cost of increased complexity and training computation.
- **Radiomics** attempts to derive quantitative diagnostic information (a **feature)** from medical images.
  - Gray level brightness, smoothness of a surface, and probability of two gray levels being next to each other are **examples of features.**
  - Features may be **derived from human expertise or created by programs** learning from a data set.
- **Convolutional neural networks** are a type of deep learning that maintains the spatial relationships of image data and learns radiomics features using image filters (convolutions).
- Supervised machine learning requires **three data sets.**
  - A large **training set** to learn features and their connections.
  - A small **validation set** to ensure the model is general enough to apply outside the data (i.e., not overfit).
  - A small **testing set** to determine the final performance.
- Popular tools to assess AI performance include **confusion matrix** (and associated metrics), receiver operator characteristic or **ROC curves** (and associated metrics), **saliency maps**, and **activation maps.**

IV.   IMAGE THEORY AND INFORMATICS

A. Decomposing Images and Frequency Space

- Any image can be **artificially decomposed into many 2D sinusoids** of differing frequency, phase, and amplitude by applying the **Fourier transform.**
  - The frequency of one of these sinusoids is called a **spatial frequency** and has units of **inverse length (e.g., 1/m).**
- These 2D sinusoid waves are simply varying gray levels and are **unrelated to radiation or sound used to create them.**
  - This decomposition can be performed on a family photo of the dog or digital drawing of a house in the exact same way as a radiograph.
- A **frequency space** (known in magnetic resonance imaging as **k-space**) image is created by plotting each sinusoid amplitude as a gray level, each frequency as a distance from image center, and each phase as an angle.
- A **large amplitude would be bright** and a **large frequency would be at the periphery of the image.**
  - **High spatial frequency** sinusoids are associated with **edges, small details, and noise.**
  - **Low spatial frequency** sinusoids are associated with image **gray level and contrast.**
- A **low-pass filter** gets rid of high frequency sinusoids to reduce noise but causes blur.

- A **high-pass filter** gets rid of high frequency sinusoids to find edges but loses all gray level information.

B. Pre- and Postprocessing

- **Raw image data** are collected by the scanner, go through **preprocessing** to create **for-processing images**, then go through **postprocessing** to create **for-display images.**
- **Preprocessing typically corrects for acquisition issues** like dead detector elements and nonuniformity.
- **Postprocessing enhances the image** in a desired way.
- **Low-pass filters blur** the image but also decrease noise.
- **Unsharp masking enhances edges** but also accentuates noise (Fig. 2.5).
  - Visibility of **tubes, lines,** and **catheters** is **improved.**
- **Segmentation outlines or otherwise identifies a group of related pixels** to create a region of interest (ROI).
  - Identifying an ROI (e.g., the kidney) is often the first step in deriving quantitative image measurements.
- **Registration aligns two images** or image series spatially.
  - Registered images are often **fused** to make a composite image (e.g., overlaying PET on top of computed tomographic images).

C. Read-Room Processing

- The radiologist can typically change window, level, and zoom using the mouse at the time of reading.

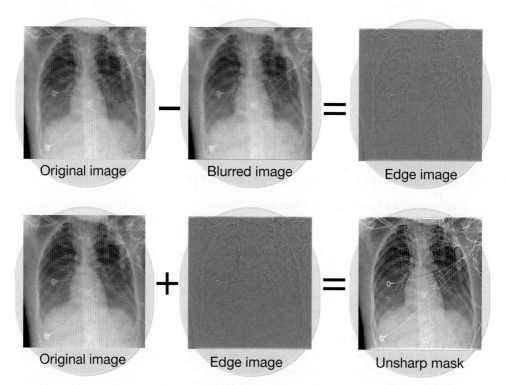

FIG 2.5 Unsharp masking to enhance edges. Top: A low-pass filter allows low spatial frequency image content to pass while filtering high spatial frequencies. This results in a blurred image with lower noise. Subtracting the blurred image from the original image leaves only high-frequency (edge and noise) data in the resultant image. Adding a weighted version of the edge image back to the original enhances the edges in the resultant image but also makes noise worse.

- Tonal qualities of any digital image can be modified by use of a **lookup table (LUT)**.
  - A simple LUT is a straight line that maps pixel values to image intensities.
- Display **window width** and **window level** settings (a type of simple LUT) can be adjusted by the operator, thus modifying image brightness and contrast.
- **Window level** (aka window center) defines the center value (middle gray) of the window width and therefore overall image **brightness.**
- **Window width** refers to how the hundreds or thousands of image values are mapped to 256 gray levels for display.
- Pixels below the window are typically set to black and those above as white.
- Image **contrast** within the window range is **increased** as **window narrows.**
- **Zoom** on the display **does not change the image resolution** but does change whether that resolution is displayed.
  - Zooming in increases the displayed resolution until it is the same as the native image resolution.
  - Further zooming increases image size and may bring small details into the **sensitive portion of the human visual system** for detection.

D. Displays

- Luminance and illuminance, grayscale standard display function (GSDF) and just noticeable difference (JND), view angle/distance.
- The **luminance** is a measure of the **brightness a monitor generates** in candelas per square meter **(cd/m^2).**
  - Maximum luminance should be at least **350 cd/m^2 for workstations** and **420 cd/m^2 for mammography** workstations.
- **Illuminance** is a measure of **light hitting the monitor** from outside sources (e.g., ambient light) and is measured in **lux.**
  - Too much illuminance **reduces contrast** on the monitor and should be limited to under 50 lux.
  - Typical home lighting produces 150 to 1,000 lux.
- **A JND** is the amount of increased luminance needed for a human to recognize a difference.
- The **human visual system is nonlinear,** so a JND requires a larger luminance difference between object and background at lower brightness.
  - It is harder for humans to see dark lesions on dark backgrounds than light regions on light backgrounds.
- The **DICOM GSDF** calibrates a monitor, so differences in image values translate into JNDs in the monitor luminance.
  - This ensures that you will see the low-contrast lesion regardless of the GSDF-calibrated monitor you view it on.
- In general, displays **lose contrast when viewed at an angle** instead of head-on.

E. Informatics Standards

- **Picture Archiving and Communications Systems (PACS)** receive, store, transfer, and display medical images.
- **Radiology Information Systems (RIS)** handle radiology department management including exam ordering, registration, billing, and reporting.
- **Hospital Information Systems (HIS)** are similar to RIS but manage the information across departments.
- **Informatics Standards** are agreed-upon methods for communicating, storing, and/or displaying information among different pieces of software and hardware.
  - Buying software conforming to a standard ensures that it can communicate with the larger ecosystem of software and computers.
- **Digital Imaging and Communications in Medicine (DICOM)** is a standard for the transferring, storing, and displaying medical images.

- The DICOM header has extensive information about study acquisition and structured reports may contain data derived from DICOM images (e.g., ultrasound size measurements).
- **Health Level 7 (HL7)** is a standard for communication among hospital systems and typically deals with nonimaging data.
- **Integrating the Healthcare Enterprise (IHE)** creates profiles detailing how overlaps between DICOM and HL7 should be handled and where gaps may need to be addressed.

Chapter 2 (Imaging) Questions

2.1 What is the ratio of scattered to primary x-rays in adult abdominal radiography?
A. 0.2:1
B. 1:1
C. 5:1
D. 25:1

2.2 What does scattered radiation degrade during image acquisition?
A. Contrast
B. Spatial resolution
C. Noise
D. Temporal resolution

2.3 What radiography examination body part is most likely to be performed without a grid?
A. Head
B. Chest
C. Abdomen
D. Extremity

2.4 What is a possible cause of grid cutoff artifact during bedside chest radiography?
A. High kV
B. Too much geometric magnification
C. Low grid ratio
D. Grid not perpendicular to beam

2.5 What grid ratio is typically used with geometric magnification?
A. No grid used
B. <10:1
C. 10:1
D. >10:1

2.6 What is the Bucky factor in adult abdominal radiography?
A. 1
B. 2
C. 5
D. 10

2.7 What is an example of preprocessing?
A. Creating a CT iodine map
B. Converting FDG concentrations to SUV
C. Interpolating over dead pixels
D. Changing window and level

2.8 What data set is typically the largest for a supervised learning algorithm?
A. Training
B. Validation
C. Testing

2.9 If illuminance is too high, what display characteristic will be degraded?
A. Contrast
B. Mottle
C. Sharpness
D. Refresh rate

2.10 An algorithm that aligns images from two different modalities (e.g., PET and CT) is an example of what type of postprocessing?
A. Segmentation
B. Registration
C. Enhancement
D. Classification

2.11 What detector should be used during fluoroscopy QC?
A. OSLD
B. Geiger counter
C. Ionization chamber
D. Well counter

2.12 Which type of detector is most likely to offer the best spatial resolution performance?
A. Photoconductor
B. Scintillator
C. Photostimulable phosphor

2.13 What informatics standard is primarily focused on transferring, storing, and displaying medical images?
A. IHE
B. DICOM
C. HL7
D. ASCII

2.14 What technique specifically utilizes image filters to automatically learn and apply features for decisions related to medical images?
A. Convolutional neural networks
B. Unsupervised machine learning
C. Artificial intelligence
D. Natural language processing

2.15 What routine imaging study takes up the most computer memory in PACS?
  A. Modified barium swallow
  B. Routine chest CT
  C. Tc 99m myocardial perfusion
  D. Screening breast tomosynthesis

2.16 How large is a 512 × 512 image with 2 byte bit depth?
  A. 1,024 bytes
  B. 512 kilobytes
  C. 0.25 megabytes
  D. 0.5 megabytes

2.17 Evaluating the performance of a diagnostic workstation would most likely use:
  A. SMPTE
  B. TCP/IP
  C. DICOM
  D. HTTP

2.18 What is the purpose of the DICOM grayscale standard display function?
  A. Ensure consistent display of image contrast
  B. Calibrate monitor pixel size
  C. Determine radiation amount to stored value relationship
  D. Assess noise under varying conditions

2.19 What pixel value will appear gray for a display with a window level of 500 and a window width of 1,000?
  A. 0
  B. 500
  C. 1,000
  D. 1,500

2.20 Which image processing algorithm is most likely to improve the visibility of tubes, lines, and catheters on bedside chest x-rays?
  A. Histogram equalization
  B. Energy subtraction
  C. Window and leveling
  D. Unsharp mask enhancement

Answers and Explanations

2.1 **C** (5:1). In abdominal radiography, about 5 scattered photons exit an adult patient for every primary photon that is transmitted.

2.2 **A** (Contrast). The presence of scattered radiation reduces (lesion) contrast.

2.3 **D** (Extremity) examinations have little scatter because of the presence of bone (high Z absorber) and the use of low tube voltages and are performed without grids.

2.4 **D** (Grid not perpendicular to beam). If the grid is not perpendicular to the beam, then the grid may block primary instead of scattered photons. This causes artificially increased opacity and may cause gridlines to be visible.

2.5 **A** (No grid used). Grids are generally not used in geometric magnification (e.g., magnification mammography) because the air gap ensures that most of the scatter emerging from the patient misses the image receptor.

2.6 **C** (5). Adding a grid increases the patient dose by a factor of 5 when the radiation intensity at the image receptor (Kair) is kept constant (i.e., Bucky factor).

2.7 **C** (Interpolating over dead pixels). Preprocessing involves correction issues with image acquisition. Uniformity correction and interpolating over dead detector elements are examples.

2.8 **A** (Training). In general, larger training sets allow for training on more diverse data and thus improve machine learning algorithm performance. Data need to also be set aside for validation and testing, but typically only a small fraction is used for these purposes. The bulk of the data is used to train the algorithm.

2.9 **A** (Contrast). Light bouncing off the monitor from ambient light interferes with light being created by the monitor and reduces the apparent contrast. At very high levels, the glare can be so bad that the image cannot be seen.

2.10 **B** (Registration). A registration algorithm takes two images and aligns them so that corresponding parts of the image overlap correctly. This allows for fusion images in SPECT/CT and PET/CT.

2.11 **C** (Ionization chamber). Ionization chambers are stable with high accuracy when measuring dose. They are the best choice when measuring a spectrum of radiation (like in x-ray imaging beams).

2.12 **A** (Photoconductor). Best resolution is achieved using photoconductors because the charge that is produced by absorbed x-rays does not disperse during the detection process as does light in scintillators.

2.13 **B** (DICOM). DICOM is the primary standard surrounding medical imaging.

2.14 **A** (Convolutional neural networks). CNNs convolve different filters over the image to derive features that are then utilized to perform a given task.

2.15 **D** (Screening breast tomosynthesis). Tomosynthesis uses the same number of pixels as mammography (larger than any other single image), involves many images for each view, and typically involves four views for screening. A tomosynthesis exam will likely be several gigabytes in size. Fluoroscopic exams could be very large, but most images are not sent to PACS for storage.

2.16 C (0.5 megabytes). Memory storage for an uncompressed image is the number of pixels times the bit depth. 512*512*2 is approximately half a megabyte.

2.17 A (SMPTE). Imaging professionals can (and should) use test patterns to evaluate monitor performance developed by the Society of Motion Picture and Television Engineers (i.e., SMPTE).

2.18 A (Ensure consistent display of image contrast). Digital pixel values (after processing) are converted into monitor brightness using the GSDF, which ensures similar contrast levels across different displays.

2.19 B (500). A pixel value of 500 will appear gray, values below 0 will appear black, and values above 1,000 will appear white.

2.20 D (Unsharp mask enhancement). Visibility of tubes, lines, and catheters in any x-ray image is markedly improved by using UME because this type of processing enhances all sharp edges.

CHAPTER

3 Foundations of Image Quality

I. CONTRAST

A. What Is Subject Contrast?

- **Subject contrast** exists if there is a difference in measurement between an object and background tissues (Fig. 3.1).
  - In x-ray imaging, a lesion **attenuates** a **different number of x-rays** compared with background tissues.
  - In ultrasound imaging, a lesion **reflects a different beam intensity** than background tissues.
  - In magnetic resonance imaging, a lesion has a different amount of transverse magnetization than background tissues.
  - In nuclear medicine, a concentrated radioisotope in a lesion emits more photons than background tissues.
- In x-ray imaging, the most **important lesion characteristic** affecting subject contrast is the **atomic number.**
  - **Density differences** will also affect **subject contrast.**
- **Subject contrast** is an **essential prerequisite** for producing **image contrast.**
- Presence of **subject contrast**, however, does **not guarantee image contrast.**
  - **Image processing** can make an image look all white and thus **display no image contrast**, even when subject contrast is present.
- **Contrast** is *always* **reduced** by the presence of **scattered radiation.**

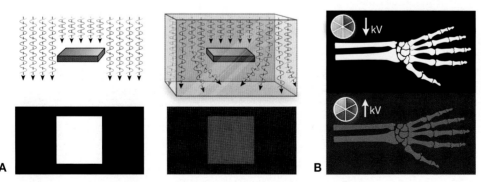

FIG 3.1 **A:** In the absence of scatter (left), lesion contrast is higher than when scatter is present (right). **B:** Use of low voltages (upper) generally results in higher contrast than use of high voltages (lower).

B. **What Is Image Contrast?**

- Changes in subject contrast typically result in a corresponding change in image contrast.
- In **digital radiography**, the image contrast is the difference in **average image brightness** of a lesion in comparison to the average image brightness of adjacent tissues.
  - A common measure of contrast is percent difference between lesion and background average values.
- **Contrast** is generally directly proportional to the **intrinsic subject contrast** of the lesion.
- Observed lesion contrast in digital imaging is also influenced by **image display** that is **controlled** by the **operator.**
- Width of the **display window** affects **image contrast**, with wide display windows reducing contrast between different types of tissue.
- Low contrast resolution is a loosely defined term associated with the ability to detect small differences in contrast
  - Conceptually, it is similar to either the contrast-to-noise ratio (CNR) or the signal-to-noise ratio (SNR) depending on the author using the term.

C. **Contrast and Photon Energy**

- In **x-ray imaging, low photon energies** result in **high subject contrast.**
- At low kV, differences in transmitted x-rays' intensities between adjacent tissues are relatively high due to photoelectric effect (Fig. 3.1).
  - **Photons hitting calcified nodules** will be absorbed much more than soft tissues when the x-ray photon **energy is low,** resulting in high subject contrast.
- **Photon x-ray energy** can be **lowered** by **reducing** the x-ray tube **voltage (kV)** or by **removing filters.**
- **Reducing** the x-ray beam average **energy** will generally result in **increased patient doses** if the same number of photons hit the patient.
  - Reducing kV is not always practical because of **insufficient patient penetration.**
- As photon energy increases, contrast decreases because of increased x-ray photon penetration (Fig. 3.1).
  - At very high energies, both calcified nodules and soft tissues transmit most incident x-rays, thereby reducing subject contrast.
- **Changes** in **lesion contrast** are strongly influenced by the **atomic number** of the **lesion.**
- **Increasing computed tomography (CT) energy** results in **modest reductions** in **soft tissue contrast** but **large reductions** in contrast of vessels containing **iodine** (Table 3.1).

D. **Latitude and Contrast**

- **Latitude** is the **range of radiation intensities (K_{air})** that result in a **satisfactory image contrast.**
- If minimum and maximum K_{air} values that show satisfactory image contrast are K_{air} (min) and K_{air} (max), respectively, **latitude** is K_{air} **(max) minus** K_{air} **(min).**
  - **Dynamic range** is the ratio K_{air}**(max):**K_{air}**(min).**

TABLE 3.1	Image Contrast of a CT Lesion in a Water Background As a Function of x-Ray Photon Energy (Normalized to 100% at 50 keV)	
X-Ray Energy (keV)	Soft Tissue Lesion (Z = 7.5)	Iodinated Vessel (Z = 53)
50	100	100
60	93	68
70	88	48
80	84	37

CT, computed tomography.
Note that contrast decreases more quickly for high-Z materials as energy increases.

- **Digital detectors'** latitude is high (e.g., **dynamic range 10,000:1)**, whereas that of **film** was low (e.g., **dynamic range 40:1)**.
- **Wide display window widths** generally have **low contrast**, whereas narrow windows permit digital image contrast to be increased.
- **Digital detectors record** images with a **wide dynamic range** receptor but present the images with a narrow window width to enhance displayed contrast.
- In **chest CT**, a **narrow window width** can offer **excellent soft tissue contrast**, but the **lungs** become **invisible** (all black).
- The use of a **wider window width** in chest CT permits **visualization** of **most tissues**, but the **contrast** between soft tissues is markedly **reduced.**

E. Contrast Agents

- **Contrast agents** including **air, barium**, and **iodine** are used to **improve subject contrast.**
- **Barium** is administered as a contrast agent for visualization of the **gastrointestinal tract** on radiographic examinations.
- Barium attenuation is high because of its high density and K-edge at 37 keV.
- Iodine is also an excellent contrast agent for reasons similar to those for barium (i.e., iodine K-edge is 33 keV).
- **Iodinated contrast agents** can be injected **intravenously** or **arterially.**
  - Dilution and the osmolar limitations of intravascular fluids limit the achievable iodine concentration.
- **Angiography** is best performed by using tube voltages of about **70 kV** where the average photon energy is slightly above the **K-edge of iodine (33 keV).**
- As the **tube voltage increases**, the **visibility** of vessels with **iodine** is progressively **reduced.**
- **Air** is a **negative contrast agent** and increases subject contrast because it is less attenuating than tissue.
  - **Carbon dioxide** is also sometimes used as a contrast agent in **angiography.**

▮▮ II. NOISE

A. What Is Noise?

- **Noise** describes the content of an image that **limits** the ability to **visualize lesions** or pathology.
  - **Noise** can be categorized as being **fixed** or **random.**
- An example of **fixed noise** is the presence of **anatomical structures** that can inhibit the visibility of lesions.
  - **Nodules** may be **masked** by the **rib cage** in chest radiographs, and this may be referred to as anatomic noise.
- X-ray images also exhibit **random variations** in image intensity.
- **Random variations** in intensity are known as **mottle**, because the resultant image has a mottled appearance (i.e., grainy).
- **Noise** is typically quantified as to fluctuations (i.e., standard deviation) expressed as **percentage** of the **mean value.**
- In many medical images, the process of image formation (e.g., **blur**) introduces a **structure (texture)** to the resultant **noise.**
- **Image reconstruction** (e.g., filtered back projection in CT) can also introduce **structure** to **noise (texture).**
- The **standard deviation σ** does **not fully characterize noise** in medical images **when correlations** are **present.**

B. Sources of Mottle

- For a flat panel detector, the **thickness** of the **scintillator** can exhibit **random fluctuations**, with higher x-ray absorption for thicker crystals.

- When **analog signals** (e.g., voltages) are **digitized**, similar signals can be allocated different digital values (**digitization noise**).
- When detected **signals** are relatively **low**, the **electronic noise** from digital detectors components **can contribute** to mottle in the resultant image.
- For a **uniform x-ray image**, adjacent pixels detect a different number of photons in a random manner resulting in **quantum mottle**.
  - Each pixel has a slightly different number of photons, and the image has a grainy appearance (perfectly uniform exposure).
- **Quantum mottle** generally depends on the **number** or concentration of **x-ray photons** used to **produce an image.**
  - Quantum mottle, also called shot noise, follows Poisson statistics, meaning that the standard deviation is the square root of the mean.
- Quantum mottle is **quantified** as the **percentage fluctuations** about the mean value (i.e., $\sigma/M \times 100\%$).
- For magnetic resonance imaging (MRI), noise may come from protons in the body outside the region of interest that randomly precess at the Larmor frequency.

C. Quantum Mottle in X-Ray Imaging

- **Quantum mottle** is the **dominant** source of **random noise** in most of x-ray imaging, which is referred to as **quantum limited imaging.**
- **Digital radiography** performed using scintillators, photoconductors, and photostimulable phosphors is **quantum mottle limited.**
- Both **analog** mammography and **digital mammography** are **quantum mottle limited**.
- Noise in **fluoroscopy** performed using image intensifiers and flat-panel detectors is **quantum mottle limited.**
- **CT** is normally **quantum mottle limited**, but electronic noise can become a problem when imaging large patients.
  - Large patients transmit very little radiation to the x-ray detectors.
- When a system is quantum mottle limited, the number of photons used to create an image is a dominant source of image mottle.
- When x-ray detectors **absorb all** of the incident x-ray photons, there is **no technical way** to **reduce mottle without increasing dose.**
  - Quantum mottle in x-ray and gamma-ray imaging is proportional to $1/\sqrt{Absorbed\ Receptor\ Dose}$.

D. Controlling Quantum Mottle

- The number of photons used to create any x-ray image is directly related to the K_{air} at the **image receptor.**
- **Increasing** the number of photons (i.e., the **mAs**) **reduces quantum mottle**, as depicted in Figure 3.2.
- Using **more photons** to reducing mottle **increases patient doses.** If the average number of **photons per pixel is 100**, the standard deviation is 10 ($100^{0.5}$), and the **mottle is 10%.**
- Increasing the average number of photons to **10,000 reduces** the **mottle to 1%** (standard deviation 100).
- **Quadrupling** the number of **photons** used to generate any x-ray image can be expected to **halve** the corresponding x-ray **mottle.**
- Image receptor **detection efficiency** affects the amount of **noise** in an **image.**
- Detectors **absorbing 50%** require **twice** the K_{air} at the image receptor to achieve the same level of mottle as **detectors absorbing 100%** of incident photons.
- **Image processing** can also be employed to **reduce image mottle.**
- Average four adjacent pixels in fluoroscopy (binning) will reduce interpixel fluctuations (noise) but also reduce the spatial resolution.
- In CT, **reconstruction kernel/filter** can **reduce image mottle** at the **price** of **reduced spatial resolution** performance.

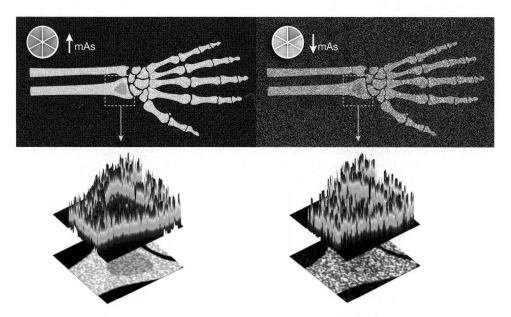

FIG 3.2 The left-hand side image was obtained using high tube current (mAs), with a large number of photons, and therefore shows little mottle. A triangular bone lesion is clearly visualized. The right-hand side image was obtained using a sixth of the mAs (i.e., 1/6th photons) and therefore has markedly increased mottle. Note loss of visibility of the bone lesion with increased noise. Lower images are surface plots (gray level plotted as height demonstrating the strength of noise compared to the subtle lesion signal strength.

E. Mottle and Image Quality

- In **photography**, the number of light photons required to expose a film is very high (e.g., $10^9/mm^2$).
  - The large number of light photons used is the reason why mottle is generally not visible in photographs.
- In **diagnostic radiography**, the number of x-ray photons used to create a radiographic image is much lower than that in photography (e.g., $10^5/mm^2$).
  - Mottle is much more notable in radiography than in photography because it uses 10,000 times fewer photons.
- In **cardiac cine imaging**, the number of photons is about $10^4/mm^2$, an order of magnitude lower than that in radiography.
  - Individual cardiac cine frames exhibit much more noise (mottle) than radiographs.
- In **fluoroscopy**, the number of photons used to generate each frame is about $10^3/mm^2$, or a hundred times lower than that in radiography.
  - Because mottle is so pronounced in fluoroscopy, these images are often not deemed to be of diagnostic quality.
- Table 3.2 shows the how the number of x-ray photons (i.e., image receptor K_{air}) varies in x-ray imaging.

TABLE 3.2	**Nominal Values of the Image Receptor K_{air} That are Commonly Used to Obtain a Single Radiographic Image (Frame)**	
Imaging Modality	**Air Kerma at Image Receptor (K_{air}) µGy**	**Relative Image Receptor K_{air}**
Fluoroscopy	0.02	1
Acquisition cine imaging	0.2	10
Photospot and radiography	2	100
Mammogram	100	5,000

- **Mammograms** use **10,000 times more x-ray photons** than **one fluoroscopy frame.**
- In **nuclear medicine**, the number of photons is very low (e.g., **10/mm²**).
  - The root cause of the highly **mottled** images in **nuclear medicine** is the **small number of photons** used.

III. RESOLUTION

A. What Is Resolution?

- **Resolution** is the ability of an imaging system to display **two adjacent objects** as **discrete entities,** as depicted in Figure 3.3.
  - Resolution is also known as **spatial resolution, high contrast resolution, detail visibility, sharpness,** or **blur.**
  - Low resolution is associated with more blur in an image.
- Two small adjacent objects such as **microcalcifications** will appear **sharp** and **distinct** in an image obtained with a system that has **good resolution.**
  - Adjacent **microcalcifications** might appear as **one blurred blob** in images obtained with a system that has **poor resolution.**
- Resolution is quantified using **spatial frequencies** expressed in **line pairs/mm (lp/mm)** or **cycles per millimeter.**
  - **High spatial frequencies** pertain to **small objects,** and vice versa.
  - Spatial frequencies are properties of an image and are NOT the same as photon or ultrasound wave frequencies.
- Resolution can be quantified using **parallel line bar phantoms** that exhibit very high intrinsic contrast.
  - Strips of **lead** absorb all the incident x-rays and **appear white,** whereas the **gaps** transmit most of the x-rays and appear **black.**
- **One line pair per millimeter** (1 lp/mm) is a bar phantom that has 0.5 mm lead bars separated by 0.5 mm of radiolucent material.
- Limiting spatial resolution is the maximum number of line pairs per millimeter that can be recorded by the imaging system.
  - **Human eyes resolve 5 lp/mm** (25 cm viewing distance).
- **Focal spot size, patient motion,** and **detector blur** all **influence** achievable spatial **resolution performance** in x-ray imaging.

B. Focal Spot Blur

- The **finite size** of a focal spot results in **blurred images.**

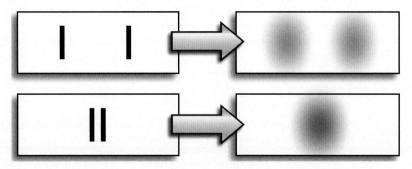

FIG 3.3 Shown on the left are test objects, which are radiopaque slabs with radiotranslucent slits. Shown on the right are resultant images. An imaging system with poor resolution will show two blurred slits when these are well separated (upper) but is unable to depict two distinct slits in the image when the objects are close to each other (bottom).

- Focal blurring is caused by x-rays emitted from slightly different locations in the focal spot depositing information from the same part of the object to different parts of the image.
- Loss of sharpness is called **focal spot blur** or **geometric unsharpness.**
- Focal spot blur increases with increasing focal spot size.
- **Large focal** spots are chosen to reduce heating and increase x-ray tube output to **reducing exposure times.**
- **Focal spot blur increases** with increasing **geometric magnification.**
  - Geometric magnification is source-to-detector distance divided by source-to-object distance.
- **Smaller focal spots are needed when magnifying to combat focal spot blur.**
- Focal spot **blur** is **minimal** in **extremity radiography** because **geometric magnification** is very **small.**
- Magnification increases focal spot blur but decreases detector blur and so may increase overall resolution if the correct amount of magnification is used.

C. **Motion Blur**
- **Patient motion** introduces blur by smearing out the object in the image.
  - **Involuntary organ motion** (e.g., heart) results in **image blur.**
- **Gross movement** of the patient, as well as movement of the imaging system relative to the patient, also results in **motion blur.**
- Patient motion can be reduced by gating or by the use of **immobilization devices** such as the **compression paddle** in mammography.
- **Motion blur** is **independent** of image **magnification.**
- For a constant x-ray tube output (mAs**), increasing the mA** will generally reduce the exposure time, thereby **minimizing motion blur.**
  - Increasing the mA may not be possible, however, because of limits on the focal spot loading of the x-ray tube.
- **Exposure times** can also be **reduced** by **increasing** the x-ray tube **voltage (kV)** because of increases in x-ray tube output and patient penetration.
  - Using **higher kV values**, however, will **reduce image contrast** and **increase scatter** radiation.
- In MRI, fewer phase encode steps, shorter repetition times, using PROPELLER, and other protocol changes can decrease acquisition times and reduce motion blur.

D. **Detector Blur and Nyquist Frequency**
- **Scintillator thickness** introduces a **limit** on the achievable spatial **resolution** performance in radiography and nuclear medicine.
  - **Light** produced by absorbed x-rays **spreads out (i.e., diffuses)** prior to detection, with the spreading increasing with thickness (Fig. 3.4).
- In all digital imaging, the **pixel size** limits the **sharpness of images**, with large pixels implying blurry edges, and vice versa.
- Using discrete **pixels** introduces "sampling" into all digital images.
  - **Sampling** is the **number** of **pixels** in **each millimeter of physical space.**
- A 500 pixel matrix along a line for a head CT (250 mm diameter) corresponds to a **pixel size of 0.5 mm** (250 mm divided by 500 pixels).
  - **Sampling frequency,** assuming 0.5 mm per pixel is 1/0.5, is **2 pixels per mm.**
- **Limiting spatial resolution** is **half** the **sampling frequency** and is referred to as the **Nyquist frequency.**
- A **sampling frequency of 2 pixels per mm** has a limiting **resolution of 1 lp/mm.**
  - One millimeter containing 2 pixels can display no better than one black and one white pixel (i.e., 1 lp/mm).
- **Nyquist frequency** defines the highest spatial frequency in an object that can be *faithfully* reproduced in digital images.
- Presence of **higher spatial frequencies** in the object results in **aliasing artifacts.**

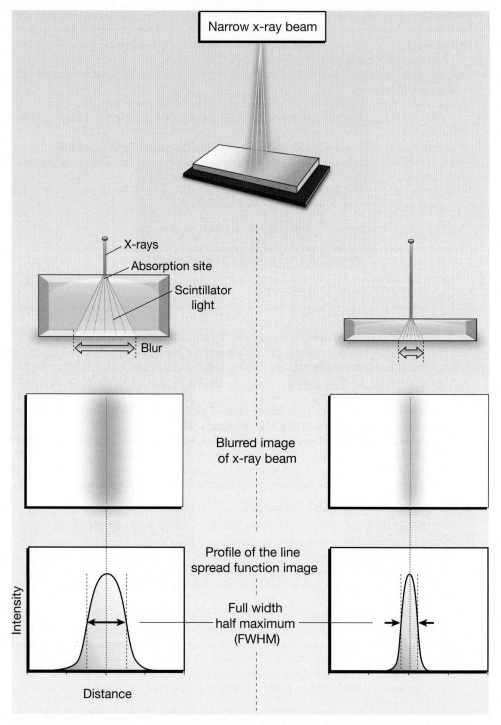

FIG 3.4 Top is an x-ray beam irradiating a radiopaque test object with a radiotranslucent slit in it. The test object is on top of a scintillator detector. The image produced is a line spread function (LSP), which is a measure of spatial resolution. Thicker scintillators (left) result in blurrier images, because of the increased spreading out of the light produced when x-rays are absorbed. Thin detectors (right) result in sharper images, but because these capture fewer x-rays, they will also likely increase patient doses. Lower images are profiles through the LSP demonstrating more blur and thus lower resolution as quantified by the full width half maximum (FWHM).

- **Aliasing artifacts** are always caused by **insufficient sampling** and are **ubiquitous** in **digital imaging.**
  - **Aliasing** artifacts are **minimized** by **increasing** the **sampling** rate (e.g., more pixels per mm).

E. LSF and MTF

- The image of a **narrow line** source is called a **line spread function (LSF),** and its width (broadening) is a measure of the system blur or resolution (Fig. 3.4).
- LSF width is measured at half the maximum value, termed **full width half maximum (FWHM),** as depicted in Figure 3.5.
- A **wide LSF** implies **poor spatial resolution.**
- **A narrow LSF** (<1 mm) is **difficult to measure,** and bar phantoms (i.e., lp/mm) are used to measure spatial resolution performance.
- **Wide LSFs (i.e., FWHM > 5 mm)** are **easy to measure** and are often used in **nuclear medicine.**
- The **modulation transfer function (MTF)** describes the spatial resolution capability of an imaging system.
  - Also called **contrast transfer function.**

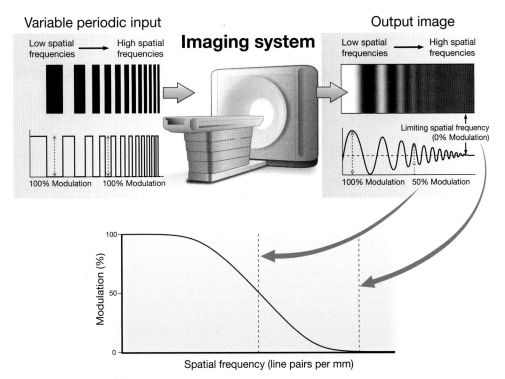

FIG 3.5 Top left is a bar phantom where radiopaque blocks are interspersed with radiotranslucent areas. The blocks and areas progressively get smaller and closer together (i.e., increase in spatial frequency). A plot of varying image values are plotted below the bar phantom—all at full (100% modulation (i.e., signal difference between radiopaque blocks and radiotranslucent areas). Imaging will result in a blurred version of the bar phantom with reduced modulation (right). Note that the output modulation is progressively reduced as spatial frequency increases (i.e., high spatial frequencies representing edges and small object are impacted more). Bottom is the modulation transfer function (MTF) is simply a plot of the output modulation produced by an imaging system as a function of the spatial frequency, and limiting resolution occurs roughly when the output modulation drops to about 10%.

TABLE 3.3	Limiting Resolution in x-Ray Imaging	
Imaging Modality	**Limiting Spatial Resolution (lp/mm)**	**Relative Resolution (%)**
Digital mammography	7	100
Extremity radiography	5	70
Chest radiography	3	45
Digital photospot (II + 1,000 line TV)	2	30
Computed tomography	0.7	10

- The MTF is the ratio of **output to input** (signal amplitude) in an imaging system at each spatial frequency (Fig. 3.5).
- **Output modulation** of all imaging systems is **less than the 100% input** because of blur introduced by the system (e.g., **focal spot**).
  - **Blur** becomes increasingly **important** as the **spatial frequency increases** (i.e., as the objects of interest get smaller).
- At **low spatial frequencies**, the **MTF is close to 1.0** and corresponds to excellent visibility of relatively large features.
  - At **high spatial frequencies**, the **MTF always falls to zero**, which corresponds to the poor visibility of small features.
  - Limiting resolution is generally taken as the lp/mm that MTF = 0.1 (i.e., 10%).
- Table 3.3 summarizes **limiting resolution performance** in diagnostic imaging modalities that use x-rays.

IV. DIAGNOSTIC PERFORMANCE

A. Diagnostic Task

- **Image quality** is always **task dependent.**
- In the **absence** of any defined **imaging task**, it is simply **not possible** to determine **"image quality."**
- A **noisy abdominal CT** image might be deemed to be of very **poor** quality when the imaging task is the detection of **low-contrast (subtle) lesions** in the liver.
  - The **same abdominal CT** image might be deemed **excellent** if the imaging task is the assessment of **diameter** of the **abdominal aorta.**
- The imaging task should always be taken into account when developing any imaging protocol.
- A **follow-up scoliosis x-ray** examination can generally be performed at **radiation intensities** that are **much lower** than that for chest x-rays.
- **Lung screening CT** examinations would use **less radiation** because the **lesions** are **high contrast** where high mottle can be tolerated.
- **Angiography** would likely require the use of **tube voltages** between **70 and 80 kV** to maximize the absorption of x-rays by iodine contrast.
  - **Barium** studies would likely use **110 kV** for adequate penetration and visualization of bowel loops.

B. Contrast-to-Noise Ratio and Signal-to-Noise Ratio

- Whether a **lesion is detected** will depend on *all* the key determinants of image quality (**contrast, mottle, and blur**).
- When the lesion contrast is high, the lesion will be generally visible irrespective of the amount of image mottle.
- When the **lesion contrast** is **lower** than the amount of **image mottle (noise)**, the lesion becomes impossible to detect.

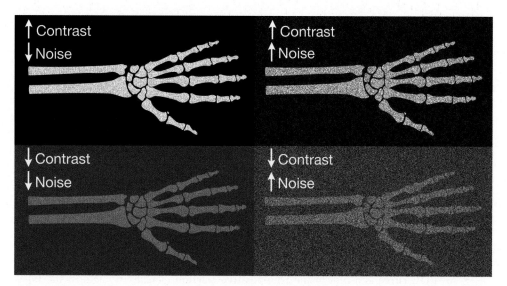

FIG 3.6 The contrast-to-noise ratio (CNR) reflects the relative visibility so that increases in CNR improve lesion visibility, and vice versa. Worst visibility occurs when contrast is low and noise is high (lower right), which can be improved by increasing contrast (upper right) or by reducing noise (lower left). The best visibility (CNR) is when contrast is high and noise is low (upper left).

- The **CNR** is a way of quantifying the *relative* **visibility** of any lesion accounting for image contrast and noise (Fig. 3.6).
- As the **CNR** is **reduced**, the **lesion** becomes more **difficult** to **detect**.
  - **Increasing the mAs increases the CNR** by decreasing noise.
  - **The CNR** in x-ray imaging **increases as** $\sqrt{Absorbed\ Receptor\ Dose}$.
- Increasing **tube voltage** decreases both mottle and contrast, so it is **unclear how the CNR is impacted** without specific measurement.
  - Clinical practice shows that **raising** the **kV** is most likely to **reduce the CNR** of **high Z objects** (e.g., angiography).
- **Visibility of a lesion** can be calculated in an **absolute** (not relative) sense using **the SNR.**
- **SNR computations** generally consider all the features of a lesion, including the **lesion contrast** and **size.**
  - **SNR computations** also account for **spatial resolution, contrast, noise**, and the response of the **human visual system.**
- An **SNR > 5** indicates that a lesion is almost **certain** to be **detected.**

C. Diagnostic Tests

- **True positives (TPs)** are positive test results in patients who have the disease.
- **True negatives (TNs)** are negative test results in patients who do not have the disease.
- **False positives (FPs)** are positive test results in patients who do not have the disease.
- **False negatives (FNs)** are negative test results in patients who have the disease.
- Table 3.4 is a **confusion matrix** that may be applied to any binary diagnostic test.
- **Sensitivity** is the ability to detect disease and is TP/(TP + FN), also known as the **true-positive fraction.**
  - A sensitive test has a low false-negative rate.
- **Specificity** is the ability to identify the absence of disease and is TN/(TN + FP), also known as the **true-negative fraction.**
  - A specific test has a low false-positive rate.
- **Accuracy** is the fraction of **correct diagnosis** and is (TP + TN)/(TP + FP + TN + FN).

TABLE 3.4	Confusion Matrix for a Binary Diagnostic Test	
Disease	**Positive Test**	**Negative Test**
Present	True positive (TP)	False negative (FN)
Absent	False positive (FP)	True negative (TN)

- **Positive predictive value** is the probability of having the disease given a positive test and is TP/(TP + FP).
- **Negative predictive value** is the probability of not having the disease given a negative test and is TN/(TN + FN).
- **Diagnostic performance** will generally depend on the **disease prevalence.**
  - Prevalence of the disease is (TP + FN)/(TP + FP + TN + FN).

D. Receiver Operator Characteristic Curve

- **Receiver operator characteristic (ROC)** curves compare performance (sensitivity and specificity) at various thresholds of interpreter confidence.
- An **ROC curve** is a plot of the **true-positive fraction** (sensitivity) against the **false-positive fraction** (1– specificity) as the **threshold criterion** is **relaxed.**
- Threshold criteria for accepting a positive diagnosis range from "strict" to "lax."
- **Strict thresholds** mean **underreading** an image, whereas **lax thresholds** mean **over-scrutinizing** an image.
  - The "strictest" threshold criterion has both sensitivity and the false-positive fraction 0, and the most "lax" criterion has these metrics 1.
- **Threshold criteria** represent different **compromises** between the need to **increase sensitivity** and **minimizing** the **number of false-positives.**
- Readers with **low sensitivities** as well as low false positives would be considered "**underreaders**."
  - Readers with **very high sensitivities** as well as corresponding **high false positives** would be considered "**overscrutinizers**."
- The **area under an ROC curve (AUC)** is a measure of overall **imaging performance** and is commonly called A_z.
  - The **maximum (best) area under the curve is 1.0** (i.e., 100%).
- For **random guessing**, the ROC curve is a straight line through the points (0,0) and (1,1), and the **area under the curve is 0.5** (i.e., 50%).
- As the imaging performance improves, the area under the ROC curve increases.
  - **ROC methods** are a good way to establish the **relative merits** of any **imaging tests.**

Chapter 3 (Image Quality) Questions

3.1 In x-ray imaging, subject contrast is dependent on what acquisition parameter?
A. Tube voltage
B. Tube current
C. Exposure time
D. Focal spot

3.2 In T2-weighted imaging, how will a small increase in echo time impact image contrast?
A. Increase
B. No change
C. Decrease

3.3 Image contrast in radiography is independent of what x-ray tube characteristic?
A. Applied voltage (kV)
B. Beam filtration (Al)
C. Relative output (mAs)

3.4 What does the large latitude (or dynamic range) of digital detectors mean?
A. Very large and very small amounts of radiation can still create image contrast.
B. Detector sensitivity on each edge of a detector is very similar.
C. A large filtration is needed to form the image.

3.5 Which atomic number (Z) is most likely to generate the highest lesion contrast relative to tissue (Z = 7.5) in chest radiography (i.e., 120 kV)?
A. 6.5 (fat)
B. 53 (iodine)
C. 56 (barium)
D. 64 (gadolinium)

3.6 The distribution of photons per pixel in a uniformly exposed digital x-ray detector is best described as being:
A. Exponential
B. Logarithmic
C. Poisson
D. Random

3.7 If a detector's x-ray absorption efficiency is halved, the number of x-ray photons required to maintain the image contrast-to-noise ratio is most likely:
A. Quartered
B. Halved
C. Doubled
D. Quadrupled

3.8 Noise reduction by the application of pixel averaging is most likely to result in _____ spatial resolution performance.
A. improved
B. the same
C. inferior

3.9 What is the quantum mottle, if the average number of counts in an NM detector element is 100?
A. 10%
B. 3%
C. 1%
D. 0.3%

3.10 What modality uses the fewest photons to construct an image?
A. Radiography
B. Mammography
C. Fluoroscopy
D. Computed tomography

3.11 Chest x-rays exhibit less mottle than NM imaging because the number of photons used is _____ times higher.
A. 5
B. 100
C. 10,000

3.12 In x-ray imaging, how is limiting spatial resolution assessed?
A. Spatial frequencies
B. Contrast-detail curves
C. ROC curves
D. SMPTE patterns

3.13 How is focal spot blur best minimized?
A. Increased source-to-image distance (SID)
B. Increased image magnification
C. Increased air gap distance
D. Increased focal spot size

3.14 How does motion blur severity change as magnification increases?
A. Increases
B. Independent
C. Decreases

3.15 If scintillator thickness increases, then how is spatial resolution impacted?
A. Increases
B. No change
C. Decreases

3.16 What is the Nyquist frequency for 0.1 mm pixels?
A. 0.1 lp/mm
B. 0.2 lp/mm
C. 5 lp/mm
D. 10 lp/mm

3.17 How does spatial resolution change as full width half maximum measurement increases?
A. Increases
B. No change
C. Decreases

3.18 What is always necessary to determine image quality?
A. Diagnostic task
B. Modulation transfer function
C. Contrast-detail curve
D. Signal-to-noise ratio

3.19 Which is the best indicator of the overall visibility of a lesion in a radiograph?
A. SNR
B. CNR
C. MTF
D. ROC

3.20 In an ROC curve, sensitivity is plotted against what quantity?
A. Specificity
B. 1+ specificity
C. 1− specificity
D. 1/specificity

Answers and Explanations

3.1 **A** (Tube voltage). The x-ray tube voltage (average photon energy) will affect subject contrast, which is independent of tube current, exposure time, and focal spot size.

3.2 **A** (Increase). T2 images show contrast through different T2 decay times. A longer echo time allows more time for T2 differences to change tissue signals and results in larger differences in signals between tissues.

3.3 **C** (Relative output (mAs)). Contrast is independent of intensity (i.e., mAs) but depends on average photon energy, which is influenced by voltage and beam filtration.

3.4 **A** (Very large and very small amounts of radiation can still create image contrast). A typical digital x-ray detector has a dynamic range of 10,000:1 or more, allowing an image contrast to be formed from both very low and very high amounts of radiation. The former will result in noisy images and the latter overdose of patient.

3.5 **D** (Z = 64). Because these have the highest K-edge energy and will absorb the highest number of incident x-rays.

3.6 **C** (Poisson). If the average number of photons per pixel is 100, there will be a Poisson distribution where the standard deviation is 10 (i.e., 1000.5). At large photon counts, the Poisson distribution is similar to a Gaussian.

3.7 **C** (Doubled). To maintain the CNR, the number of detected photons used to create an image must be maintained, which requires doubling the incident number of x-rays when a detector only detects one half of these photons.

3.8 **C** (inferior). Random noise can be reduced by averaging the detected counts in adjacent pixels, but this will most likely result in a blurrier image.

3.9 **A** (10%). The mottle is *always* expressed as the fluctuation (10) as percentage about the mean (100), or 10%. This is representative of NM, where pixel-to-pixel fluctuations are 10%, and why NM images are poor (i.e., mottled).

3.10 **C** (Fluoroscopy). Low doses for each fluoroscopy frame are needed to keep from harming the patient.

3.11 **C** (10,000). Radiographs use 10^5 light photons per mm^2 to create an image, 10,000× higher than the 10 gamma rays per mm^2 used to make planar NM images.

3.12 **A** (Spatial frequencies). Resolution performance can be assessed using line pair phantoms containing a range of spatial frequencies (lines pairs per millimeter); low spatial frequencies are "large" objects, whereas high spatial frequencies are small objects.

3.13 **A** (Increased SID). Increasing the SID will generally reduce image magnification and the corresponding amount of focal spot blur, whereas all the other factors increase image blur.

3.14 **B** (Independent). Motion blur is independent of magnification. If the image is magnified, this affects both the blur and size of the image exactly the same amount.

3.15 **C** (Decreases). Light spread will increase, as it needs to travel longer distances through the scintillator. This spread adds blur to the image.

3.16 **C** (5 lp/mm). With 0.1 mm pixels, there are 10 in each mm (i.e., sampling frequency), which means that 5 can be "black" and 5 can be white, corresponding to a best possible spatial frequency of 5 line pairs per mm (1 black + 1 white pixel is a line pair).

3.17 **C** (Decreases). A large FWHM means there is more blur and thus lower spatial resolution.

3.18 A (Diagnostic task). Without a defined imaging task, it is (literally) impossible to define any kind of meaningful image quality.

3.19 A (SNR). The signal-to-noise ratio (SNR) is a number that provides the best indication of whether a lesion would be detected (imaging scientists consider that an SNR > 5 means the lesion is definitely visible).

3.20 C (1 – specificity). An ROC curve plots sensitivity versus false-positive fraction (i.e., 1– specificity).

Patient Dosimetry

I. INCIDENT AND ABSORBED RADIATION

A. **Kerma**

- **Kerma** is the ability of the x-ray beam to transfer energy to electrons in a given material.
  - Kerma can be specified in **tissue**, **air**, or other materials.
- Specification of the tube voltage (kV) and intensity (mAs) is insufficient to characterize the radiation incident on the patient or receptor.
  - X-ray beam **output** also **depends** on x-ray **tube design** as well as x-ray beam **filtration**.
  - K_{air} is proportional to the "**number of x-ray photons per mm^2.**"
- **X-ray intensity** (i.e., K_{air} **in a given time period**) falls off with **increasing distance** from an x-ray source according to the **inverse square law.**
  - **Doubling the distance** from a source reduces K_{air} to **a quarter.**
- K_{air} is generally **proportional** to the **selected mAs** and increases in a **supralinear** manner with x-ray **tube voltage** in radiography and CT.
  - When tube voltages increase by 10%, K_{air} at a given point will generally increase by much more than 10%.
- **Increasing** x-ray tube **filtration reduces K_{air}.**
  - **Adding 3 mm aluminum** to a typical radiographic x-ray beam (80 kV) is likely to **reduce K_{air} by 50%.**
- X-ray output (K_{air} or **quantity**) and x-ray beam penetrating power (**half-value layer [HVL] in mm Al** or **quality**) are *both* required to characterize the radiation incident on a patient.
- **Tissue kerma is ~10% greater than air kerma** because tissue is denser than air, so there are more interactions for the same number of photons.
- Table 4.1 shows **typical dose metrics and their units**.

B. **Entrance K_{air}**

- The radiation **incident** on a **patient** is referred to as the **entrance K_{air}.**
- **Entrance K_{air}**, when combined with beam quality information, can be used by physicists to estimate the **pattern** of **energy deposition** in the **patient.**
- Patient attenuation, source-to-image distance (SID), beam energy, and percentage of x-rays absorbed in the receptor are important **determinants** of entrance K_{air}.
- **Entrance K_{air}** for an adult lateral skull **radiograph** is **~1 mGy.**
  - **Entrance K_{air}** can be much **lower** for a posteroanterior (PA) **chest** x-ray (**e.g., 0.1 mGy**) and much **higher** for a **lateral lumbar** spine x-ray (**e.g., 10 mGy**).
- In **fluoroscopy** examinations on a typical adult patient, the **entrance K_{air} rate** is **roughly 10 mGy/min.**

TABLE 4.1	Common Dose Metrics		
Quantity	**Units**	**Definition**	**Common Use in Radiology**
Kerma	Gray (Gy) or rad[a] (old units)	Energy per kilogram given to charged particles	Amount of radiation incident on person or detector
Exposure	Coulombs per kilogram (C/kg) or Roentgen (R)	Charge ionized per kilogram of air	Like air kerma, no longer used
Absorbed dose	Gy or rad[a] (old units)	Energy per kilogram deposited locally	Radiation absorbed in an organ or some area of the patient
Equivalent dose	Sv or rem[a] (old units)	Absorbed dose accounting for ability of a radiation type to damage tissue	Risk of tissue damage when radiation is not a photon or electron
Effective dose	Sv or rem[a] (old units)	Whole-body equivalent dose giving same patient detriment as the scan of interest	Compare stochastic risk across different scans

[a]rad and rem are old units that have generally been replaced by Gy and Sv. 1 rad is 10 mGy and 1 rem is 10 mSv.

- Fluoroscopy **entrance K_{air} rates** can **vary** markedly depending on the **field of view**, **frame rate, selected dose level, and SID**.
- **Entrance K_{air}** always depends on patient **size** (i.e., attenuation) and beam **quality** (i.e., penetration).

C. Kerma-Area Product

- The quantity that takes into account the *total* amount of **radiation incident** on the patient is the **kerma-area product (KAP).**
  - **Dose-area product (or DAP)** is often used instead of KAP, and the two terms are synonymous.
- **KAP** is the product of the **entrance K_{air}** and the corresponding cross-sectional **area** of the **x-ray beam** (exposed area).
- An **entrance K_{air}** of **10 mGy**, with a corresponding x-ray beam **area** of **1,000 cm²**, results in a **KAP** of **10 Gy-cm²**.
  - **KAP** is **independent** of the **measurement location**.
- **KAP** incident on the patient is the **key input metric** for all **subsequent patient dose** computations such as effective dose.
- The median **KAP** in **radiographic imaging** is **1 Gy-cm²**.
- For fluoroscopy-guided **gastrointestinal (GI) studies** and **urological** procedures, the median **KAP** is **20 Gy-cm²**.
  - Patient doses and risks in fluoroscopy-guided **GI/genitourinary (GU)** studies can be expected to be **20 times higher** than that in **radiographic examinations**.
- The median **KAP** in **interventional radiology** is **200 Gy-cm²**.
  - Patient doses and risks in **interventional radiology** can be expected to be **10 times higher** than that in fluoroscopy-guided **GI/GU studies**.
- KAP use is problematical for radiologists because vendors use different varying units, which results in confusion as to the amount of radiation delivered.

D. Absorbed Dose

- **Absorbed dose (D)** measures the amount of **radiation energy (E) locally absorbed per unit mass (M)** of a medium.
- **Absorbed dose** is specified in **gray (Gy)**, where 1 gray is equal to 1 J of energy deposited per kilogram.
  - 1 Gy is 1,000 mGy, and 1 mGy is 1,000 µGy.
- For the **same air kerma**, **absorbed dose depends** on the **material or tissue** that is placed into the x-ray beam.

- An **air kerma** of 1 mGy **deposits more** energy **into bone than soft tissue** because bone has a higher atomic number (12.5 vs 7.5).
- The **skin absorbed dose** is used to estimate the **likelihood** of **skin injury.**
- **Eye lens absorbed dose** is used to estimate the **likelihood** of **cataract induction.**
- **Organ absorbed doses** (e.g., lung or breast) can be used to estimate the **risk** of a radiation-induced **cancer.**
- **Embryo and fetal doses** are used to estimate the **likelihood** of **harm.**
- Absorbed dose in tissue is **strictly less than or equal to** tissue kerma.
- In **radiology,** the low energies mean tissue absorbed dose and tissue kerma are **usually the same.**
  - Energy transferred to charged particles in tissue is also deposited locally.

II. PATIENT ABSORBED DOSES

A. Superficial Doses

- **Superficial doses** relates to doses absorbed by the **skin, scalp,** and **eye lens.**
- **Peak** (not average) **absorbed dose** best **predicts** the **likelihood** of the relevant bio effects (i.e., **erythema, epilation, cataracts**).
- Radiations incident on any patient (i.e., **entrance K_{air} and KAP**) are generally **easy to calculate** and/or **measure.**
- An **entrance K_{air} of 1 mGy** can result in a superficial **skin dose** of up to **1.5 mGy** depending on the x-ray beam area and quality.
  - Tissue absorbs about **10% more than air** (higher Z), and the presence of **backscatter** can **increase superficial tissue doses** by up to **40%.**
- **Exit skin doses** for head examinations are about **1%** of the **entrance dose.**
  - When the **exit dose** is **1%,** the dose in the **middle** is the geometric mean of the entrance and exit doses (i.e., 100% and 1%), or **10%.**
- **Skin doses** in **radiography** are generally **very low (<10 mGy).**
- For **fluoroscopy-guided** procedures, **skin doses** are generally **below 500 mGy.**
  - Skin doses in radiography and fluoroscopy-guided procedures are well below the threshold for inducing radiation burns.
- In **interventional radiology, superficial** absorbed **doses** often **exceed 500 mGy,** so **radiation-induced burns** and **eye cataracts** are **possible.**

B. Organ Doses

- **Organ absorbed doses** also depend on the **location, size,** and the **fraction** of the organ being **irradiated.**
- The **average organ dose** (e.g., lung) is used to predict the lung stochastic **(cancer) risk.**
  - When half the lung is exposed to 3 mGy, and the other half to 1 mGy, the average lung dose (i.e., 2 mGy) is used to predict the lung cancer risk.
- For a **given** irradiation **geometry, mean organ doses** in x-ray imaging are generally directly **proportional** to entrance K_{air} **(and KAP).**
- **Superficial organs** will have doses that **approach** the **skin dose.**
- **Organs close** to the **patient exit** will have organ **doses** that are **much lower** because exit doses are much lower (e.g., 1%).
- Mean **organ doses** generally **increase** with **increasing beam quality.**
  - Higher beam qualities can penetrate further into the patient, thereby increasing the relative doses of deeper lying organs.
- **Organs** that are **not in** the **direct field** of view are only subject to scatter radiation and will generally receive **very low radiation doses.**

C. Embryo Doses

- When the x-ray beam does **not directly irradiate** the **embryo** (i.e., uterus) in any x-ray examination, the corresponding **dose will be very low.**
  - Embryo dose for examinations of the head and extremities are negligible.
- For an **abdominal or pelvic radiograph** in a standard-sized patient (**anteroposterior [AP] projection**), the embryo dose is about 1/3 the entrance K_{air}.

- An adult **AP abdomen** has an **entrance K$_{air}$** of about **3 mGy**, so the corresponding **embryo dose** would likely be **1 mGy**.
- For PA projections and lateral projections, embryo doses are about 1/6 and 1/20 of the entrance K$_{air}$, respectively.
- **Embryo doses** in radiography are **cumulative**, and directly proportional to the number of images obtained.
- In **fluoroscopy**, for a **PA projection**, the **dose rate** at the **embryo** (i.e., uterus) will be about **1.5 mGy/min** in a normal-sized patient.
- In **abdominal/pelvic computed tomography (CT)**, embryo doses are expected to be about **25 mGy**.
- **Embryo doses** in a **chest CT** are **low** and typically about **0.1 mGy**.
- **Internal scatter** is the main source of embryo dose during chest CT, and placing **lead aprons** on the **abdomen** results in **negligible dose benefit**.
  - Although **lead aprons** during head and chest CT provide little dose or risk benefit, these can **reassure patients**.

D. **Gonad and Integral Dose**
- **Genetically significant doses (GSD)** are dose metrics that quantify potential genetic damage.
- **GSD** takes into account the **dose** received by the **gonads** and the number of **offspring** an **individual** is likely to **produce**.
  - **GSD** in the United States was estimated at **0.3 mGy in 1980**.
- Gonad doses are now of little concern in diagnostic radiology.
- Use of **gonad shields** is not recommended due to potential interference with diagnostic performance and limited dose reduction.
- The **integral dose** measures the **total energy (mJ) imparted** to a patient (i.e., absorbed).
- A **chest x-ray** radiograph imparts **~0.002 J** of energy to the patient and an **abdominal radiograph** imparts **~0.02 J**.
  - A **head CT** scan imparts **~0.15 J** of energy, and a **body CT** scan imparts **~0.5 J**.
- **Integral dose** to patients may be used as an approximate **indicator** of **relative risk**.
  - Increasing energy imparted likely increases patient risk.

III. BIOLOGICAL DOSES

A. **Cell Survival Curves**
- **Radiobiologists measure** the ability of **radiation** to **kill cells.**
- When a given amount of **radiation kills 90%** of the cells, the **surviving fraction** is **one-tenth (10%)**.
- A **cell survival curve** plots the **surviving faction** as a function of radiation **dose,** as depicted in Figure 4.1.
- Figure 4.1 shows that for fixed amount of energy deposited in these cells (i.e., absorbed dose D), alpha particles kill many more cells than x-rays.
  - At a dose of **2 Gy**, for example, **99% of cells** are **killed** by **alpha particles**, whereas only **5%** of the same cells are **killed** by **x-rays.**
- Figure 4.1 clearly demonstrates that energy absorbed by cells (i.e., absorbed dose D) is insufficient to predict biological consequences.
  - At the **same dose, alpha particles** cause much **more biological damage** than **do x-rays.**

B. **Radiation Weighting Factors**
- For the same energy deposited in cells, **alpha particles** are more **biologically damaging than x-rays.**
- The reason for this is that the **pattern of energy deposition** for alpha particle irradiation differs from the corresponding pattern for x-rays.
- Figure 4.2 shows **alpha particles** result in a more **concentrated pattern** of **energy deposition** than x-rays, which are more diffuse.

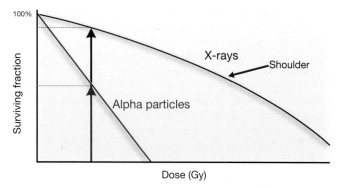

FIG 4.1 For the same dose, alpha particles are much more damaging biologically because lesions produced are clustered together. Radiobiologists quantify this denser pattern of energy deposition by alpha particles using linear energy transfer (LET), where alpha particles have a much higher LET than do x-rays. The shoulder is where single-strand breaks start mimicking double-strand breaks resulting in a steeper curve slope and less cell survival.

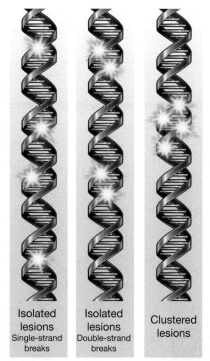

FIG 4.2 Pattern of energy deposition is diffuse for x-rays (left) causing damage that can be faithfully repaired. Damage to both strands (middle) may lead to mutation or cell death. When energy deposition is dense (high linear energy transfer [LET]) cluster damage (right) occurs and is most likely to lead to cell death. This is more likely using heavy charged particles like alpha and very high dose rates of photons and lighter particles. For the same total energy deposited, the concentrated pattern (high LET) results in a greater amount of biological damage (harm).

- The **concentration of energy** deposition is technically characterized by the **linear energy transfer (LET).**
  - **LET** is measured in **keV/μm,** the **energy deposited** in a given **distance.**
- **Alpha particles** are an example of **high LET** radiation (e.g., 100 keV/μm).
- **X-rays, gamma rays,** and **beta particles** are all examples of **low LET** radiation (e.g., 1 keV/μm).

- For radiation protection purposes, all radiations are allocated a radiation **weighting factor (W_R),** which reflects their specific LET values.
  - **Higher LET** values generally result in **higher W_R** values.
- **X-rays, gamma rays,** and **beta particles** have a W_R of 1.
- W_R is 2 for **protons** and 20 for **alpha particles.**
- Neutrons' W_R depends on their energy and can be as **high as 20.**
- **Higher radiation weighing factors** indicate **more biological damage** at the same absorbed dose.

C. Equivalent Dose

- **Equivalent dose (H)** is a dosimetry metric that attempts to quantify **biological damage** by **different types** of **radiation** (Fig. 4.3).
- The **equivalent dose** is the **absorbed dose (D)** multiplied by the **W_R** of the radiation **($H = D \times W_R$).**
- **Equivalent dose** is expressed in **Sievert (Sv),** where 1 Sv is 1,000 mSv, and 1 mSv is 1,000 μSv.
- When the liver absorbs 1 mJ of energy per kg, the absorbed dose to the liver is *always* 1 mGy.
  - At this **dose of 1 mGy,** the liver **equivalent dose is 1 mSv** for **x-ray radiation** and **20 mSv** for **alpha radiation.**
- **Equivalent dose** is primarily used for **radiation protection purposes.**
  - Use of **W_R permits comparisons** of effects of **different types of radiation** on a common scale.
- **Equivalent doses** are **only approximate indicators** of potential **biological harm.**

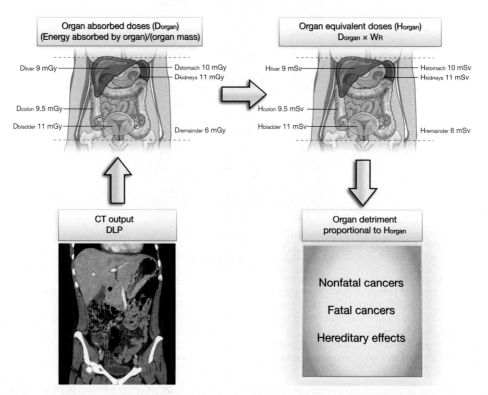

FIG 4.3 From DLP to organ detriment. Bottom left: A CT scan delivers radiation to the abdomen and pelvis of a patient. The output of the CT scanner is measured as DLP. Top Left: Conversion factors can be used to determine the absorbed radiation dose (in mGy) for each organ irradiated. Top right: Multiplying each absorbed dose by the W_R produces and equivalent dose for each organ (in mSv). Bottom right: The amount of organ detriment is proportional to the organ equivalent dose and can be used to calculate organ risks. CT, computed tomographic; DLP, dose-length product; W_R, radiation weighting factor.

D. Tissue Weighting Factors

- For a **uniform whole-body irradiation**, every organ and tissue receives exactly the same absorbed dose.
- A **10 mGy uniform whole-body x-ray** dose delivers **10 mGy to every organ** and tissue.
  - Each organ receives an equivalent dose of 10 mSv.
- At a dose of 10 mGy, patients may be harmed because of **fatal cancers, nonfatal cancers**, and **genetic effects** in the offspring of irradiated individuals.
- The amount of **harm** will depend on the **age** and **sex** of the **exposed individuals.**
  - Cancer induction risks are higher in younger people, and genetic effects only occur in individuals capable of producing offspring.
- **Radiation detriment** has been defined by the **International Commission on Radiological Protection (ICRP).**
  - **Radiation detriment** involves **judgments** of the **relative importance** of fatal cancers, nonfatal cancers, and genetic effects in future generations.
- The **tissue weighting factor (W_T)** is the **fractional contribution** of each **organ** to the **total detriment (uniform whole-body radiation).**
  - W_T values are **age** and **sex averages.**
- Table 4.2 shows the current values used by the ICRP for W_T for radiation protection purposes.
  - The **remainder organs** include the adrenals, gallbladder, heart, kidney, pancreas, prostate, small intestine, spleen, thymus, and uterus/cervix.
- W_T values are very approximate **indicators** of the **relative radiosensitivity** of any **organ** (i.e., age/sex averaged).
  - Values of W_T undergo periodic **revisions** and change with time.

E. Effective Dose

- Most **radiological examinations** result in a **nonuniform dose distribution** within the patient.
- Organ doses (mGy) for common radiographic and CT examinations are listed in Tables 4.3 and 4.4.
  - **Dosimetry software packages** can easily generate a long **list of organ absorbed doses.**
- **Interpretation** and **comprehension** of organ doses as listed in Tables 4.3 and 4.4 is problematical.
  - **Lists of organ doses** do not help practitioners understand "**how much radiation patients receive**" in any radiological examination.
- **Effective dose (E)** considers the **equivalent dose** to **every organ**, as well as each **organ's relative radiosensitivity (i.e., W_T).**
- E is obtained by multiplying equivalent dose (H) to an organ by the organ's W_T, summed for all irradiated organs.
  - **Effective doses** are confusingly also expressed in **mSv** like equivalent dose.
- The **effective dose E** is the **uniform whole-body equivalent dose** that results in the **same patient detriment** as the exam of interest (Fig. 4.3).

TABLE 4.2	Tissue Weighting Factors (W_T) Currently Used by the International Commission on Radiological Protection (ICRP) as given in ICRP Publication 103	
Tissue Weighting Factor (W_T)	**Organs and Tissues**	**Detriment**[a]
0.12	Red bone marrow; colon; lung; stomach; breast; remainder	Cancer[a]
0.08	Gonads	Hereditary
0.04	Bladder; liver; esophagus; thyroid	Cancer[a]
0.01	Skin; bone surfaces; salivary glands; brain	Cancer[a]

[a]Fatal and nonfatal.

TABLE 4.3	Selected organ doses (mGy) or equivalent doses (mSv) for Three Common Radiographic Examinations		
Organ	Lateral Skull	Posteroanterior Chest	Anteroposterior Abdomen
Red bone marrow	0.05	0.02	0.2
Lungs	<0.01	0.06	0.02
Stomach	<0.01	0.01	1.3
Colon	<0.01	<0.01	1.3
Breast	<0.01	0.01	0.01
Gonads[a]	<0.01	<0.01	0.60
Effective dose (mSv)	0.03	0.015	0.5

Only organs with W_T values > 0.04 are shown, but effective dose (mSv) accounted for all organs listed in Table 4.2.
[a]Average of male and female.

- **Patient detriment** from a **CT** depicted in Figure 4.4 scan is **comparable** to the *same patient* receiving a uniform **whole-body equivalent dose** of **5 mSv** (or 5 mGy of absorbed dose in the case of photons with $W_R = 1$).
- Effective dose is an educational aid that helps the radiological community to quantitatively understand "how much radiation a patient received."

IV. EFFECTIVE DOSES IN RADIOLOGY

A. Effective Doses in Radiology

- The **effective dose** is used to deal with the **nonuniform dose distributions** that occur in **radiological examinations**.
- **Effective doses compare radiation** pattern deposited in the same patient from various **types of examinations using ionizing radiation**.
- Effective doses less than **0.1 mSv** are categorized as "**very low**."
  - A PA chest x-ray is generally very low (<0.1 mSv).
- **Effective doses between 0.1 and 1 mSv** are categorized as "**low**."
  - Most body radiographic examinations have low effective doses.
- **Effective doses between 1 and 10 mSv** are categorized as "**moderate**."
  - GI studies and CT scan of the major parts of the body have moderate effective doses.
- **Effective doses in excess of 10 mSv** are categorized as "**high**."
  - Highest patient doses occur generally occur in complex interventional radiology procedures.

TABLE 4.4	Selected organ doses (mGy) or Equivalent Doses (mSv) for Three Common Computed Tomographic Examinations		
Organ	Head Computed Tomography	Chest Computed Tomography	Abdomen/Pelvic Computed Tomography
Red bone marrow	2.2	3.6	5,0
Lungs	0.1	12	1.5
Stomach	<0.1	2.5	12
Colon	<0.1	0.1	11
Breast	<0.1	10	0.4
Remainder	2.9	4.0	7.0
Gonads[a]	<0.1	<0.1	6.6
Effective dose (mSv)	1.5	5	6

Only organs with W_T values > 0.04 are shown, but effective dose computation accounted for all organs listed in Table 4.2.
[a]Average of male and female.

- Since children are ~3× more radiosensitive than adults, similar categories would have threshold at about one-third those listed for adults.
- Table 4.5 gives examples of each category of effective dose in radiology.
- **Effective dose** permits direct **comparisons** of radiation exposures in radiology **with natural background** doses.
  - **Radiological effective doses** can also be compared with **regulatory dose limits.**

B. Ubiquitous Natural Background

- All Americans are exposed **ubiquitous natural background** radiation, of **cosmic, internal**, and **terrestrial radioactivity.**
- **Cosmic radiation** from outer space and internal primordial radionuclides like ^{40}K both give an average E of **0.4 mSv/y.**
- **Terrestrial radioactivity** such as ^{226}Ra results in an average E of **0.3 mSv/y.**
- In the United States, the **average ubiquitous background annual dose** is **1 mSv.**
- A **transcontinental US flight** results in a dose of approximately **0.03 mSv.**
- **Radon (^{222}Rn)** is a radioactive gas formed during the decay of radium and **emits alpha particles.**
- The **progeny of radon** are also **radioactive** and **attach** to **aerosols** that are inhaled and **deposited** in the **lungs.**
  - In the United States, the **U.S. Environmental Protection Agency believes** that up to **15% of lung cancers** are a result of **domestic exposure** to **radon.**
- The current average annual **effective dose** from **radon exposure** in America is estimated to be **2 mSv/y.**
- The **average American** thus receives about **3 mSv** from **natural background** each year.

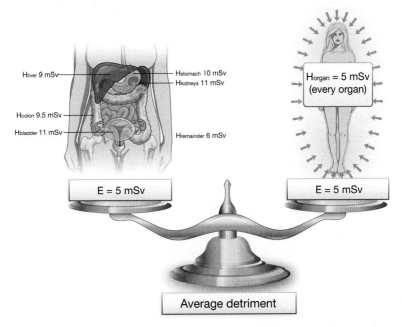

FIG 4.4 A patient's detriment can be determined from the individual organ equivalent doses. The patient detriment (total harm) can be estimated by multiplying each organ equivalent dose by its organ-specific tissue weighting factor and then summing up all the resulting values. This is called the effective dose. The detriment from the equivalent organ doses on the left side of the scale is comparable to a uniform whole-body x-ray dose of 5 mGy, which corresponds to an effective dose of 5 mSv. Effective dose is thus the uniform whole-body x-ray dose that results in the same patient detriment as any pattern of nonuniform exposure and enables simple intercomparisons of the radiation used in any radiological examination.

TABLE 4.5	Representative Values of Effective Doses for Adult Radiological Examinations	
Category	**Effective Dose (mSv)**	**Examples of Radiological Examinations [Nominal Effective Doses in mSv]**
None	0	Ultrasound and Magnetic Resonance Studies
Very low	<0.1	Dual x-ray absorptiometry (DEXA) [0.001]; CT x-ray absorptiometry [0.04]; intraoral radiograph [0.005]; panoramic radiograph [0.01]; shoulder x-ray [0.01]; knee x-ray [0.005]; extremity x-rays [0.001]; posteroanterior chest x-ray [0.02]
Low	0.1-1	Skull examinations [0.1]; cervical spine [0.2]; screening mammogram [0.4]; video fluoroscopic swallow study (0.4); abdomen x-ray [0.5]; pelvis or hip [0.6]
		Thoracic and lumbar spine examinations [1]
Moderate	1-10	Upper gastrointestinal series [6]; small-bowel series [5]; barium enemas [8]; intravenous urography examinations [3]; endoscopic retrograde cholangiopancreatography [4]; head CT [2]; neck CT [3]; chest CT [5]; abdomen/pelvic CT [6]; Tc 99m-labeled pharmaceuticals [4]
High	>10	Chest/abdomen/pelvis CT [10]; multiphase studies (e.g., 3-phase liver) [15]; retrospectively gated cardiac CT [20]; abdominal angiography or aortography [10]; coronary percutaneous transluminal angioplasty, stent placement, or radiofrequency ablation [15]; pelvic vein embolization [60] transjugular intrahepatic portosystemic shunt placement [70];

CT, computed tomography.

- **One-third** of the 3 mSv background radiation is from **ubiquitous sources**, and **two-thirds** from **radon.**

C. Effective Dose and Risk

- The **ICRP** estimates **risk** and **detriment** associated with any exposure using **effective dose (mSv).**
  - **ICRP risk estimates** provided are always **averaged** over both **gender** and **age.**
- Population averaged incidence of **fatal cancer** from radiation is currently estimated to be ~**4% per Sv.**
  - **Cancer incidence** (i.e., fatal + non-fatal) is ~**10% per Sv.**
- ICRP estimates radiation detriment by adjusting for lethality and impact on quality of life.
- Nominal **cancer detriment**, when averaged over age and sex, is ~**5.5% per Sv.**
  - The corresponding **total radiation detriment** (cancer + hereditary effects) is ~**6% per Sv.**
- **ICRP risk estimates** are for **populations** (not individuals) and are for radiation protection purposes (**not individual risk** estimation).

D. Interpreting Effective Doses

- Effective dose must not be directly converted in quantitative individual risks.
  - **Effective doses** do *not account* for **patient age, sex, or other conditions** that affect patient risks.
- The **same effective dose** has a higher **risk** in a **newborn** than in a **retiree.**
- **Individual subject risk** must always be based on **organ doses** and take into account subject **age** and **sex.**
  - Preexisting conditions may also play a role in risk.

- Equivalent doses to individual organs and patient effective dose both use the same dosimetry quantity (i.e., mSv), which is often a **source of confusion.**
  - For electrons, x-rays, and gamma rays, organ doses have the same numerical value, irrespective of whether absorbed dose or equivalent dose is being used.
- Choosing to express **organ absorbed doses in mGy**, and **patient effective doses in mSv**, is **helpful to avoid confusion.**

Chapter 4 (Dosimetry) Questions

4.1 What are the units for air kerma?
   A. Gray
   B. Roentgen
   C. Sievert
   D. Rad

4.2 What is the entrance K_{air} for a normal-sized adult undergoing a lateral skull x-ray examination?
   A. 0.1 mGy
   B. 1 mGy
   C. 10 mGy
   D. 100 mGy

4.3 What is a reasonable general fluoroscopy entrance K_{air} rate for a typical adult (AP abdomen)?
   A. 0.1 mGy/min
   B. 1 mGy/min
   C. 10 mGy/min
   D. 100 mGy/min

4.4 What is a typical KAP for a complete radiographic examination (e.g., skull AP + lateral)?
   A. 0.1 Gy-cm^2
   B. 1 Gy-cm^2
   C. 10 Gy-cm^2
   D. 100 Gy-cm^2

4.5 Controlling the skin dose during fluoroscopy is the responsibility of which medical professional?
   A. Radiologist
   B. Medical physicist
   C. Technologist
   D. Radiology manager

4.6 What is the organ absorbed dose when a liver (mass 2 kg) absorbs 0.002 joules of energy?
   A. 1 mGy
   B. 10 mGy
   C. 100 mGy
   D. 1,000 mGy

4.7 For the same incident K_{air}, which tissue will receive the highest absorbed radiation dose?
   A. Fat (Z = 6.5)
   B. CSF (Z = 7.5)
   C. Muscle (Z = 7.5)
   D. Bone (Z = 12)

4.8 What is likely the highest skin dose for single radiograph for typical adult study?
   A. 1 mGy
   B. 10 mGy
   C. 100 mGy
   D. >100 mGy

4.9 For an AP abdomen x-ray examination with an entrance K_{air} of 3 mGy, the average liver dose is most likely:
   A. <0.03 mGy
   B. 0.03 mGy
   C. 0.3 mGy
   D. >0.3 mGy

4.10 Which CT examination will likely result in the highest genetically significant dose in a 20-year-old woman?
   A. Head
   B. Chest
   C. Abdomen
   D. Pelvis

4.11 Compared to energy deposited in heating a chicken in a 500 W microwave oven (1 minute), energy deposited in a patient undergoing a TIPS procedure is most likely:
   A. Lower
   B. Comparable
   C. Higher

4.12 For the same dose, which type of radiation most likely kills the most cells?
   A. Alpha
   B. Beta
   C. X-ray
   D. Gamma

4.13 For a whole-body CT, how does the bone equivalent dose compare to the bone absorbed dose?
   A. Higher
   B. Equal
   C. Lower

4.14 What organ has the lowest tissue weighting factor (W_T)?
   A. Breast
   B. Red bone marrow
   C. Lung
   D. Brain

4.15 In a chest, abdomen, and pelvis CT scan where all directly irradiated organs receive 10 mGy, what is the patient effective dose?
A. <10 mSv
B. 10 mSv
C. >10 mSv

4.16 The effective dose of a screening mammogram would most likely be classified as:
A. Very low (<0.1 mSv)
B. Low (0.1-1 mSv)
C. Moderate (1-10 mSv)
D. High (>10 mSv).

4.17 What yearly dose is delivered on average from ubiquitous background exposure (i.e., excluding radon) in the United States?
A. 0.1 mSv/y
B. 0.3 mSv/y
C. 1 mSv/y
D. 3 mSv/y

4.18 What yearly dose is delivered on average from exposure to radon (+daughters) in the United States?
A. 0.1 mSv/y
B. 0.5 mSv/y
C. 2 mSv/y
D. >2 mSv/y

4.19 A population exposed to a uniform whole-body dose of 10 mGy (effective dose of 10 mSv) potentially results in what percentage of additional radiation induced cancers.
A. 0.001%
B. 0.01%
C. 0.1%
D. 1%

4.20 Effective doses *are not* indicators of individual patient risk because these fail to account for what?
A. Dose rates
B. Patient demographics
C. Examination type
D. Risk uncertainties

Answers and Explanations

4.1 A (Gray). The SI unit of air kerma is the Gy, which was measured in roentgen in the non-SI system (1 R ~ 10 mGy). The SI unit for equivalent dose is the Sv and the non-SI unit for absorbed dose is the rad (1 rad = 10 mGy).

4.2 B (1 mGy). A typical entrance K_{air} for a lateral skull radiograph is 1 mGy.

4.3 C (10 mGy/min). 10 mGy/min is a typical entrance K_{air} rate during fluoroscopy of 23 cm of tissue (i.e., AP abdomen) but this can vary markedly depending on FOV, pulse rate, as well as selected dose level.

4.4 B (1 Gy-cm²). A typical value of the total radiation intensity incident on an adult patient undergoing a complete radiographic examination is 1 Gy-cm².

4.5 A (Radiologist). The dose delivered to the patient is the responsibility of the radiologist.

4.6 A (1 mGy). Dose is the absorbed energy (0.002 J) divided by organ mass (2 kg), which is 0.001 Gy or 1 mGy.

4.7 D (Bone). For the same incident radiation, bone absorbs much more radiation because it has a much higher atomic number and absorbs more radiation.

4.8 B (10 mGy). 10 mGy is likely the highest skin dose (mGy) in any normal-sized adult having a single radiograph (e.g., lateral lumbar radiograph).

4.9 C (0.3 mGy [which is 10% of entrance K_{air}]). In radiography, the radiation at the abdomen exit is ~1% of the radiation entrance. "Middle" gets ~10% because radiation is attenuated exponentially (i.e., a tenth to the middle and another tenth to the exit).

4.10 D (Pelvis). GSD is highest radiation dose during a pelvic CT because the female gonads are directly irradiated and will receive the highest dose (by far).

4.11 A (Lower). A 500 W microwave oven deposits 30,000 joules in a minute, whereas a patient undergoing a TIPS procedure (100 mSv) absorbs less than 10 joules. X-rays heating effects are negligible, and risks arise because of the ionizing nature of this type of radiation.

4.12 A (Alpha). For the same deposited energy (dose), alpha particles are much more damaging than beta/x-ray/gamma rays.

4.13 B (Equal). In all of diagnostic radiology using x-rays or gamma rays, absorbed organ doses (mGy) are always numerically equal to the organ equivalent dose (mSv).

4.14 D (Brain). The brain has the lowest tissue weighting factor (W_T) of 0.01, whereas the breast, RBM, and lung each have a high tissue weighting factor (W_T) of 0.12.

4.15 A (<10 mSv). When the *whole body* gets 10 mGy, the patient effective dose is 10 mSv, so a CAP that excludes the head and legs must be less than 10 mSv.

4.16 A (Low (0.1-1 mSv)). A screening mammogram has an effective dose of ~0.4 mSv (Table 4.5).

4.17 C (1 mSv/y). US natural background exposure from cosmic radiation, internal primordial radionuclides, and terrestrial activity but excluding radon exposure is 1 mSv/y.

4.18 C (2 mSv/y). Average US exposure to radon (+daughters) is 2 mSv/y.

4.19 C (0.1%). Following a whole-body dose of 10 mGy to a population (effective dose 10 mSv), there will be expected to be 0.1% additional radiation-induced cancers.

4.20 B (Patient demographics). Organ doses can be used to compute effective doses and risks, but the latter always requires patient demographic information.

Radiation Risks

I. RADIATION BIOLOGY

A. Biological Damage

- When **ionizing radiation interacts** with atoms in tissues, energetic recoil **Compton electrons** and **photoelectrons** are **produced.**
- **Direct action** occurs when **Compton electrons and photoelectrons ionize molecules.**
- **Indirect action** occurs when Compton electrons/photoelectrons interact with water to **produce free radicals** that are **chemically reactive.**
  - **Hydroxyl radicals** are the most important and exist long enough to diffuse to, and **damage**, target **molecules.**
- About **two-thirds** of the **biologic damage** by x-rays is caused by **indirect** action and the remaining third by direct action.
- Energy deposited in cells can damage biologically important molecules (e.g., DNA).
  - The **greater** the **DNA** content, the **easier** it is to **inactivate biological systems.**
- **Mammalian cells** are much **easier to kill** than **bacteria**, because they have more DNA (i.e., bigger target).
- In turn, **bacteria** are much **easier to kill** than **viruses** because of differences in DNA (or RNA) content.
  - Massive radiation doses (e.g., **20,000 Gy**) are required for **sterilization** purposes.

B. Basic Radiobiology

- **Radiobiology** studies the effects of ionizing radiation in cells and animal models.
- Energy from x-rays is deposited unevenly and can produce **single-strand** and **double-strand DNA breaks.**
- **Single strand** breaks are **repaired with high fidelity**, whereas **double-strand** breaks may **result** in cell **death, carcinogenesis**, and **mutations.**
  - **Chromosome breaks** and **aberrations** are examples of biological damage that can be caused by radiation.
- **Damaged DNA** may result in a **modification** of cellular **function** or **cell death.**
- At **lower doses**, cells are more likely to undergo **modification**, whereas at **higher doses**, cells are more likely to be **killed.**
  - **Health consequences** of **cell death** occur on a time scale measured in **hours** and **weeks.**
- **Damaged somatic** cells can result in the induction of **cancer.**
  - Induction of **cancer** by radiation takes **years** and **decades** to develop.
- **Damaged** sperm and eggs (i.e., **germ cells**) can result in **hereditary effects** (mutations).
- **Changes** in the **genetic code** of a germ cell can **affect future generations.**

C. **Cell Sensitivity**

- **Biological effects** of radiation depend on the total energy deposited in the cell (i.e., **absorbed dose**).
- **Radiation type** is also an important **determinant** of **biological damage**, where alpha particles (i.e., **high linear energy transfer [LET]**) are **more damaging** than x-rays (i.e., **low LET**).
- For a constant total dose, **reduced dose rates** generally **reduce cell killing.**
  - Damage **repair** can **occur** when the radiation delivery is **protracted.**
- **Fractionated** exposures, as occurs in radiotherapy, also reduce cell killing.
  - Fractionated radiotherapy helps protect normal tissues.
- **Law of Bergonie and Tribondeau** states that **highest sensitivities** occur when cells are **undifferentiated and** have **high mitotic rates.**
- Rapidly proliferating cells (e.g., bone marrow stem cells) are very sensitive.
- Highly **differentiated** and **nonproliferating** cells (e.g., neurons) are **least sensitive.**
  - An **exception is peripheral lymphocytes** that are sensitive to radiation, even though they are differentiated and do not divide.
- **Oxygenated cells** are generally two to three times **more sensitive** when irradiated by x-rays than are anoxic cells.
  - An **oxygen enhancement ratio** of 2 means it takes a 2× dose to kill hypoxic cells compared to oxygenated cells.
  - **Oxygen prolongs the lifetime** of free radicals, promoting bond breaking.

D. **Tissue and Stochastic Effects**

- **Tissue effects (aka deterministic effects)** have a **threshold dose** ($D_{threshold}$).
- **Below** its $D_{threshold}$ value, deterministic **effects** do **not occur**, whereas above $D_{threshold}$, tissue effects are possible (but not definite).
  - For doses **well above** $D_{threshold}$, **deterministic effects** are expected to occur in **all exposed individuals.**
- **Erythema, epilation, eye cataracts,** and **sterility** are **tissue effects.**
- Deterministic effects occur at high doses (e.g., >1 Gy) and generally are the result of cell killing.
- **The severity** of deterministic effects **may increase** with **increasing dose** (e.g., temporary vs permanent epilation).
- **Stochastic effects** of radiation have **no threshold dose** (i.e., $D_{threshold} = 0$).
  - Stochastic means random or probabilistic.
- In radiology, **stochastic effects** pertain to **carcinogenesis** and induction of **hereditary effects** in the offspring of irradiated individuals.
- **The severity** of radiation-induced **stochastic** effects is **independent** of **radiation dose.**
  - The **radiation dose** only **affects** the **probability** of the stochastic effect occurring.

E. **Whole-Body Irradiation**

- **Uniform whole-body** doses of **5 Gy** and above are likely **lethal.**
  - The lethal whole-body dose to kill 50% of the population (**LD$_{50}$) is 3 to 5 Gy** depending on whether they receive treatment.
  - A peak skin dose of 5 Gy in interventional radiology is never lethal but could result in localized erythema.
- **Radiologists** do **not encounter** high whole-body doses in **clinical practice** but may become involved during **medical emergencies.**
- **Peripheral lymphocyte count** is used to triage the severity of acute radiation exposures.
  - Immediate diarrhea, fever, and hypotension are indications of a (very) highly lethal whole-body exposure to radiation.
- **Acute radiation syndrome** is caused by whole-body doses above a Gray and manifests in three distinct ways (Table 5.1).

TABLE 5.1	Acute Radiation Syndrome (ARS)		
Type	**Dose Threshold**	**Time to Death**	**Major Effects Leading to Death**
Hematopoietic syndrome	1-2 Gy	One or more months (recovery possible under 8 Gy)	Drop in blood cell counts; hemorrhage; infection
Gastrointestinal syndrome	10 Gy	One or more weeks	Loss of crypt cells leading to infection, dehydration, and electrolyte imbalance
Cardiovascular (CV) or central nervous system (CNS) syndrome	50 Gy	One or more days	Collapse of circulatory system and increased brain pressure from edema, vasculitis, and meningitis

- Whole-body doses of above **2 Gy** sterilize stem cells, reducing circulating blood elements within two or 3 weeks (i.e., **hematopoietic syndrome**).
  - At whole body doses **above 8 Gy**, **survival** is extremely **unlikely.**
  - Death occurs about **a month** after exposure if the patient does not recover.
- Whole-body doses of ~**10 Gy** would **kill** everyone in about **a week** due to loss of epithelial lining of the gastrointestinal tract (i.e., **gastrointestinal syndrome**).
- Whole-body doses of ~**50 Gy kill** everyone in about **a day** from permeability changes in brain blood vessels (i.e., **cerebrovascular syndrome**).

■ II. DETERMINISTIC RISKS

A. Skin Doses <10 Gy

- Highest skin doses generally occur where the x-ray beam enters the patient.
- Skin reactions below 10 Gy are typically level 1 according to the National Cancer Institute (NCI) skin reaction grading system
- The **peak skin dose** (D_{peak}) is the dosimetry metric that is used to predict the likelihood of a skin injury that occurs at the timescales listed in Table 5.2.
  - Exposed **skin area** is not considered in predicting skin injury, but larger areas take longer time to heal.
- **Below** peak skin doses of **2 Gy**, **no effects** are observed.
- At peak skin doses between **2 and 5 Gy**, **erythema** is possible (**prompt and/or early phases**).
  - The patient should be advised that erythema may be observed but should fade with time and to report back if skin changes cause physical discomfort.
- At peak skin doses between **5 and 10 Gy**, **erythema** will **occur** within 8 weeks.
- **Prolonged erythema** may occur **within 40 weeks**, with **dermal atrophy** or **induration long term**, but full recovery is generally expected.
  - The patient should be advised perform self-examination (2-10 weeks) where skin effects would most likely occur, and report back if erythema occurs.

TABLE 5.2	Time Scales for Onset of Skin Deterministic Effects
Descriptor	**Time Scale**
Prompt	<2 wk
Early	2-8 wk
Midterm	6-52 wk
Long Term	>40 wk

B. **Skin Doses >10 Gy**

- At peak skin doses between **10 and 15 Gy**, transient erythema occurs within 2 weeks, followed by **erythema** as well as **dry** or **moist desquamation** within 8 weeks.
- **Midterm effects** relate to prolonged **erythema**, whereas **long-term effects** include **telangiectasia**, **dermal atrophy** or **induration**, and **weak skin.**
  - Medical follow-up is appropriate, and prophylactic treatment for infection may be required.
- At peak skin doses in **excess of 15 Gy**, signs include transient erythema and **possibly edema** and **acute ulceration** within 2 weeks.
- **Early effects** (<8 weeks) pertain to erythema and **moist desquamation.**
- **Midterm** effects (<52 weeks) include **dermal atrophy, secondary ulceration**, and **dermal necrosis**, all of which may require surgical intervention at higher doses.
- **Long-term effects** include telangiectasia, dermal atrophy or induration, with possible late skin breakdown, likely requiring **surgical intervention.**
  - Medical follow-up is essential, and the treating physician needs informing that the wound could progress to ulceration or necrosis.
- Table 5.3 provides a summary of the current **NCI categorization** of **radiation-induced skin injuries.**

C. **Epilation**

- **Epilation** can occur in diagnostic radiology following irradiation in high-dose procedures (e.g., **interventional neuroradiology**).
- Below a peak skin dose of 3 Gy, epilation is not expected.
- For scalp doses of **3 to 5 Gy, temporary epilation** can occur.
  - The **onset** of epilation occurs after **2 to 3 weeks.**
- **Regrowth** of hair usually occurs **2 months** after irradiation and is expected to be completed 6 to 12 months post exposure.
  - Hair that grows **after** a radiation-induced **epilation** may be coarse and/or a **different color.**
- At doses in excess of **7 Gy, epilation** is likely to be **permanent.**

D. **Cataracts**

- **Cataracts** are opacifications of the eye lens that is normally transparent.
  - The eye lens has no method of removing dead or damaged cells.
- Cataracts appearing at the **posterior pole** of the lens of exposed individuals would **suggest** that the cataract has been caused by **radiation (e.g., posterior subcapsular).**
- Up to **2011**, threshold doses for radiation-induced cataracts were taken to be ~2 Gy for **acute** x-ray exposure and ~5 Gy for **chronic** x-ray exposure.
- **International Commission on Radiological Protection (ICRP)** now considers the **threshold dose** for **cataract** induction to be **0.5 Gy.**
  - This new ICRP threshold pertains to **acute** and **chronic exposures.**

TABLE 5.3	National Cancer Institute (NCI) Categorization of Radiation-Induced Skin Injuries	
NCI Toxicity Grade	**Skin Dose Range (Gy)**	**Descriptor**
1	2-10	Faint erythema or dry desquamation
2	5-15	Moderate erythema; patchy moist desquamation mainly in skin folds; moderate edema
3	>10	Moist desquamation in areas other than skin folds and creases; bleeding from minor abrasion
4	>15	Skin necrosis or ulceration of full-thickness dermis; spontaneous bleeding

- **Latency** periods for **cataracts** are reported of **several years** after eye lens doses of a few Grays.
  - As **doses increase**, **latent periods** may get **shorter**.
- Radiation eye damage has been observed in interventional radiologists, interventional cardiologists, and astronauts.
- **Cataract induction** is a possibility for **patients** with high or chronic eye exposures.

E. **Sterility**

- In men, low doses of 0.2 Gy can produce a diminished sperm count.
- Doses **above 0.5 Gy** can result in **azoospermia** (temporary sterility).
  - Recovery time from temporary sterility is dose dependent and can be as long as 3 years.
- **Permanent sterility** requires a single dose of **6 Gy in men**.
- In men, **fractionated exposure** to the gonads produces **more damage** than does **acute exposure**.
- Permanent sterility can result from 3 Gy fractionated over a few weeks.
- In women, radiation can induce permanent ovarian failure.
- The dose for **female sterility** is highly **dependent** on **age**.
- The dose required for permanent sterility in ovaries is reported to be as high as 10 Gy in prepuberty.
- A dose of **2 Gy** can result **permanent sterility** in **premenopausal women**.

III. CARCINOGENIC RISKS

A. **Ionizing Radiation and Cancer**

- **Below** the **threshold** for induction of **deterministic** effects, **carcinogenesis** is the **main concern** following doses of ionizing radiations.
- The link between exposure and ionizing radiations has been established using **epidemiological studies**.
- **Epidemiological studies** of radiation-induced carcinogenesis require **large cohort size(s)** and also adequate **control group(s)**.
- **Long follow-up** periods (decades) are **essential** for observing solid tumors.
- Epidemiological data on radiation-induced cancers are available by studying **atomic bomb survivors and radiation workers**.
- Data are available by studying **patients** exposed to high organ doses associated with **therapeutic** applications of **x-rays**.
- At high radiation doses (above 100 mSv), it is generally accepted that radiation exposure may result in cancer.
- At lower doses, there is uncertainty as to whether radiation causes cancer.

TABLE 5.4	Evidence of Organ Radiosensitivity (Cancer) in High-Dose (Therapeutic) Uses of Ionizing Radiations
Organ	**Medical Studies Showing Radiation-Induced Cancers**
RBM	Patients treated for ankylosing spondylitis
Breast	Women treated for postpartum mastitis at doses up to 6 Gy
Thyroid	Children treated for enlarged thymus treated for cancer/tonsils
Lung	Patients treated for ankylosing spondylitis (corrected for smoking)
Bone	Patients injected with ^{224}Ra to treat tuberculosis or ankylosing spondylitis
Skin	Children epilated with x-rays for treatment of *tinea capitis*

RBM, red bone marrow.

B. High-Dose Studies

- The largest group studied for radiation-induced cancer is the survivors of the atomic bomb survivors of **Hiroshima** and **Nagasaki.**
- Excess **cancer deaths** depend on **dose, age at exposure**, time since exposure, and **gender.**
- Excesses of **lung cancer** have been observed in **miners** in Colorado (uranium), Czechoslovakia (uranium), Canada (fluorspar), and Sweden (nonuranium).
- **Bone sarcomas** and carcinomas of the epithelial cells lining the nasopharynx have been observed in **dial painters** who ingested **radium.**
- Radiation-induced skin cancers have also been reported in radiologists, dentists, technologists working in the early 20th century when radiation safety was lax.
- A **significant excess** of **cancers** has been observed following **radiotherapy** for Hodgkin lymphoma, prostate cancer, and carcinoma of the cervix.
- Excess thyroid cancers in children were seen in the aftermath of **Chernobyl** due to radioactive iodine released in the air and concentrated in cow milk.
- **Secondary cancers** have also been seen following **radiation therapy** for **childhood malignancies.**
- Studies (Nova Scotia and Massachusetts) showed increased **breast cancer** in women who underwent **fractionated diagnostic fluoroscopy.**
- Table 5.4 lists radiation-induced cancers in specified organs at high doses during therapy.

C. Low-Dose Studies

- Children scalps **treated** for **tinea capitis** by **radiation** had a significant excess of **thyroid cancer** because of exposure to low levels of scattered x-rays.
- Low radiation doses (**10 mGy**) received by the **fetus** in utero in the 1950s are now generally accepted as **increasing childhood cancer.**
- Small but statistically significant **cancer risks** have been observed in **atomic bomb** survivors exposed to relatively **low doses (e.g., ~30 mSv).**
- Studies of **UK radiation workers** provide quantitative radiation risks estimates for leukemia and solid tumors **comparable to** those of **atomic bomb survivors.**
- A study of **breast cancer mortality** in **children** exposed for **scoliosis** showed significant **excess relative risks** similar to those of **atomic bomb survivors.**
- A UK study (2012) of children who underwent **computed tomographic (CT)** scans showed evidence of **increases** in **leukemia** and **brain tumors.**
- An Australian study (2013) showed **increased cancer** incidence with increasing number of **pediatric CT scans.**

D. Cancer Risks

- **Radiation-induced malignancies** are **similar** to **natural malignancies** of the same type and appear at similar ages.
  - There is **no characteristic neoplasm** due to radiation.
- Stochastic risks are dependent on age at exposure.
  - Overall, children are more susceptible to radiation in about 25% of cancers, less in 10% of cancers, equivalent in 15% of cancers, and unknown in the rest.
- Cancer risks are dependent on sex, with **radiation-induced thyroid cancer more likely in women.**
- **Bone marrow, colon, lung, female breast, stomach, and childhood thyroid** are the organs that are **most susceptible** to radiation-induced malignancy.
- **Bladder, liver, and esophagus** are **moderately radiosensitive.**
- **Latency** refers to the time interval between irradiation and the appearance of the malignancy.
- Cancer induction has a **short latency** period 5 to 7 years for **leukemia.**
  - Leukemia incidence is age dependent, with a peak at 15 years (average).

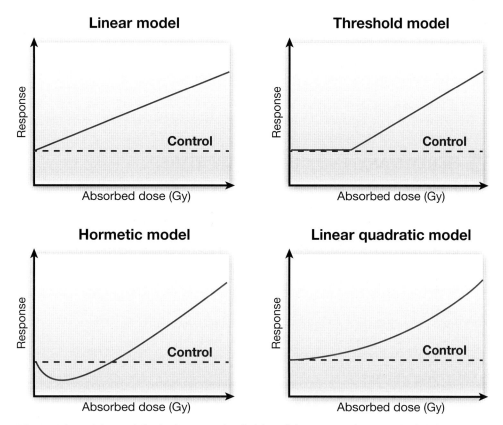

FIG 5.1 Risk models. Top left: The linear no threshold model assumes risk is increased with any increase in radiation. This is the current radioprotection model used for radiation induced solid tumors. Top right: The threshold model assumes there is no risk up to a certain dose. Once enough tissue is damaged, effects begin. This is the current model for tissue (deterministic) effects. Bottom left: The hormetic model assumes small amounts of radiation stimulate the immune system causing decreased risk until a threshold dose where risk increases. Bottom right: The linear quadratic model is used to model radiation induction of leukemia for radiation protection purposes.

- **Latency** for **solid tumors** is much **longer** and is often measured in **decades**.
- Most cancer radiation risk estimates at doses encountered in diagnostic imaging are based on a **linear no-threshold (LNT)** model (Fig. 5.1).

E.   Quantitative Cancer Risks

- The US National Academy of Sciences Committee on the **Biological Effects of Ionizing Radiation (BEIR)** provides detailed information on radiation risks.
- Both the **UN Scientific Committee on the Effects of Atomic Radiation (UNSCEAR)** and the **ICRP** also study risks.
  - Radiation **risk estimates** from BEIR, UNSCEAR, and ICRP are **similar.**
- Figure 5.2A shows how radiation risk of fatal and nonfatal breast cancer varies with age in women.
  - Figure 5.2B shows the importance of age and sex for the induction of cancer following a uniform whole-body dose of 100 mGy.
- The average **25-year-old** US adult cancer risk for undergoing a uniform whole-body x-ray exposure of **10 mSv** is **0.1% (1 in a 1000).**
- Overall, **women** are about **70% more radiosensitive** (cancer) than men.
  - Breast cancer accounts for almost all of the gender differences in radiosensitivity.
- **Newborns** are about **three times more radiosensitive** (cancer) than are **25-year-olds.**

- On average, **70-year-olds** are about **three times less radiosensitive** (cancer) than are **25-year-olds.**
- Current **radiation risk estimates** have **large uncertainties**, and true risks could be over-estimated.
  - Radiation risks at low doses may also be zero (threshold).
- In the **absence** of any **radiation exposures**, the average American has a **40% chance** of getting **cancer** in their lifetime.
  - Figure 5.3 shows graphically how radiation exposure increases the cancer induction relative to the background incidence.

IV. **HEREDITARY AND CONCEPTUS RISKS**

A. Hereditary Effects

- Irradiation of **germ cells** involved in reproduction can result in **hereditary effects.**
- Induction of **hereditary effects** is a **stochastic** process with **no threshold.**
- Radiation increases the incidence of the mutations that occur spontaneously. There is **no epidemiological evidence** of hereditary effects in exposed **humans.**
  - Studies of children born to the atomic bomb survivors (>40,000) have not shown any significant increased hereditary effects.
- Information on the **hereditary effects** of radiation comes almost entirely from **animal experiments.**
- Mutation rates have been measured in studies on the **fruit fly.**
- Mutation rates have also been measured in mice, in a study using ~7 million mice (**MegaMouse** Project) at Oak Ridge National Laboratory in the late 1940s.

B. Hereditary Risks

- **Hereditary effects** (i.e., Mendelian, chromosomal, and multifactorial) depend on the **demographics** of the exposed populations.
  - **Older populations** have **lower risks** than younger populations for the same exposure.
- In the 1950s and 1960s, hereditary effects were considered the most important risk of radiation exposure.
  - Nowadays, **concern** about **hereditary effects** is **much lower.**
- The current **ICRP hereditary risk estimate** is **0.2% per Gy** up to the second generation for a whole population.
  - In a **working population**, the hereditary **risk estimate** is **lower** (0.1%), because this group excludes children.

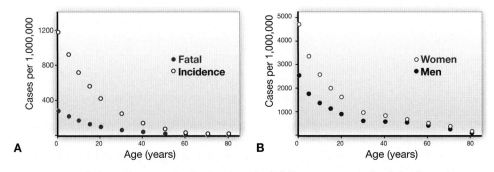

FIG 5.2 A: Female breast cancer risks (fatal and nonfatal) following a mean glandular dose of 10 mGy. **B:** Cancer incidence in men and women following uniform whole-body x-ray doses of 10 mGy (i.e., effective dose of 10 mSv), resulting in a risk of 0.1% (i.e., 1,000 cases per million exposed individuals) in an average 25-year-old.

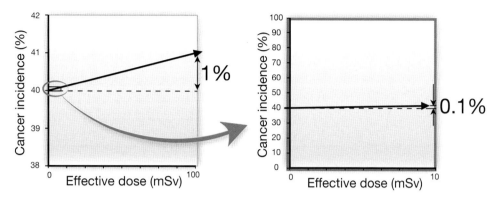

FIG 5.3 Radiation risk estimates for cancer induction by uniform whole-body x-ray exposures (100 and 10 mSv) based on BEIR VII risk estimates, where the background cancer incidence in the United States is taken to be 40%. BEIR, Biological Effects of Ionizing Radiation.

- Only a **few percent of spontaneous mutations** in humans may be ascribed to natural **background radiation.**
- The **doubling dose** is the absorbed dose to the gonads of the whole population that would double the spontaneous mutation incidence.
  - **Doubling dose** is currently estimated to be **between 1 and 2 Gy.**
- ICRP (2007) states that **hereditary effects** account for about **8%** of **total detriment** when populations are irradiated (whole-body doses).

C. Radiation and the Conceptus

- Radiation **risks** during **pregnancy** have been extensively studied using **animals** (e.g., mice).
  - These risks are **deterministic** with the exception of carcinogenesis.
- **Limited data** is also available in humans (e.g., **atomic bomb survivors**).
- Gestation in humans is divided into **preimplantation (conception to 9 days), organogenesis (10 days to 6 weeks)**, and **fetal (6 weeks to term).**
- Exposure to diagnostic x-rays prior to fertilization is not expected to have any detrimental effects.
- **Radiation** during preimplantation can result in **spontaneous abortion.**
- **Congenital malformations** are also associated with radiation exposure during **organogenesis.**
- **Growth retardation** and functional effects (e.g., **intellectual deficit**) may occur following radiation exposure.
  - Risk estimates during pregnancy depend on gestational age and the amount of radiation received (embryo dose or fetal dose).
- **Background incidence** of **congenital abnormalities** in the United States, in the absence of any radiation, is believed to be about **5%.**
  - This high background makes detection of radiation induced abnormalities problematical.

D. Conceptus Deterministic Risks

- **Below 50 mGy**, it is believed that there is **no risk** of **embryonic death** (preimplantation) or **major malformation** during organogenesis.
  - At these low doses, there is also no risk of growth retardation or functional impairment during the fetal period.
- **Between 50 and 100 mGy**, embryo and fetal effects are **scientifically uncertain.**
  - At these doses (i.e., 50-100 mGy), it is believed that any effects would likely be too subtle to be clinically detected.

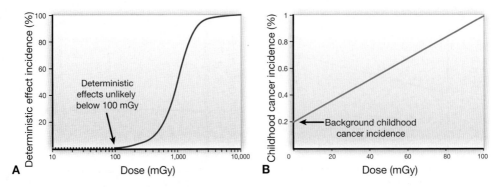

FIG 5.4 Schematic representation of deterministic (A) and stochastic risks (B) in embryo and fetus that are currently employed for radiation protection practice purposes.

- **Above 100 mGy, deterministic** effects **may occur.**
- Embryo death during preimplantation leads to resorption and is deemed an "all or nothing" type of event.
- **Major malformations** are primarily **expected** to occur during **organogenesis.**
- Reduced head size and mental impairment are most likely to occur at the gestational age of 8 to 15 weeks, with a much lower risk of these effects at 16 to 25 weeks.

E. **Conceptus Carcinogenic Risks**
- The primary concern beyond 25 weeks is carcinogenesis.
- Empirical data on the **carcinogenic** effects of embryonic and **fetal exposure** have been obtained in the UK (**Stewart and Kneale**) and the United States (**MacMahon**).
  - Whether x-rays are the causative agent has been debated for 50 years.
- Many now accept that **doses as low as 10 mGy** increase the **risk of childhood cancer**, especially during the third trimester.
- For a dose of 25 mGy, a **risk of 1 in 500 (0.2%)** of childhood cancer is used for radiation protection purposes.
- This **risk estimate** is likely **conservative** when applied to exposures during the first and second **trimesters.**
  - Fetal cancer risk estimates are broadly comparable to those obtained from atomic bomb survivors.
- In the **absence** of any **radiation exposure**, the background incidence of **childhood cancer** is **1 in 500 (0.2%).**
- An abdominal pelvic **CT** scan, which delivers an absorbed dose of **25 mGy** to the fetus, is thus taken to **double** the **likelihood** of **childhood cancer.**
- Figure 5.4 shows **schematic graphs** of our **current understanding** of **embryonic** and **fetal radiation effects.**

Chapter 5 (Radiation Risks) Questions

5.1 Which organism is likely to be easiest to "kill" with ionizing radiation?
  A. Virus
  B. Bacteria
  C. Human cells

5.2 What radiation-induced effect is least likely to occur from a head CT exam?
  A. Cell death
  B. Fatal cancer
  C. Nonfatal cancer
  D. Genetic effects

5.3 What effect is normally associated with a threshold dose?
  A. Genetic effect
  B. Fatal cancer
  C. Nonfatal cancer
  D. Sterility

5.4 What is the threshold for cerebrovascular syndrome?
  A. 0.5 Gy
  B. 5 Gy
  C. 50 Gy
  D. 500 Gy

5.5 Dermal atrophy and induration are most likely observed (long term) at peak skin doses of:
  A. 0.5 Gy
  B. 2 Gy
  C. 10 Gy
  D. 25 Gy

5.6 What is the threshold dose for temporary epilation?
  A. 2 mGy
  B. 50 mGy
  C. 3 Gy
  D. 15 Gy

5.7 When is radiation-induced skin erythema most likely to be observed?
  A. 10 minutes
  B. 10 hours
  C. 10 days
  D. 10 weeks

5.8 What is the current threshold dose for cataract induction?
  A. 0.5 Gy
  B. 2 Gy
  C. 5 Gy
  D. >5 Gy

5.9 What is the characteristic difference between a radiation-induced cancer and a natural cancer?
  A. Age of occurrence
  B. Lethality
  C. Treatment response
  D. None

5.10 Radiation-induced cancers have not been observed in what group?
  A. Uranium miners
  B. Watch dial painters
  C. Postpartum mastitis patients
  D. Nuclear medicine technologists

5.11 What is the typical latent period for induction of leukemia?
  A. 1 years
  B. 7 years
  C. 25 years
  D. 50 years

5.12 What is the model for radiation-induced solid tumor carcinogenesis used for radiation protection purposes?
  A. Threshold
  B. Linear no threshold
  C. Supralinear no threshold
  D. Hormesis

5.13 What is the baseline chance of getting cancer for an American?
  A. 5%
  B. 20%
  C. 40%
  D. 75%

5.14 The cancer sensitivity of a 65-year-old is most likely _____ times lower than that of a 25-year-old.
  A. 1.5
  B. 3
  C. 6
  D. >6

5.15 What is the most likely genetic doubling dose in humans?
  A. 1 mGy
  B. 1 Gy
  C. 20 mGy
  D. 20 Gy

5.16 Deterministic effects due to radiation are generally not discussed with a patient below what fetal dose?
A. 0 mGy
B. 10 mGy
C. 100 mGy
D. 1000 mGy

5.17 What effect is not associated with high fetal/embryo doses of radiation?
A. Congenital abnormality
B. Embryonic death
C. Mental retardation
D. Atrial septal defect

5.18 What is the increased cancer risk when a 25-year-old undergoes a TIPS procedure (effective dose 100 mSv)?
A. 0.01%
B. 0.1%
C. 1%
D. 10%

5.19 For a population exposed to uniform whole-body doses, genetic effects are currently estimated to contribute what percentage to the total detriment?
A. <1%
B. 1%
C. 8%
D. 25%

5.20 What is the typical time to death for gastrointestinal syndrome?
A. A day
B. A week
C. A month
D. A year

Answers and Explanations

5.1 **C** (Human cells). It is easier to kill human cells because they contain much more DNA (or RNA).

5.2 **D** (Genetic effects). For genetic effects to occur, energy must be deposited in the gametes (eggs or sperms), not somatic cells.

5.3 **D** (Sterility). Sterility is a deterministic effect with a threshold dose that depends on the sex of the exposed individual, as well as their age.

5.4 **C** (50 Gy). Cerebrovascular syndrome occurs for acute whole-body doses of about 50 Gy.

5.5 **C** (10 Gy). Dermal atrophy and induration are most likely observed as long term at peak skin doses approaching 10 Gy.

5.6 **C** (3 Gy). Currently accepted values for the threshold dose are 3 and 7 Gy for temporary epilation and permanent epilation, respectively.

5.7 **C** (Days). Radiation-induced erythema is most likely to be observed 10 days after the skin has been irradiated and is likely at peak skin doses of 5 Gy or more.

5.8 **A** (0.5 Gy). In 2011, ICRP stated that there is a 0.5 Gy threshold dose for cataract induction, applicable for both chronic and acute eye exposures.

5.9 **D** (None). There is no difference between radiation-induced and other types of cancer, with radiation increasing the rate at which cancers occur.

5.10 **D** (Nuclear medicine technologists). No radiation-induced cancers have ever been observed in any group of technologists.

5.11 **B** (7 years). Excess leukemia from radiation is seen as early as 2 years after exposure, but peaks 5 to 7 years after. Solid tumors begin to appear roughly 10 years after exposure, but take decades.

5.12 **B** (Linear no threshold). For practical radiation protection purposes, most radiation protection organizations recommend the use of a linear no threshold (LNT) model for radiation-induced carcinogenesis of solid tumors. Leukemia follows the linear quadratic model.

5.13 **D** (40%). About 40% of Americans will get cancer in their lifetime unrelated to radiation exposure.

5.14 **B** (3 times lower). A 65-year-old is most likely three times less sensitive than is a 25-year-old in terms of radiation-induced carcinogenesis.

5.15 **B** (1 Gy). Current estimates of the genetic doubling dose in humans are generally between 1 and 2 Gy.

5.16 **B** (100 mGy). Although animal models have shown possible spontaneous abortion at 50 mGy, this has not been shown in humans. It is generally accepted that fetal deterministic effects will not occur below 100 mGy.

5.17 **D** (Atrial septal defect). Atrial septal defects are not associated with radiation exposures, whereas congenital abnormalities, embryonic death, and mental retardation are all observed at high doses (e.g. 1 Gy).

5.18 **C** (1%). Average cancer risk increase from 100 mSv is about 1%, though this is may be a conservative estimate.

5.19 **C** (8%). The gonad tissue weighting factor (W_T) is currently assigned a value of 0.08 by the ICRP, which implies 8% of the detriment is due to genetic effects.

5.20 **B** (A week). GI syndrome will result in death to a human in about a week.

CHAPTER

6

Radiation Protection

I. MEASURING RADIATION

A. Solid-State Dosimeters

- Solid-state materials (crystals) may store energy absorbed during x-ray exposure in "electron traps."
- In **thermoluminescent dosimeters (TLDs)**, these energetic electrons are released by the **application of heat (i.e., baking), emitting visible light** (Fig. 6.1).
- **Lithium fluoride (LiF)** is a TLD used in diagnostic radiology because it **simulates** the absorption of x-rays by **soft tissues.**
  - LiF has a response (sensitivity) that is independent of x-ray energy and is typically found in ring dosimeters and is often used to measure patient dose.
- **Optically stimulated luminescence dosimeters (OSLDs)** use **laser light** to **release stored energy** and are typically used in personnel radiation badges (Fig. 6.1).
  - OSLDs can be read out several times, whereas TLDs can only be read out once.
- Solid-state dosimeters can measure doses as low as 0.01 mGy, or as high as 10,000 mGy (10 Gy).

B. Ionization Chambers

- **Ionization chambers** detect ionizing radiation by **measuring** the **charge (electrons) liberated** when x-ray photons ionize the gas inside.
- Ionization chambers need a positive voltage at the collecting electrode (anode), which attracts the liberated electrons.
  - The applied voltage should be high enough to collect all the liberated electrons.
- Figure 6.2A shows a schematic of the components of an ionization chamber.
- **Charge liberated** in the chamber is collected and used to **determine** the air kerma (K_{air}) or exposure (**Roentgen**).
- **Ionization chambers** are **very accurate** even in a spectrum and are used to measure x-ray tube outputs and injected dosages.
- **Ionization chambers** are **not very sensitive** and are **useless** for detecting small amounts of **radioactive contamination.**

C. Geiger Counters

- A **Geiger (or Geiger-Muller) counter** is an ionization chamber with a **very high voltage** across the chamber.
  - It counts interacting particles instead of recording energy deposited.
- The voltage causes each ionized electron to go on and ionize even more electrons (**avalanche**) as depicted in Figure 6.2B.
- *Any* detected incident beta **particle or photon** results in a **similar signal** (i.e., electron avalanche).

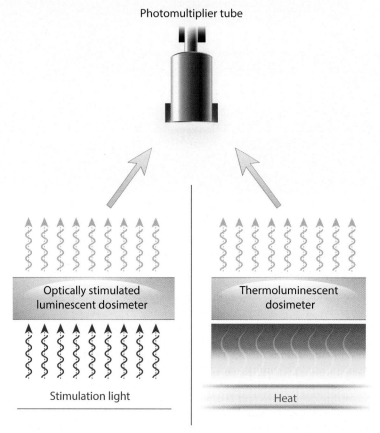

Photomultiplier tube

Optically stimulated luminescent dosimeter

Thermoluminescent dosimeter

Stimulation light

Heat

FIG 6.1 For both optically stimulated luminescent dosimeters (OSLDs) and thermoluminescent dosimeters (TLDs), radiation interacts with the detector and excites electrons, which get trapped in an excited state. The more radiation hitting the dosimeter, the more electrons are trapped. Left: In OSLDs scan the detector with a laser, which knocks some of the trapped electrons into their ground state. As they drop to their ground state, they emit photons, which are collected. More photons mean more trapped electrons and thus more radiation must have hit. Right: For TLDs, the dosimeter is baked. The heat knocks the electrons out of their traps and causes them to omit photons. Again, more photons mean more trapped electrons and thus more radiation must have hit the dosimeter. OSLDs have an advantage in that they can be read out several times and still give an accurate reading.

- **Geiger counters** are extremely **sensitive** and are used to detect low levels of **radioactive contamination.**
  - Each **detected photon** results in the **"click"** generally heard when using the Geiger counter.
- **Geiger** counters **cannot accurately** measure dose rates (i.e., **mGy/min**) or x-ray tube outputs (i.e., **mGy/mAs**).
  - A crude dose rate estimate can be calculated if the system is calibrated to the specific photon energy.

D. Personnel Dosimetry

- **Radiation workers** such as radiologists are monitored to ensure that their radiation exposures are within **regulatory limits.**
- Commercial laboratories provide dose values for the skin dose ("shallow"), the eye lens dose, and the **"deep" dose** corresponding to **penetrating** radiations.
  - Because current US regulations use non-SI units (mrem), reports express effective and equivalent doses in mrem (100 mrem is 1 mSv).

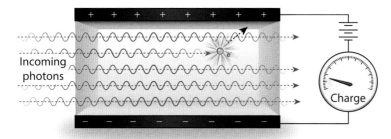

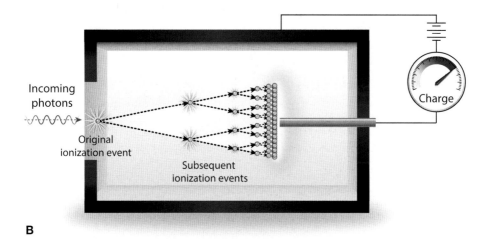

FIG 6.2 A: Ionization chamber where only electrons liberated by x-rays during photoelectric and Compton interactions are collected, and which requires a large number of x-ray photons (i.e., poor sensitivity and high accuracy). **B:** Geiger counter where an initial electron is amplified in an avalanche process to result in a massive electronic signal producing an audible "click" for each detected photon (i.e., high sensitivity and low accuracy).

- **Operator exposures** are provided for the **current period** (e.g., 1 month), **current quarter, current year,** and **lifetime** exposure.
- The National Committee on Radiological Protection and Measurements (**NCRP**) recommends that the operator **effective dose** be taken to be 0.18 of the dose recorded by a dosimeter worn on the collar (H_{collar}).
- **Interventional radiologists** may wear **one dosimeter outside** the lead apron (H_{collar}), and **another under** their **lead apron** (H_{waist}).
  - Operator effective dose is estimated by $[1.5 \times H_{waist} + 0.04 \times H_{collar}]$.
- **Dosimeters** may be worn on a **finger** to assess **extremity doses**, or on **glasses** to estimate eye **lens doses**.

II. REGULATORY LIMITS

A. Organizations

- The **International Commission on Radiological Units and Measurements (ICRU)** advises on issues such as measurement units in radiology (e.g., kerma).
- The **United Nations Scientific Committee on the Effects of Atomic Radiation (UNSCEAR)** scientifically evaluates radiation risks.
- The **National Academy of Sciences (NAS) committee Biological Effects of Ionizing Radiation (BEIR)** estimates radiation risks applicable to the United States.

- The **International Commission on Radiological Protection (ICRP)** provides recommendations for radiation workers, patients, and members of the public.
- In the United States, the foremost radiation protection body is the **NCRP.**
  - NCRP advises federal and state regulators on radiation protection.
- The US federal **Nuclear Regulatory Commission (NRC)** is responsible for regulating radioactive materials.
  - **Agreement states** arrange with the NRC to self-regulate medically related licensing and inspection requirements for nuclear materials.
- The **Food and Drug Administration (FDA)** has oversight of manufacture of x-ray equipment and production of radioactive drugs.
- In the United States, individual states are responsible for regulating x-ray emitting devices.
- US states coordinate state-level regulations through the **Conference of Radiation Control Program Directors (CRCPD).**
- In the United States, organization can either be advisory or regulatory (i.e., are governmental may create regulations and levy consequences if they are not followed).
  - **Regulatory:** FDA, NRC, EPA, agreement states, and others
  - **Advisory:** ICRU, NAS, ICRP, NCRP, CRCPD, ACR, AAPM, and others

B. Occupational (Effective Dose)

- Individuals **occupationally exposed** to radiation are generally **monitored** using personnel dosimeter (**OSLD**).
  - **Personnel dosimeters** are worn to ensure **regulatory dose limits** are not exceeded.
- **Occupational dose limits** *exclude* doses from **medical** procedures and **natural background** radiation.
- In the United States, the **regulatory** (i.e., legal) effective **dose limit** for **radiation workers** is **50 mSv/y**
  - **NCRP** also recommends a lifetime effective dose limit of **ten times** the **individual's age (mSv),** but this is not a regulation.
- **Radiation workers** are **unlikely** to receive regular annual effective doses **higher than ~5 mSv.**
  - **Occupational effective doses** are all **well below regulatory limits (i.e., ≤10%).**
- **Emergency occupational exposures** can exceed these dose limits if **lifesaving** actions are involved.
- The radiation badge quantity associated with this dose limit is either the **deep dose equivalent** or **total effective dose equivalent.**
  - These values only differ if the worker also intakes nuclear material during the course of their job (**committed dose**) as may happen from volatile liquid I-131.

C. Occupational (Other Doses)

- The US **eye lens dose limit** for occupational exposed workers is **150 mSv/y,** to prevent the induction of eye cataracts over a working lifetime.
  - To date, the United States has not reduced occupational lens dose limits despite the substantially reduced cataract induction limit published by ICRP in 2011.
- Skin and extremity dose limits have been designed to prevent the induction of deterministic effects.
  - Skin tolerates therapy fractionated doses of 20 Sv (20 Gy), so a limit of 500 mSv/y guarantees lifetime doses below this value.
- The dose limit to the **skin** of a radiation worker is **500 mSv/y.**
  - The radiation badge quantity associated with skin dose is **shallow dose equivalent.**
- Dose limit for **extremities** (e.g., hands) of radiation workers is **500 mSv/y**

D. Public Doses

- **Dose limit** for **members of the public** is **1 mSv/y**
  - All **dose limits** to members of the public **exclude** natural **background radiation,** which is unavoidable.

- In addition, **dose limits** to members of the **public exclude medical exposures**.
  - Exclusion of medical x-rays is justified because diagnostic information from radiological examinations confers a benefit to the exposed individual.
- **X-ray facilities** must be designed to **ensure** that exposure to members of the **public** does **not exceed 1 mSv/y**.
- **Public dose limits** are **conservative** to account for the possibility of **multiple sources** of exposure.
- **Public exposures** from **radiological activities** are normally **negligible.**

E. **Pregnant Workers**
- A worker must declare their pregnancy in writing to the radiation safety committee for extra regulatory protection measures to take effect.
  - At any time, a worker may undeclare in writing to stop with extra regulatory protections.
- **US maximum fetal dose of 5 mSv** during pregnancy is thus **higher** than the **public limit (1 mSv).**
  - Dose should be spread throughout the pregnancy if possible (e.g., **~0.05 mSv/mo**).
- Setting the fetal dose limit same as public (1 mSv) would have deprived women of reproductive capacity employment as radiation workers.
  - A dose limit of 0.5 mSv/mo permits women of reproductive capacity to seek employment as radiation workers (e.g., nuclear medicine technologists).
- **Declared pregnant radiation workers** are monitored by an extra **dosimeter** worn on the **abdomen under lead apron.**

III. PROTECTING PATIENTS

A. **Medical Patient Doses**
- Approximately **691 million diagnostic and interventional examinations** using ionizing radiation are performed **annually** in the **United States.**
- Table 6.1 shows the types of examinations that were performed, together with the average effective dose per patient examination, and per capita dose.
- In **2016**, the **US population average effective dose** from **medical** examinations and procedures was **2.16 mSv.**
  - In the **1980s**, the US population average effective dose from medical examinations and procedures was **0.6 mSv and in 2006 it was roughly 3 mSv.**
- In 2006, **average effective dose to Americans was roughly 6 mSv**, but this **decreased to ~5 mSv** in 2016 **due to reduction of medical dose.**
- **Population** doses from **diagnostic radiology increased sixfold** in one generation, but dose reduction measures have reversed this trend in the past decade.
- **CT** scans account for **11%** of ionizing radiation **exams**, but **63%** of the **population medical dose (the largest contributor).**
  - Nuclear medicine is the second largest contributor with cardiac studies being the biggest part of that.

TABLE 6.1	Approximate Number of Radiological Examinations Performed Annually in the United States (2016)		
Type of Examination	**Examinations Performed (Millions)**	**Average Effective Dose per Patient Examination (mSv)**	**Per Capita Dose (mSv)**
Radiography	275	0.3	0.22
Noncardiac interventional fluoroscopy	4	10	0.12
Computed tomography	74	6	1.37
Nuclear medicine	14	8	0.32

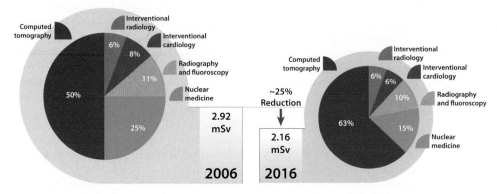

FIG 6.3 Annual effective dose from medical procedures. Left: In 2006, annual effective dose from medical procedures was comparable to natural background. CT was the largest contributor followed by nuclear medicine. Right: Annual effective dose decreased in 2016 despite the increase in the number of procedures. The ranking of contributors did not change, but per procedure doses did generally decrease.

- - CT dose has **dropped 6%** since 2006 despite a 20% increase in exams.
- • Figure 6.3 compares annual medical doses and their contributors between 2006 and 2016.
- • **Average pediatric effective dose** from medical examinations and procedures is **0.3 mSv**.
  - - Radiography is 86% of exams, but **CT is the highest pediatric medical dose contributor (83%).**

B. **Protection Philosophy**
- • **Principles of radiation protection** include **justification, optimization, and dose limits.**
  - - Justification and optimization apply to everyone, but dose limits only apply to occupational workers and members of the public (not patients).
- • **Justification** is selecting the "right exam" or no exam if there is no net benefit.
  - - ACR Appropriateness Criteria can aid in exam selection.
  - - Referring physicians need to practice ".DAM" (**D**on't **O**rder **T**ests [dot] that **D**on't **A**ffect **M**anagement [DAM]).
- • Radiation exposures involve risk, so **patient doses** should always be **optimized.**
  - - **ALARA (as low as reasonably achievable)**—no more radiation should be used than is necessary to obtain the required diagnostic information.
  - - For patients with implants, magnetic resonance (MR) heating and other risks must be optimized.
- • **Occupational and public dose limits** are written in the Code of Federal Regulations.
  - - **Diagnostic (dose) reference levels and achievable doses** are NOT dose limits; they are merely guidance on what peer institutions are doing.

C. **Justification**
- • **Justification** requires a **net benefit** where the value of diagnostic information obtained is greater than any radiation risks.
- • **Practitioners** need to understand the magnitude of **radiation risks to identify indicated examinations (benefit > risk).**
  - - It is not possible to perform any kind of benefit/risk analysis when the magnitude of the risk is unknown.

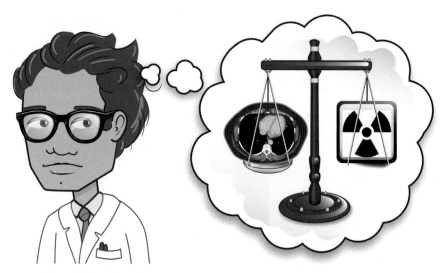

FIG 6.4 Weighing the benefits of patient risks and corresponding benefits of performing radiologic examinations is essential for identifying indicated examinations where there is a net benefit (benefit minus risk). This requires radiologists to have a quantitative understanding of radiation risks and the use of professional judgments as risks and benefits are generally incommensurate.

- In medical imaging, **radiologists** need to have an understanding of the patient **risks**, as well as the **corresponding uncertainties.**
- A **uniform whole-body dose of 10 mSv** in a **25-year**-old carries a nominal **radiation risk** of the order of **0.1% (1 in 1,000).**
  - Corresponding radiation risks in **infants** would be about **three times higher**, and risks in **retirees** would be about **three times lower.**
- Other risks include MR safety risks and overdiagnosis risks.
  - Device implant labeling can help guide discussions of MR risks to patients.
- Balancing risks and benefits in medical imaging generally requires the use of value judgments as depicted in Figure 6.4.
  - **Radiologists** generally **have an idea** whether they would choose to perform any given **diagnostic test** on a **family member** to solve a clinical problem.

D. ALARA

- **ALARA** requires **elimination** of **unnecessary radiation** in medical imaging.
- Using **too much radiation** is unlikely to incur any image quality penalty, but **unnecessarily irradiates** the **patient.**
  - Using **too little radiation** increases mottle and may **reduce diagnostic performance.**
- Following ALARA also reduces occupational dose for fluoroscopy operators and the public (e.g., lead wall shielding).
- **ALARA** requires **tailoring techniques** to the **diagnostic task.**
- Appropriate **time, distance, and shielding** help to keep doses ALARA for workers, the public, and the patient.
- ALARA allows for consideration of societal and financial factors.
  - Leaded glasses could block negligible (but nonzero) amounts of scatter for x-ray techs, but are expensive so they are not routinely used (we as a society accept the negligible risk).
- Table 6.2 lists examples of how imaging protocols might be adjusted to account for diagnostic imaging task.

TABLE 6.2	Examples of Imaging Protocol Modifications That Take Into Account the Imaging Task	
X-Ray Modality	**Diagnostic Task**	**Protocol Design Consideration**
Radiography	Scoliosis follow-up examinations	Reduce mAs by 90% as spine curvature changes are easy to see even when mottle is increased
Mammography	Ductal carcinoma in situ (DCIS) microcalcifications	Perform magnification imaging to help characterize microcalcifications
Fluoroscopy	Swallowed coin by child	High-contrast lesion so increased kV makes x-ray beam more penetrating and reduces dose (AEC[a])
Digital spot imaging	Dynamic imaging of carotid arteries	To see vasculature requires iodine contrast, and use of ~70 kV maximizes x-ray absorption by iodine. Note the neck is "thin" and easy to penetrate
CT	Lung cancer screening	Reduce radiographic techniques to reduce doses in asymptomatic patients. High-contrast lesion in lung will not be affected by the increase in mottle

[a]Automatic exposure control, which ensures a constant radiation at image receptor irrespective of the kV (penetrating power) used.

E. **Exposure of Pregnant Patients**
- Before a pregnant patient is exposed to x-rays, the magnitude of the fetal or embryo doses and risks should be considered.
  - A **qualified medical physicist** should be **consulted if fetal/embryo dose could exceed 50 mSv** and a dose **calculation should be requested if fetal/embryo dose could exceed 100 mSv.**
- When the **x-ray beam does not directly irradiate the fetus or embryo**, the corresponding **dose will be low**, and clinically unimportant.
- **No medical action** is needed at unintended **doses up to 100 mGy**, as any risks would be deemed to be low compared with normal risks of pregnancy.
- A **conceptus dose** of **100 mGy**, extremely rare in diagnostic imaging, **triggers consideration** of possible **medical intervention.**
  - **High doses** (risk) during organogenesis from an Interventional Radiology (IR) procedure or Nuclear Medicine (NM) therapy, for example, **might warrant consideration** of a **therapeutic abortion.**
- Consideration of medical intervention needs to take into account all clinical aspects, as well as social conditions of the patient.

IV. PROTECTING WORKERS

A. **General**
- Radiation **protection of workers** is designed to **prevent deterministic effects** and **minimize stochastic risks.**
  - **Minimization** of **stochastic risks** needs to be "**reasonable,**" and take into account any **benefits gained** by the radiation **workers.**
- X-ray personnel only receive significant exposures when they are standing close to the patient undergoing the x-ray examination (i.e., in the same room).
- **Operator doses** are generally directly **proportional** to **patient doses** and can be readily estimated.
- As a general rule, the **scatter** dose level from **patients at 1 m** is approximately **0.1%** of the **entrance skin dose**, as illustrated in Table 6.3.

TABLE 6.3	Representative Entrance K_{air} Values in Diagnostic Imaging, and the Corresponding Scatter Radiation	
Examination	**Patient Skin Doses (mGy)**	**Air Kerma @ 1 m (µGy)**
Lateral skull x-ray	1	1
Body fluoroscopy (1 min)	10	10
Head CT scan	40	40

- Radiation workers should not routinely hold a patient for a study, because doses from many examinations could be substantial.
  - A parent or relative should position the patient and be given a lead apron to wear.
- Methods of **controlling radiation dose** are decreasing **exposure time**, **increasing distance** from the radiation source, and using appropriate **shielding.**
- Radiation workers are also subject to annual dose limits established by the federal government and discussed earlier in this chapter.

B. Time and Distance

- **Fluoroscopy time** should always be **optimized** and **last image hold (LIH)/last cine loop** capabilities used whenever possible.
  - Viewing images in these modes delivers no dose to patients.
- **Pulsed fluoroscopy** rates (e.g., 15 frames per second) or less should be used where this is technically feasible and clinically desirable.
- The **"5-minute"** alarm (federal regulation) in fluoroscopy **reminds** the **operators** of increasing patient exposures.
- Like fluoroscopy time, the number of **spot images**, and **photospot images** acquired should be **optimized.**
  - **Reducing exposure** times and exposures must **never be** at the **expense** of **diagnostic performance.**
- During fluoroscopy, workers should not be in the room if not necessary.
- Because **radiation intensity** falls off as the **inverse square of the distance,** doubling the distance reduces doses fourfold.
  - If the **distance** from a radiation source **increases** by **X,** the radiation **intensity** is **reduced** by a factor of X^2, and vice versa.
- Operators should **maximize** the **distance** between them and the patient **without impeding patient safety** or the **diagnostic information.**
- For portable examinations, the operator should stand **at least 6 ft (2 m)** from patients.
- **Increasing** the **distance** from a source of radiation is generally **more effective** at reducing operator doses than **reducing** the **exposure time.**
  - Doubling the distance from a source reduces operator doses by 75%, whereas halving the exposure time reduces operator doses by 50%.

C. Shielding

- X-ray attenuation by lead is high because of its high density and atomic number.

TABLE 6.4	Approximate Values of Lead (Pb) Half-Value Layers (HVL) and Tenth-Value Layers (TVL) as a Function of X-Ray Tube Voltage (kV)	
Tube Voltage (keV)	**Pb HVL (mm)**	**Pb TVL (mm)**
30	0.02	0.07
40	0.04	0.14
140	0.2	1
511	4	13

Decreased efficacy of lead at nuclear medicine energies.

- **Protective effect** of **lead** is highly **dependent** on **photon energy** (Table 6.4), and it becomes less effective as energy increases.
- **Lead aprons** may use from **lead-impregnated vinyl or other materials that are lighter, although they are often still referred to as "lead" aprons.**
- **Aprons** used in diagnostic radiology must be at least **0.25 mm** of lead equivalence.
  - Aprons made from materials lighter than lead often show lower protection than actual lead.
- **Aprons** must be worn at all times during fluoroscopy and are expected to **attenuate at least 90%** of an incident x-ray beam.
  - **Aprons** should be hung on appropriate racks, as folding them can produce cracks, and they should be **tested annually.**
- A **neck shield** can significantly reduce the dose to the **thyroid.**
- **Leaded glasses** should be worn to **reduce eye lens doses (~60%-70%).**
- Lead-impregnated latex **gloves** may be used to minimize extremity dose, but are only effective when hands are outside the beam.
- **Leaded surgical caps only reduce head dose a few percent** due to scatter through the neck and face.
- **Shielding** and table skirts are generally **0.5 mm lead equivalent.**
  - Shields should be **tight to the operator and to the patient body** and oriented to block scatter from the **patient entrance surface.**
- All shielding combined reduces operator dose >99%.
- Figure 6.5 shows **protection devices** used by operators to **minimize** their **exposure** to radiation.

D. Radiation Worker Doses

- Most **x-ray technologists** receive relatively **low effective doses.**
  - Shielding of x-ray rooms and booth housing the x-ray controls offers a high degree of attenuation of the x-ray beams.

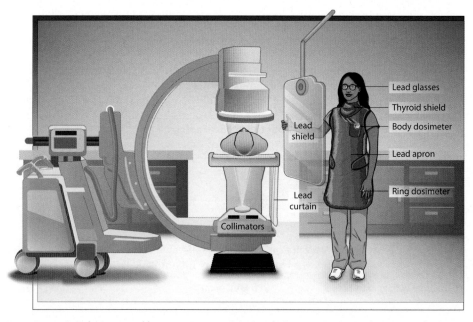

FIG 6.5 Protection devices used by operators to minimize their exposures to radiation are shown. Operators should also maximize the distance to the patient (source of scatter radiation), and minimize the amount of radiation used, while ensuring satisfactory diagnostic performance.

- Doses to 90% of x-ray technologists will be below the detection limit of the radiation badges used.
- Average monthly badge reading for **radiology** residents is **0.07 mSv.**
  - **75%** of **residents'** badges are **below** the **detection limit.**
- Sources of **operator doses** in diagnostic radiology include **general fluoroscopy, interventional radiology,** and **nuclear medicine.**
- Operator effective doses recorded by staff working in **general fluoroscopy** procedures (GI/GU) are modest, and **unlikely** to exceed 1 mSv.
- Technologists working in **nuclear medicine** are expected to receive effective doses of **2 to 3 mSv each year.**
- **Aprons** are **less effective** at energies used in NM (e.g., **140 keV**) and are **impractical** in the vicinity of **"radioactive patients."**
  - **Sources are shielded in thick lead** (L-blocks and pigs).
- **IR fellows** typically receive annual effective doses of **a few mSv.**
- IR physicians with high workloads may approach annual dose limits, but this is the minority.

Chapter 6 (Radiation Protection) Questions

6.1 What is the best detector to find low-level contamination (e.g., 40 kBq of ^{99m}Tc) in an NM department?
A. Ionization chamber
B. Geiger counter
C. Thermoluminescent dosimeter
D. Thyroid probe

6.2 Where should a GI radiologist wear their dosimeter to assess occupational exposure?
A. At collar level
B. Under the Pb apron
C. On their wrist
D. Glass frame (eyes)

6.3 What group coordinates US States radiation protection regulations?
A. BEIR
B. UNSCEAR
C. CRCPD
D. NCRP

6.4 Who regulates the use of radioactive materials in the United States?
A. BEIR
B. NRC
C. CRCPD
D. NCRP

6.5 What is the US regulatory dose limit for the annual effective dose to radiation workers?
A. 1 mSv
B. 5 mSv
C. 20 mSv
D. 50 mSv

6.6 What is the current annual US regulatory dose limit for the eye lens?
A. 5 mSv
B. 50 mSv
C. 150 mSv
D. 500 mSv

6.7 What is the current annual US dose limit for members of the public?
A. < 1 mSv
B. 1 mSv
C. 5 mSv
D. 20 mSv

6.8 US regulatory dose limits would most likely include exposures from:
A. Cosmic radiation
B. Scatter from patients
C. Diagnostic x-rays
D. NM Studies

6.9 What is the current monthly US regulatory dose limit to the fetus for a declared pregnant worker?
A. 0.1 mSv
B. 0.2 mSv
C. 0.5 mSv
D. 1 mSv

6.10 How has the average effective dose from medical exposures changed between 2006 and 2016?
A. +100%
B. +25%
C. −25%
D. −50%

6.11 What body regulates manufacture of fluoroscopy equipment?
A. EPA
B. NRC
C. NCRP
D. FDA

6.12 Per capita medical doses in the United States are _____ natural background doses.
A. lower than
B. comparable to
C. greater than

6.13 Which imaging modality contributes the most to US medical doses for children?
A. Nuclear medicine
B. CT
C. Interventional radiology
D. Radiography and fluoroscopy

6.14 What is the best advice a radiologist can offer a patient concerned about radiation?
A. The exam is worthwhile
B. The dose is low
C. The exam is painless
D. The monetary cost is low

6.15 What is the meaning of ALARA in radiology?
A. Keeping patient doses low
B. Eliminating unnecessary radiation
C. Ensuring costs are minimized
D. Ensuring exams are cost-effective

6.16 What embryo/fetal radiation dose
would likely trigger consideration of
possible medical intervention?
A. 1 mGy
B. 10 mGy
C. 30 mGy
D. 100 mGy

6.17 The scattered radiation a meter from
a patient undergoing fluoroscopy is
most likely:
A. 0.1 μGy/min
B. 1 μGy/min
C. 10 μGy/min
D. 100 μGy/min

6.18 When a radiologist increases the
distance to a patient from 50 to
150 cm, how does their radiation dose
change?
A. 9×
B. 3×
C. 1/3×
D. 1/9×

6.19. What is the minimum regulatory lead
equivalent lead apron thickness?
A. 0.1 mm
B. 0.25 mm
C. 0.75 mm
D. No minimum value

6.20 How much do glasses likely reduce
eye dose?
A. 20%
B. 60%
C. 80%
D. 99%

Answers and Explanations

6.1 B (Geiger counter). Only Geiger counters have the sensitivity to detect low levels of radioactivity.

6.2 A (At collar level). A single personal dosimeter would normally be worn *above* the lead apron at the level of the collar.

6.3 C (CRCPD). The Conference of Radiation Control Program Directors meets each year to coordinate regulations in all 50 US states.

6.4 B (NRC). The Nuclear Regulatory Commission (NRC) regulates the use of radioactive materials (e.g., Nuclear Medicine) in the United States.

6.5 D (50 mSv). The current regulatory effective dose limit to radiation workers in the United States is 50 mSv/y.

6.6 C (150 mSv). The current US regulatory dose limit for the eye lens is 150 mSv/y, and this is designed to prevent the induction of cataracts.

6.7 B (1 mSv). The current regulator dose limit for members of the public in the United States is 1 mSv/y.

6.8 B (Scatter from patients). Scatter from patients hitting a worker is an occupational exposure. *Natural* background radiation and diagnostic examinations to the worker are excluded from all regulatory dose limits.

6.9 C (0.5 mSv/mo). The current US regulatory dose limit to the fetus of a radiation worker is 5 mSv/y (~0.5 mSv each month).

6.10 C (−25%). Average effective dose for medical exposures went from 2.92 to 2.15 mSv.

6.11 D (FDA). The FDA sets regulations on the manufacture of medical equipment.

6.12 A (lower than). In 2006 they were similar, but more recent data from 2016 show they are about 30% lower than dose from natural sources (~3 mSv).

6.13 B (CT). CT is the primary source of medical dose for both children and adults.

6.14 A (The exam is worthwhile). Worthwhile exams are those where the patient benefits are expected to exceed (any) corresponding risks, including those associated with radiation.

6.15 B (Eliminating unnecessary radiation). An excellent definition of ALARA in diagnostic imaging is eliminating unnecessary radiation to obtain the required diagnostic information.

6.16 D (100 mGy). An embryo/fetal dose of 100 mGy would normally trigger consideration (though not necessarily execution of) medical intervention.

6.17 C (10 µGy/min). Scatter at 1 m is 0.1% of the entrance K_{air} rate, which is about 10 mGy/min.

6.18 D (1/9×). According to the inverse square law, tripling the distance from a radiation source (scatter from patient) reduces exposures by a factor of 9 (i.e., X 1/9).

6.19 B (0.25 mm). The minimum regulatory thickness is 0.25 mm Pb (or equivalent), although most operators would use 0.5 mm.

6.20 B (60%). Dose may still scatter into the eye from the head, face, and neck. This brings glass protection from >90% down to ~60% to 70%.

X-Ray Imaging
Modalities

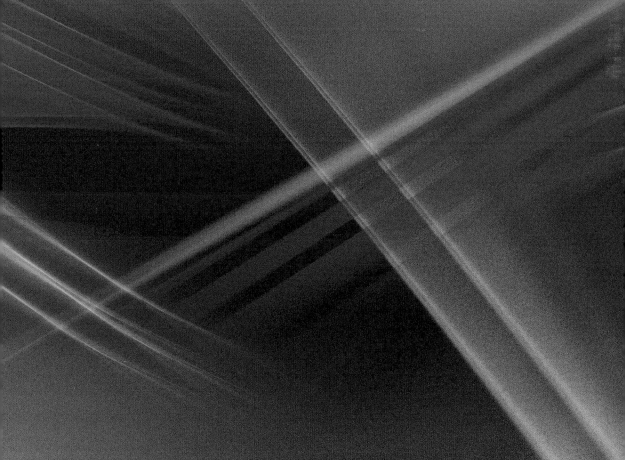

CHAPTER 7

Radiography

I. X-RAY TUBES

A. **Tube Design**
- **X-ray tubes** have a **negative cathode** containing the filament that serves as an **electron source** (Fig. 7.1A).
- A **positive anode** contains a **target**, usually made of **tungsten**, where **x-rays are produced.**
- The **target/anode** is angled at about **15°** (Fig. 7.1B), which exhibits the **line focus principle.**
  - Electrons hit a large area of the target, which helps with cooling, but x-rays appear to come from a "small" area when viewed at an angle (i.e., from the patient's perspective).
- The **area generating x-rays** is known as the **focal spot** and is characterized by a focal spot diameter.
- The anode and cathode are contained in an **evacuated envelope**, surrounded by a tube housing that **shields staff from radiation.**
- **Primary x-ray** beams go through the x-ray tube **window**, which is directed toward the patient to produce radiographic images (i.e., **useful x-ray beam**).

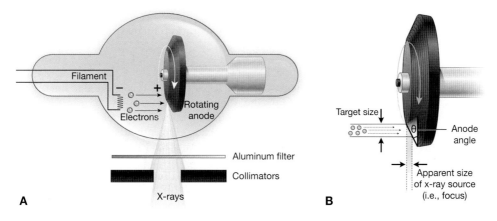

FIG 7.1 A: Schematic of an x-ray tube showing a heated filament that produces electrons (cathode), which are then accelerated into the rotating anode that contains a tungsten target as depicted in Figure 1.2. **B:** A small anode angle (e.g., 15°) permits a large target area to be irradiated that reduces heating problems, while resulting in a *narrow source of x-rays* (focus) as seen from the patient's perspective below.

- **Leakage radiation** is transmitted through the x-ray tube housing.
  - Regulations require **leakage K_{air}** be less than **1 mGy per hour at 1 m.**
- **Scattered radiation** has been deviated in direction after leaving the tube.
  - The patient is the largest source of scattered radiation.
- **Secondary radiation** is the sum of the leakage and scattered radiation, resulting in exposure to any personnel in the x-ray room (radiologists, technologists, etc.).

B. **Targets and Anodes**
- **Energetic electrons** striking the target **produce heat** and **x-rays.**
- **X-rays produced per electron increase** with increasing electron energy (i.e., **kV**) and increasing target material atomic number (**Z**).
- The target is embedded in an **anode** material, which temporarily stores the **heat energy** deposited in the target.
- Heat **energy deposited** in the **focal spot,** and which is immediately conducted to the anode, is known as **tube loading.**
  - X-ray **tube loading** increases with tube **voltage,** tube **current,** and exposure **time.**
- **Modern anodes** are circular and **rotate** at high speeds (e.g., 10,000 rpm) to **spread heat** loading over a large area.
- Total energy deposited in the anode also depends on the number of exposures.
- Heat energy is temporarily stored in the **anode,** which has a **heat capacity** of **several hundred thousand Joules.**
  - When the **anode** is "**full,**" no more exposures can be made until the anode **cools down.**

C. **Focal Power Rating**
- The total energy put into the **focal spot** must ensure it does **not overheat** and melt.
- X-ray tube techniques (i.e., kV, mA, s) are constrained by the x-ray tube design.
  - **Computers** limit technique selection and ensure **focal spots do not overheat.**
- **Power rating** is the maximum kilowatts (**kW**) that a focal spot can tolerate in a specified exposure time.
  - A tube with a rating of **100 kW (100,000 W)** could tolerate **100 kV** and **1,000 mA** for an exposure lasting **0.1 second.**
- In radiography, **power rating** is ~**100 kW** for a **large focal spot** size and ~**25 kW** for a **small focal spot.**
- At **100 kW, 100,000 J** of energy are deposited in the target every **second.**
  - In 0.1 second, **10,000 J** will be **deposited** in the **target**, with virtually all of this heat **energy** immediately **transferred** into the **anode.**
- Achieving the **required x-ray tube output** may require an **increase** in **exposure time** to reduce power loading.

D. **Heat Dissipation**
- Virtually all (**99%**) **electrical energy** supplied to x-ray tubes is converted to **heat.**
  - Only about 1% is turned into x-rays in radiology.
- Heat loading into the anode and x-ray tube housing must ensure neither overheats.
  - **X-ray tubes** are **expensive,** as they are designed to efficiently **dissipate heat.**
- **Heat** is **transferred** from the focal spot by **radiation** to the tube housing and **conduction** into the anode, as depicted in Figure 7.2.
- **Anodes get white hot** during the x-ray exposure and **lose** their **energy** by emitting light photons, **radiating** the heat away similar to our sun.
- X-ray tubes are usually **immersed** in **oil,** which aids heat dissipation by convection.
  - **Air fans** are sometimes used to increase the rate of heat loss.
- Taking a **large number** of radiographs can **saturate** the **anode** heat capacity.
- When the anode heat capacity is reached, **anodes must cool** down before additional exposures are allowed.
- It generally takes **several minutes** for a **hot x-ray tube anode** to **cool.**

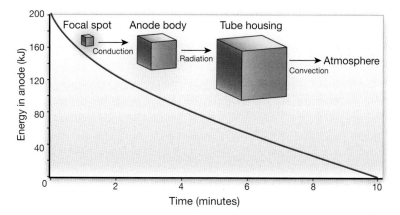

FIG 7.2 Anode ray tube cooling curve (red) illustrating that it takes several minutes to cool a saturated anode. Energy deposited in the focal spot appears as heat, which has to be limited to prevent the target melting. Energy from the focal spot is conducted into the anode body, which gets "white hot," and is subsequently radiated (via light) to the tube housing.

E. Heel Effect

- X-rays produced within the anode travel equally in all directions (**isotropic**).
- Since x-rays are produced within the anode, they **must pass** through a **portion** of the **target** and are therefore **attenuated** on their way out of the target.
- The **target** is normally **tungsten (Z = 74),** which has attenuation properties similar to those of **lead (Z = 82).**
- **Attenuation** of x-rays is **greater** in the **anode direction** than in the cathode direction because of differences in the path length within the target (Fig. 7.3).
- This results in **higher x-ray intensity** at the **cathode end** and lower x-ray intensity at the anode end of the beam, called the **Heel effect.**
- To **reduce** the **Heel effect**, the **anode angle** should be **increased, source-to-image distance (SID) increased,** and **field size decreased.**
- The **Heel effect** can be taken **advantage** of by placing **more attenuating parts** of the body at the **cathode side** and less attenuating parts at the anode side of the beam (Fig. 7.3).

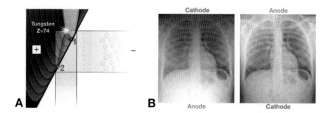

FIG 7.3 **A:** Heel effect is a result of x-rays traveling in the anode direction (path length 2) being attenuated more than those traveling in the cathode direction (path length 1). Tungsten targets attenuate x-rays almost as much as lead, resulting in noticeable decrease in x-ray intensity at the anode side of an x-ray tube. **B:** Radiograph images produced with anode pointing at the upper (left) and lower (right) portions of the body. Shading indicates photons reaching the detector. The number of photons reaching the detector is more uniform when the cathode is aligned with thicker anatomy.

TABLE 7.1	X-Ray Tube Beam Quality and X-Ray Tube Output Versus X-Ray Tube Voltage (kV)	
X-Ray Tube Voltage (kV)	Half-Value Layer (mm Al)	Tube Output at 1 m (mGy/100 mAs)
60	2.0	3.5
80	2.9	6.7
100	3.7	11
120	4.5	15

II. RADIOGRAPHIC IMAGING

A. Tube Voltage (kV)

- Table 7.1 shows how tube voltage (kV) affects beam quality (i.e., HVL) and beam quantity (i.e., mGy/mAs) in radiography.
- **Low x-ray tube voltages** in radiography range between **50 and 65 kV.**
  - **Low tube voltages** are associated with low average x-ray photon energies, and thereby **limited penetration** through tissues.
- **Low tube voltages** are used for imaging the **extremities,** where bone ensures that photoelectric effects are the dominant mode of interaction.
  - Imaging very **thin body parts** such as infants also uses **low tube voltages.**
- Most of **radiographic imaging** is performed using intermediate x-ray tube voltages ranging between **70 and 90 kV.**
  - Intermediate voltages have higher average photon energies, which increases patient **penetration.**
- **High voltages** (120 kV) are used in examinations such as **chest** x-rays.
- **High tube voltages reduce** the radiation **latitude (dynamic range),** which is the difference in number of photons transmitted through different body parts.
  - At 120 kV, penetration through rib and mediastinum is better.
- **Reducing the latitude** of the transmitted radiation through a patient results in a narrower range of detected signals that is easier to capture, process, and display.
  - **High kVs** that reduce the transmitted latitude also **reduce patient doses** when K_{air} at the image receptor is kept constant (i.e., more penetrating beam).
- The impact of kV changes on image quality is given with clinical examples in Table 7.2.

B. Tube Output (mAs) and Focal Spots

- At a given x-ray tube voltage, the **beam intensity (tube output)** is **proportional** to both the **tube current (mA)** and the exposure **time (seconds).**
- **Tube currents** are a **few hundred mA** in radiography.
- **Exposure times** in radiography are generally **very short (<10 ms)** or **short (<100 ms).**
- A **chest x-ray** would likely use a tube current of 200 mA, an exposure time of 5 ms, corresponding to **1 mAs** (500 mA × 0.002 ms).

TABLE 7.2	Effect of *Increasing* the X-Ray Tube Voltage in Radiographic Examinations	
Parameter	Effect	Clinical Use (Example)
Penetration	Increases	High kV to penetrate bowel contrast media
Image contrast	Reduces	Low kV used to increase bone contrast
Scatter	Increases	Low kV used in bedside (nongrid) radiography
Patient dose	Reduces	High kV permits big reduction of mAs for screening examinations

- An **abdominal radiograph** would likely use a tube current of 400 mA and an exposure time of 50 ms, corresponding to **20 mAs.**
- **Focal spot** sizes in radiography are **0.6 mm (small)** and **1.2 mm (large).**
- **Small focal spots** produce **sharp images** (high resolution), whereas **large focal spots** can tolerate a **high heat loading** and reduce exposure times.
  - Choice of the **focal spot** size is achieved by balancing the **conflicting need** for **sharp images**, and being able to tolerate **high heat loadings.**
- **Large focal spots** are favored when a **short exposure** time is important.
  - **Small focal spots** are needed to obtain the **best spatial resolution.**

C. Irradiation Geometry

- The distance from the x-ray tube source (i.e., focal spot) to the image receptor is the **SID.**
- The distance from the source (focus) to an object is the **source-to-object distance (SOD).**
- **Geometric magnification** is the **SID divided** by the **SOD.**
- Very "thin" objects located at the image receptor have virtually no geometric magnification.
  - **Objects halfway** between the **source** and **image receptor** have a **2× magnification.**
- **Geometric magnification varies** with **patient depth**, introducing **distortion.**
- Shorter SIDs increase skin doses as well as geometric magnification.
- **More radiation** is **required** with **longer SIDs**, increasing exposure times and any corresponding motion blur.
- The **most common SID** in radiography is **100 cm (40 in).**
  - Exceptions to this rule include chest x-rays and C-spine examinations (180 cm/72 in).
- **Magnification imaging** is generally **not used** in **radiography** because of the associated increase in focal spot blur.

D. Grids and Detectors

- Table 7.3 shows how patient thickness and x-ray beam area affect scatter in radiography.
  - **Scatter** intensities in **radiography** are generally **much greater** than **primary** intensities reaching the detector (i.e., scatter-to-primary ratios greater than 1).
- **Grid lines** are generally aligned along the **anode-cathode axis.**
- Most radiography uses **scatter removal grids**, with a grid ratio of about **10:1.**
  - Virtual grids use modeling and image processing to remove some scatter from images but generally are less effective than physical grids.
- For very **thin body parts**, generally below about **12 cm**, grids are **optional.**
  - When a **grid** is **added** to image an extremity, **image quality (contrast) slightly improves** at the cost of an **increase** in **patient dose.**
- Virtually all **radiography** is performed using **digital x-ray detectors**, consisting of mainly **scintillators and less often photoconductors and photostimulable phosphors.**
- **Cassettes** that use **photostimulable phosphors** need to be taken to a **reader**, analogous to films developed in a film processor.

TABLE 7.3	Scatter-to-Primary Ratios in Abdominal Radiography as a Function of Field of View and Patient Thickness		
Anteroposterior Thickness (cm)	**Field of View (cm)**		
	5 × 5	**10 × 10**	**20 × 20**
10	0.9	1.2	1.4
20	2.2	3.0	3.4
30	4.2	5.3	6.0

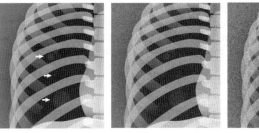

High mAs	Average mAs	Low mAs

FIG 7.4 Simulated radiographs showing the impact of mAs. Left: High mAs demonstrates all lesions clearly but may use more patient dose than necessary. Middle: Lesions are still visible at lower mAs (and patient dose). Right: Dropping mAs too low increases the noise making lesions much more difficult to detect.

E. Pediatric

- **Dedicated pediatric x-ray units** may include added **copper filtration (0.1-0.2 mm)** to make the x-ray beam more penetrating.
- More penetrating (i.e., filtered) beams reduce patient doses when AEC is used.
    - High filtration is tolerable because less radiation is required to penetrate smaller patients (pediatric).
- **Pediatric radiography** needs to **minimize exposure times** to **reduce motion blur**, and use of large focal spots (100 kW power) offers short exposure times.
    - Because children are small, magnification is relatively low, and focal spot blur is minimal.
- For smaller **patients less** than **12 cm** of tissue equivalence, the use of a **grid** is generally **optional.**
- X-ray tube voltages for a **1-year-old** chest/abdomen would be ~**60 kV**, and for a **5-year-old** would increase to ~**65 kV.**
    - Younger children may be radiographed tabletop (i.e., no grid).
- A **10-year-old** child would likely have the x-ray tube voltage increased to ~**85 kV**, and performed using a **standard Bucky (10:1 grid).**
- **EI** values for body radiographs in **children** are generally **similar** to those used in **adults.**

IV. IMAGE QUALITY AND DOSE

A. Penetration, Contrast, and Noise

- When the voltage is set to (just) penetrate a patient, lesion contrast is maximized.
    - **Lower voltages will not penetrate**, and **higher voltages reduce contrast.**
- Table 7.4 shows how patient penetration varies with photon energy and patient size.
- The **atomic number (Z)** of the **lesion** affects the change in contrast with photon energy.
- When lesion Z is similar to tissue, reductions in lesion contrast with increasing photon energy will be modest.
- When **lesion Z differs markedly from that of tissue, reducing** the **photon energy** will dramatically **improve** the **visibility** of the lesion.
- At a fixed tube voltage, choice of the **mAs impacts** the image **noise (mottle).**
- When the **mAs quadruples,** patient dose also quadruples and **image mottle** is **halved.**
- The (lesion) **contrast-to-noise ratio (CNR)** is dependent on the operator's choices of x-ray tube **voltage (kV)** and x-ray tube **output (mAs).**
- Figure 7.4 shows the impact of reduced mAs on noise and detectability.

Penetration (%) of Monoenergetic Photons Through Varying Patient Thicknesses (Water or Soft Tissues) Simulating Adults Patients			
Patient Tissue Thickness (cm)	**Patient Penetration (%) at Photon Energy (keV) of:**		
	40	**50**	**60**
18	0.82	1.7	2.5
23	0.22	0.54	0.88
28	0.06	0.17	0.31

TABLE 7.4

B. Resolution

- In most of radiography, a large focal spot is used, and the resultant focal spot blur is clinically acceptable.
  - A **small focal spot** is used where **sharp images** are important (e.g., **extremity radiography**).
- For **scintillators**, increasing **detector thickness** generally reduces image spatial resolution because of the increasing spread (diffusion) of light.
- For **photostimulable phosphors**, increasing detector thickness increases **scatter** of the **incident readout laser** light into adjacent pixels, which **reduces spatial resolution.**
- Se-based **photoconductors** would offer **the best spatial resolution.**
- A **35 × 43 cm detector** (2k × 2.5k matrix size) has pixels of **175 µm** (i.e., sampling rate of 6 pixels per millimeter) and a limiting resolution of **3 line pairs per millimeter.**
  - A **20 × 24** detector (2k × 2.5k matrix size), has pixels of **100 µm** (i.e., sampling rate of 10 pixels per millimeter) and a limiting resolution of **5 line pairs per millimeter.**
- In radiography, reducing exposure time minimizes motion blur.
- Spatial resolution in radiography is important in musculoskeletal, pediatric, and chest imaging.

C. Artifacts

- Objects worn by patients (**false teeth, necklaces, hairpins**) can mask important anatomy.
- Uniformity correction ensures AEC dosimeters are not visible and each detector element gives the same response for the same amount of radiation.
- **Grids** need to be correctly **aligned** to transmit primary x-rays over the whole image.
- **Grid cutoff** artifact can occur when the SID does not match that of the grid, or when the grid is not aligned correctly.
  - This is typically visualized as unilateral attenuation increase with "grid lines" visible.
- When a region of an image has received an unexpectedly high (or low) exposure, this area can have a different sensitivity for a short period after the exposure (ghosting).
  - A **ghost** of a **metallic implant** may appear in images obtained subsequent to a radiograph on a patient with this implant.
  - **Ghosting** can be **minimized** by waiting for **digital detectors** to **"recover"** from an unusually high or low exposure.
- **Dead pixels or pixel lines** will result in bright dots or lines in the image and require detector calibration to interpolate over them.
- **Patient motion** during acquisition causes blur and may be addressed using restraints or reducing exposure time.
- **Electromagnetic interference** occurs when the electromagnetic fields of other devices are picked up by digital detectors and cause image artifacts similar to grid line interference.
  - Shielding the detector, turning off the device, or moving the device further from the detector can all help mitigate this artifact.
- Figure 7.5 shows a few image artifacts in radiography.

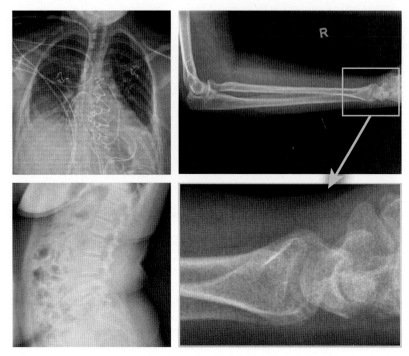

FIG 7.5 A few common artifacts in radiography. Bottom-Left: Motion artifact occurs when the patient moves during the exposure and results in blurring (here in the abdomen) that can decrease detectability. Right: Grid lines can interfere with the discrete pixels in a detector and cause low frequency lines throughout the image (here in an extremity). Both full-image and zoomed-in versions are shown to demonstrate how the artifact may slightly change depending on zoom. Checking the Bucky motor and confirming software grid suppression is functioning properly can help. Top-Left: Electromagnetic interference may cause artifact similar to grid lines (here in a chest). As in this case, it may not cover the whole image but only the portion of the image close to the device causing interference (here an external pacemaker located outside the field of view inferiorly).

D. Doses and Risks

- **Skin doses** in **radiography** are very low **(<10 mGy)** and of no clinical importance.
- When the embryo/fetus is in the field of view (or FOV) it will get a few mGy.
  - Outside the FOV, fetal dose is negligible.
  - Lumbar spines give the highest fetal dose in radiography.
  - Fetal dose also increases with gestational age.
- Patient **effective doses** in **radiography** are very low **(<0.1 mSv)** or low **(0.1-1 mSv)**.
- Examples of radiographic examinations with **very low effective doses** include the **extremities** and **chest x-rays.**
- Examples of radiographic examinations with **low effective doses** include the **skull, cervical spine, abdomen,** and **pelvis/hip.**
  - **Highest radiographic examinations** (e.g., thoracic and lumbar spine) examinations have **effective doses approaching 1 mSv.**
- A **25-year-old** adult exposed to an effective dose of **1 mSv** might have an increase in (any) **cancer risk** from **40%** to **40.01%.**

Chapter 7 (Radiography) Questions

7.1 What is a typical x-ray tube target anode angle (°)?
A. 15
B. 45
C. 75
D. >90

7.2 What type of radiation that escapes through the protective lead of an x-ray tube?
A. Scatter
B. Leakage
C. Primary
D. Secondary

7.3 The ideal x-ray tube target would possess a _____ atomic number and a _____ melting point.
A. high; high
B. high; low
C. low; high
D. low; low

7.4 If we switch to a small focal spot (0.6 mm) in W targets, how much will power loading likely be reduced (%)?
A. 90
B. 50
C. 25
D. 10

7.5 When energy is deposited at a rate of 100 kW into x-ray tube anodes, the anode heat dissipation rate is most likely (kW):
A. 10
B. 30
C. 60
D. 90

7.6 Where should the anode be directed in a chest x-ray?
A. Upper chest
B. Upper abdomen
C. Left lung (heart)
D. Right lung

7.7 Which radiographic examination most likely uses the highest x-ray tube voltage?
A. Extremity
B. Chest (diagnostic)
C. Chest (ICU)
D. Abdomen

7.8 The tube output (i.e., mAs) for an abdominal radiograph is likely how many times that of a chest x-ray (1 mAs)?
A. 2
B. 5
C. 10
D. >10

7.9 Which radiography examination would most likely use a small focal spot?
A. Chest x-ray (ICU)
B. Extremity (tibia)
C. Abdomen (pediatric)
D. Abdomen (adult)

7.10 What radiographic examination is most likely to use a SID of 50 cm?
A. Extremity
B. Pediatric
C. C-spine
D. Not used

7.11 Above what patient thickness (cm) is a grid required (i.e., not optional)?
A. 1
B. 5
C. 12
D. 20

7.12 What is the exposure index (EI) when a chest x-ray is performed with radiation intensity (K_{air}) of 3 µGy at the image receptor?
A. 0.3
B. 3
C. 30
D. 300

7.13 In radiographic imaging, what is the optimal deviation index?
A. Positive
B. Zero
C. Negative

7.14 What acquisition parameter is "wrong" for a diagnostic (departmental) chest radiograph?
A. 60 kV
B. 1 mAs
C. 10:1 grid ratio
D. 300 EI

7.15 What is an incorrect acquisition parameter for an extremity radiograph?
A. 55 kV
B. <1 mAs
C. No grid
D. 10 EI

7.16 What fetal dose is received during a lateral radiography of the mother's head?
A. >30 mGy
B. 10 mGy
C. 1 mGy
D. <0.1 mGy

7.17 In radiography, the contrast-to-noise ratio is most likely highest when tube voltages (kV) are kept _____ and tube intensities (mAs) are kept _____.

A. high; high
B. high; low

C. low; high
D. low; low

7.18 How does extremity radiography limiting resolution compare to the human eye spatial resolution at a normal viewing distance (25 cm).
A. Better
B. Comparable
C. Worse

7.19 What is a typical KAP in a skull examination (AP + lateral) (Gy-cm^2)?
A. 0.1
B. 1
C. 10
D. 100

7.20 In contact chest radiography, how does magnification change as the x-ray tube is pulled away from the patient?
A. More magnification
B. No change in magnification
C. Less magnification

Answers and Explanations

7.1 A A (15). The most likely x-ray tube anode angle is 15°, which is the reason for the Heel effect in x-ray imaging.

7.2 B (Leakage). Radiation is transmitted through the x-ray tube housing is called leakage and is limited to 1 mGy/h at a meter by law.

7.3 A (high; high). Targets in x-ray tubes need a high atomic number (Z) to maximize bremsstrahlung x-ray production and a high melting point to tolerate massive power loadings (e.g., 100 kW).

7.4 C (25%). A large focus (1.2 mm) on a W target will generally tolerate 100 kW, whereas a small focus will tolerate 25 kW (i.e., 25%).

7.5 A (10 kW). A typical x-ray tube anode heat dissipation rate is 10 kW and explains why in IR and CT x-ray tubes heating may become a problem.

7.6 A (Upper chest). Because of the heel effect, the anode is directed toward the (least attenuating) upper chest because the x-ray tube output is lower (Heel effect).

7.7 B (Chest (diagnostic)). Diagnostic chest x-rays are obtained using dedicated systems operated at 120 kV (or even higher).

7.8 D (>10). An abdominal radiograph would likely use 20 mAs, or 20 times higher than a chest x-ray.

7.9 B (Extremity). To get the best resolution for detection of hair line fractures, extremity x-rays would use a small focal spot. In pediatric abdomen, short exposures are critical, which requires large focal loadings and therefore large focal spots.

7.10 D (Not used). 100 cm is the SID for the overwhelming majority of x-ray radiographs, but longer distances may be used for chest x-rays and C-spines. SIDs less than 100 cm are not used in radiography, although 65 cm is used in mammography.

7.11 C (12 cm). The thickness at which scatter becomes so important that grids are considered essential is 12 cm.

7.12 D (300). A K_{air} of 3 µGy at the image receptor corresponds to an exposure index of 300.

7.13 B (Zero). A deviation index (DI) of zero means that the target amount of radiation was incident on the image receptor.

7.14 A (60 kV). 120 kV would be the most likely choice of x-ray tube voltage to perform any departmental chest radiograph on a dedicated chest x-ray system.

7.15 D (10 for exposure index). The exposure index in extremity imaging is typically 1,000, or three times higher than that in body radiography (low energy x rays deposit less energy in detectors, which is why a higher EI is used).

7.16 D (<0.1 mGy). When the fetus is outside the field of view, all dose comes from internal scatter. As a result, the dose is essentially negligible.

7.17 C (low; high). The tube voltage should be as low as possible to increase contrast, and the tube intensity should be as high as possible to reduce noise (mottle).

7.18 B (Comparable). Both the human eye (at 25 cm) and extremity radiography have limiting spatial resolutions of about 5 line pairs/mm.

7.19 B (1). The most likely Kerma area product value for a complete x-ray examination (e.g., AP + lateral skull radiographs) is about 1 Gy-cm².

7.20 C (Less magnification). As the tube is pulled further from the patient, both the SID and SOD increase. However, the SOD increases faster, resulting in a lower magnification.

CHAPTER 8
Mammography

I. DIGITAL MAMMOGRAPHY I

A. Breast Cancer and Mammography

- **One in eight (13%) US women** develop invasive **breast cancer** during their **lifetime.**
- In **2022**, the American Cancer Society estimated nearly **291,000 new cases** of invasive breast cancer and about **44,000 breast cancer deaths** in women.
- **Breast cancer** is the **second leading cause** of **cancer death** in women, exceeded only by lung cancer.
- **Mammography** is a **low-cost** and **low-dose** procedure that can detect early-stage breast cancer.
- **Cancer detection rates** in screening mammography are about **4 per 1,000** patients.
  - Because most patients (i.e., >99%) are normal, **radiation doses (risks)** in mammography **must** be kept **low.**
- **Mammography, by law,** is performed using **dedicated imaging systems** that are only used for mammography.
  - **Screening mammography** examinations include a **craniocaudal** and a **mediolateral oblique** view of each breast.
- **Breast cancer death rates** have been **declining since** about **1990**, with larger decreases in women younger than 50.
  - These decreases in mortality are likely a result of earlier detection as well as improved treatment.

B. Detection Tasks

- An **average compressed breast** is **60 mm thick** with **15% glandularity.**
- Table 8.1 summarizes the key physical properties of the major breast tissues and cancer (i.e., **density, attenuation coefficient,** and **half-value layer [HVL]**).
- **Microcalcifications** are specks of calcium hydroxyapatite with diameters as small as 0.1 mm that have very high x-ray attenuation coefficients (Table 8.1).
- **Detection** and **characterization** of **microcalcifications** is **difficult** because of their **small dimensions.**
  - Spatial **resolution** in **mammography** is **exceptional (7-10 lp/mm)**, and *superior* to the human eye at 25 cm viewing distance (~5 lp/mm).
- X-ray **attenuation** of **breast cancer** is **similar** to **normal fibroglandular tissue** (Table 8.1), so imaging systems are designed to maximize image contrast.
  - **Mammography contrast** is **increased** by using **low-energy photons (~20 keV).**
- High contrast-to-noise ratio for low-contrast masses requires noise to be minimized.
  - **Noise** is **reduced** by using **much higher radiation intensities at** the image receptor than that in conventional radiography.

TABLE 8.1	Properties of Tissues in the Breast, Including Density, Linear Attenuation Coefficient (at 20 keV), and the Corresponding Tissue Half-Value Layer		
Tissue	Density (g/cm³)	Attenuation (µ) (mm⁻¹)	Half-Value Layer (mm)
Adipose	0.93	0.045	15
Fibroglandular	1.04	0.080	8.7
Carcinoma	1.05	0.085	8.2
Calcification	2.20	1.250	0.55

- **Digital mammography** contrast, noise, and resolution are all **superior** to those of any other medical x-ray imaging modality.

C. X-Ray Tubes

- Figure 8.1 shows the x-ray production process (bremsstrahlung + characteristic x-rays), and the resultant spectrum.
- Targets in mammography may be Mo, Rh, or W.
- When **Mo or Rh targets** are used, **K-shell characteristic x-rays** are a significant, but not majority, component of the resultant x-ray beam spectra (Fig. 8.2A).
  - Rh has higher energy characteristic x-rays than that of Mo.
  - Tungsten characteristic K-shell x-rays are a minor contributor to the total spectrum.

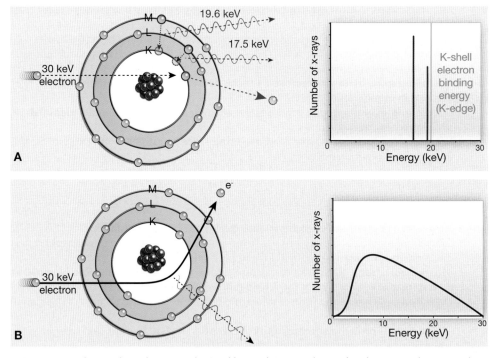

FIG 8.1 A: Incident 30 keV electrons, obtained by applying a voltage of 30 kV across the x-ray tube, produce characteristic x-rays by ejecting Mo target K-shell electrons (left) with the resultant vacancies filled by outer shell electrons. The characteristic x-ray spectrum (right) has (two) discrete energies (purple and red peaks) just below the Mo K-shell binding energy (green line at 20 keV). **B:** Bremsstrahlung x-rays are produced when 30 keV electrons are decelerated close to the Mo target nuclei (left), resulting in a continuous spectrum (right). The bremsstrahlung spectrum has energies up to the maximum electron kinetic energy (i.e., 30 keV).

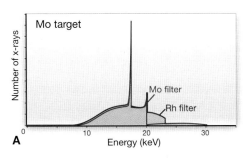 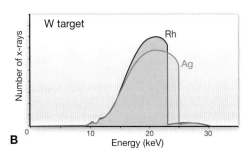

FIG 8.2 Mammography x-ray spectra illustrating how choice of K-edge filters (Mo, Rh, and Ag), rather than tube voltage (30 kV), is the key factor for determining x-ray beam quality (i.e., average energy). **A:** Mo target with Mo filter (red) and Rh filter (purple), showing that replacing the Mo filter by a Rh filter increases the average photon energy because the Rh k-edge energy (23 keV) is higher than that of Mo (20 keV); **B:** W target and Rh filter (purple) and Ag filter (green) showing that replacing the Rh filter with an Ag filter increases the average photon energy because of the higher Ag k-edge energy (25 keV).

- **Modern mammography** systems are increasingly using **tungsten targets**, with no characteristic x-rays in the resultant spectra.
  - **Tungsten (Z = 74)** is a **better target** material than **molybdenum (Z = 42)**, with more bremsstrahlung production and a higher melting point.
- Standard **focal spot** size is **(0.3 mm)**, which is much smaller than that in conventional radiography (1.2 mm).
  - A **small focal spot (0.1 mm)** is used for **magnification mammography.**
- A **beryllium (Z = 4) x-ray tube window** is used to minimize x-ray beam attenuation as the low-energy beam leaves the tube.
- **Heel effect** provides an **increase** in radiation **intensity** to **chest wall** by pointing the cathodes side in this direction, and the anode toward the nipple.
- The x-ray tube is tilted into **half-beam geometry.**
  - This allows visualization of tissue near the chest wall and reduces unused radiation going into the chest.
- **Spectral shape** is obtained using **K-edge filters (Mo, Rh, Ag)** as depicted in Figure 8.2.

D. Tube Parameters and Output

- **Tube voltages** in mammography are low (~30 kV).
  - Tube voltages in conventional radiography are much higher than in mammography (e.g., 80 kV in abdominal radiographs).
- In mammography, the **tube voltage (kV)** has a very **minor influence** on the average x-ray beam energy.
  - In conventional radiography, the average x-ray beam energy is controlled by the choice of x-ray tube voltage (kV).
- **Tube currents** in contact mammography are fixed at ~**100 mA** and do not change.
  - In magnification mammography, tube current is reduced ¼ to ½.
- **Exposure times** are **very long** in mammography (e.g., **0.5-1 second**) and control the total radiation, since mA is fixed.
  - These long exposures make mammography especially susceptible to motion artifact.
  - Chest radiographs use tube currents up to 1,000 mA, very short exposure times (<0.01 s), and an x-ray technique of 1 mAs.

E. Filters

- **Filters** in **mammography** may be **molybdenum, rhodium, or silver (in order of increasing K-edge energy).**
- All **filters primarily remove very low–energy X-rays** that only contribute to patient dose.

TABLE 8.2	X-Ray Tube Voltages are Generally About 30 kV, and Have Very Modest Influence on the Resultant Beam Quality (<10%)	
Target-Filter Combination	Breast Thickness (mm)	Nominal Half-Value Layer (mm Al)
Mo/Mo	<65	0.35
Mo/Rh	>65	0.45
W/Rh	<65	0.50
W/Ag	>65	0.60

- For a **Mo target**, an x-ray beam **filter** that is also **Mo (K-edge 20 keV)** will attenuate most of the very low x-ray photons and photons *above* the K-edge energy.
- **Replacing** the **Mo filter** with a **Rh filter (k-edge 23 keV)** **increases beam energy and transmission for medium or thick breasts** (Fig. 8.2A).
  - A Rh target with a Mo filter is not used, since the Mo would knock out the high-energy photons we want from the Rh target.
- **Tungsten targets** are typically used with filters of **Rh or Ag (K-edge 25 keV),** as depicted in Figure 8.2B.
  - **Rh** or **Ag** filters **remove** both **very low–energy** photons and those **above** their **K-edges.**
- The average energy of transmitted photons is always "slightly less than" the K-edge energy of the filter (i.e., Rh or Ag).
  - **The average energy** and HVL of a **W/Ag** combination is **higher than** those of a **W/Rh** combination, and **W/Ag** combination is used for thicker/denser breasts.
- Table 8.2 summarizes **beam qualities (HVLs)** of the most common clinical **target and filter** combinations for imaging **thin and thick breasts.**
  - In comparison, **radiography** performed at **80 kV** has a **HVL** of **3 mm Al.**

II. DIGITAL MAMMOGRAPHY II

A. Geometry and Compression

- **Source-to-image receptor distance** (SID) in most commercial systems is **65 to 70 cm**, shorter than the 100 cm SID used in most of radiography.
  - **Shorter SIDs** would **increase** focal spot **blur** and **distortion**, and **longer SIDs** would result in unacceptably **long exposure times.**
- Optimal mammography requires the use of **breast compression**, achieved by using radiolucent paddles.
- With the **breast immobilized, motion blur** is **minimized.**
  - Breast tissues are also spread out to **decrease tissue overlap.**
- **Compression** also brings the breast closer to the image plane, minimizing image magnification and **reducing focal spot blur.**
- **The compressed thickness reduces scatter, dose, and exposure times.**
- **Compression force** is normally between 111 and 200 Newton (25 and 45 lb), which can result in **brief patient discomfort.**
  - Initial power-driven compression must be between 111 and 200 Newtons by law.

B. Grids

- **Scatter-to-primary** ratios in mammography are typically **1:1,** much lower than the 5:1 ratio encountered in abdominal radiography.
  - **Mammograms** have **more photoelectric interactions** than Compton scatter, the reverse of body radiography.
- **Mammography** imaging systems use **grids** with ratios of **~5:1** and linear grid line densities of ~50 lines per centimeter (Fig. 8.3).
  - Radiographic imaging is generally performed with a 10:1 grid.

- One manufacturer produces a **high transmission cellular (HTC) grid**, with a honeycomb pattern and an air-interspace material (Fig. 8.3).
- **HTC grids** improve scatter removal because of its **two-dimensional structure.**
  - HTC grids also improve primary transmission because the **interspace material** is **air** with negligible attenuation.
- Using a **grid doubles** the **patient dose** relative to nongrid examination.
  - Mammography grids have a Bucky factor (BF) of ~2.
- Benefits of **contrast outweigh** (any) risks associated with **higher doses.**
- Only physical grids are used in mammography.

C. Detectors

- In the United States, **almost all systems are digital and the majority have tomosynthesis capability.**
- **Digital mammography** can use **scintillators (CsI)** or **photoconductors (Se).**
- Both CsI and Se have **excellent x-ray absorption (>90%)** at the low x-ray photon energies used in mammography.
- **CsI** scintillators are **faster** and more **reliable**, whereas **Se** photoconductors offer better resolution (i.e., **sharper images**).
- **Photostimulable phosphors** have been used for digital mammography but are **technically inferior** (e.g., worse resolution).
- **Detector element sizes** in digital mammography range between **50** and **100 μm,** resulting in high spatial resolution and large matrix sizes.
  - A typical **digital mammogram** contains about **15 million pixels.**
- **Digital mammography** is performed using **automatic exposure control (AEC).**
  - Mammography AEC may alter kV, mAs, and filtration.

E. Displays

- **5 MP monitors** are essential for viewing digital mammograms, but these cannot display all the pixels in a mammogram.
  - **Maximum resolution** (1 image pixel per 1 display pixel) requires the use of "**zoom**" that only displays part of one image.
  - Radiologists are required to view the image in this "native resolution" as part of their read.
- Monitors should have a **maximum luminance above 420 cd/m²**.
  - Monitors with **low luminance** make reading conditions susceptible to **poor ambient lighting** and illuminance.

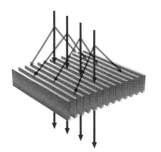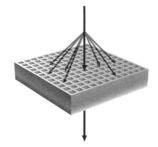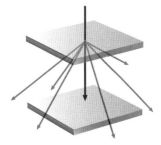

FIG 8.3 Scatter removal may be achieved by the use of a conventional linear grid (left), a two-dimensional (cellular) grid (middle), or by the air gap present in magnification mammography (right). Use of a linear grid generally doubles the patient dose (i.e., Bucky factor is 2) for examinations that use automatic exposure control. Two-dimensional cellular grids are more effective at removing scatter, and reduce primary photon losses because the intergrid material is air, not graphite as in linear grids. Air gaps permit a reduction of 30% radiation intensity (mAs) because primary photon losses in grids are eliminated (i.e., no grid required).

TABLE 8.3	Comparison of Mammography and Nonmammography Display Technologies	
Property	Mammography Workstation	Nonmammography Diagnostic Workstation
Megapixels	>5 MP	>3 MP
Ambient Illuminance	25-75 lux	25-75 lux
Maximum luminance	>420 cd/m²	>350 cd/m²
Compression for final interpretation images	Lossless only	Lossy or Lossless
Tomosynthesis considerations	Technology to reduce blur while rapidly scrolling through series	-

- Digital mammograms should be viewed in a **dark reading room (illuminance < 50 lux).**
- Typical workstations have two or more large format portrait LCD monitors (2 k × 2.5 k) with a **high contrast ratio (>300:1).**
  - **Contrast ratio** is ratio of **brightest to darkest pixel.**
- The optimal viewing distance is about 50 cm, which is slightly less than an arm's length.
- Monitors should be calibrated using the **DICOM (**Digital Imaging and Communications in Medicine) **grayscale standard display function** to ensure consistent display contrast.
  - To optimize **workflow,** automated **mammography-specific hanging protocols** are **essential.**
- Table 8.3 summarizes characterizes typical display parameters ?? display of mammography and nonmammography images.

III. MAMMOGRAPHY ADJUNCTS

A. Magnification Mammography

- **Magnification** is achieved by moving the **breast away from** the **detector,** as depicted in Figure 8.4.
- By law, magnification must be between 1.4× and 2×.
- An **air gap reduces** the amount of **scatter** reaching the detector and **eliminates** the need for a **grid** (see Fig. 8.3).
  - **Removing girds** eliminates loss of primary photons and permits the technique to be reduced from **~100 mAs to ~70 mAs.**
- **Small focal spots (0.1 mm)** are essential to minimize geometric unsharpness.
- The small focal spot requires **reduced** x-ray tube **currents (25 mA-50 mA).**
- **Exposure times > 1 second** are needed to achieve a technique of 70 mAs.
  - **Longer exposure times** increase the chance of **patient motion (blur).**
- **Magnification mammography improves** visualization of **mass margins** and **fine calcifications.**

B. Digital Breast Tomosynthesis

- **Overlapping** of the breast **tissue** reduces lesion visibility and may cause artifactual lesions to appear.
- **Digital breast tomosynthesis (DBT)** creates 1 mm slices through the breast, which improves lesion visibility, as depicted in Figure 8.5.
- A **conventional digital mammography imaging chain** is used to **generate tomographic images.**
- **DBT** acquires 5 to 15 projection images, each at a different angle.
- **X-ray tubes move** in a 15° to 50° **arc** around the breast.

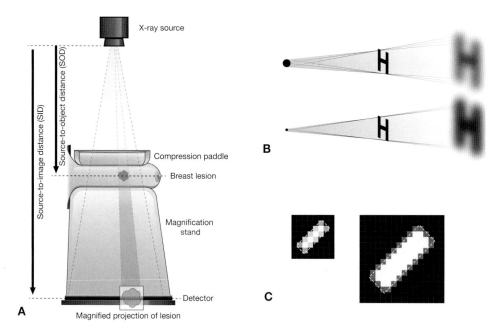

FIG 8.4 A: In magnification mammography, the breast is moved closer to the x-ray tube so that the source-to-object distance (SOD) is about half the source-to-image receptor distance (SID). In magnification mammography, only part of the breast is irradiated, and lesions appear twice as large. **B:** Magnification impacts the focal spot as well, so mammography machines switch to a smaller focal spot to limit magnified focal spot blur. **C:** The magnified image size utilizes 4× more detector elements and so decreases detector blur. Overall resolution is improved (blur decreased) in magnification mammography.

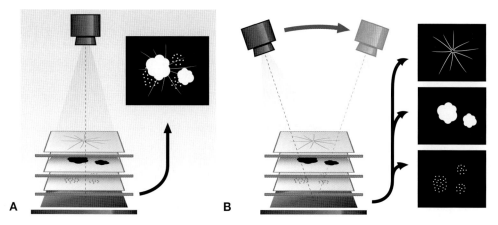

FIG 8.5 A: Projection radiography superimposes all structures (masses, microcalcification clusters, and linear structures) onto the same image, even though these structures are at different depths in the patient. This superposition of lesions results in "clutter" and very poor lesion contrast. **B:** Breast tomosynthesis shows only those lesions in a given plane, thereby minimizing clutter and markedly improving lesion contrast.

- **Examination times** are typically **5 to 20 seconds** and **require compression** to minimize motion artifacts.
- A synthetic mammogram is a mammogram simulated from tomosynthesis data.
  - It allows for tomosynthesis only, instead of mammography and tomosynthesis.
  - Image quality differs from conventional mammograms, but specifically how depends on the vendor and software version.
- Radiation **dose in DBT** is **comparable** to a **contact mammogram** on a digital system.

C. DBT Performance and Artifacts

- Almost half of all units in the United States had DBT in 2022.
- **Cancer detection rates** in screening mammography with tomosynthesis are about **6 per 1,000** patients.
  - Studies suggest that **DBT reduces** patient **recall** rate by **15%.**
- **DBT** offers similar in-plane **resolution** as conventional **2D imaging.**
- As arc angle increases, through-plane resolution increases.
- Accordion artifact is artificial elongation of the object as you move to slices further from the object.
  - It may cause artifactual skin thickening.
- If the beam intersects the breast, but is not in the reconstructed volume, it may cause artifactually increased attenuation at the image edge (e.g., axilla).

D. Biopsies

- **Traditional biopsy systems** have the patient lying **prone** on a **table.**
- Digital imaging systems have a 5 × 5 cm field of view, with pixels of 50 µm.
- **Two views** of the breast are normally acquired (**±15° from the normal**).
- Images of the lesion will shift by an amount that depends on the lesion depth, which permits a three-dimensional localization of the lesion.
- A **biopsy needle gun** is positioned and fired to capture a tissue sample.
- **Benefits** of **core needle** over open biopsies are a **short procedure time, reduced cost** and **risk,** and **improved cosmesis.**
- **Upright biopsy systems** are becoming popular using DBT systems that permit the x-ray tube to be rotated ±15° from the normal.
  - In the upright configuration, x-ray tube moves automatically from one angle to the other, or may move in tomographic mode.
- **Advantages** of upright biopsy include **improved lesion visibility, faster lesion targeting,** and **reduced patient procedure time.**
- Stereotactic biopsy delivers 10× dose to the tissue in the FOV than screening mammography, but this is acceptable due to the diagnostic information gained.
  - Tomosynthesis biopsy delivers ~5× the dose of screening mammography to the tissues in the FOV and allows direct location of the lesion.

E. CAD and Contrast-Enhanced Mammography

- **Computer-aided detection (CAD$_e$)** and **diagnosis (CAD$_x$)** use algorithms to flag possible findings and diagnosis malignancy, respectively.
  - **CAD$_e$ software** has been shown to have **sensitivities** as high as **90%,** but have a high **false-positive rate** of up to 1 or **2 false positives per image.**
- **Contrast-enhanced mammography (CEM)** utilized iodine contrast agent to locate and characterize lesions due to their leaky vessels.
- Contrast is injected followed by low and high energy mammograms at each view.
  - Combining low- and high-energy acquisitions results in an image primarily iodine contrast (similar to digital subtraction angiography).
  - CEM dose is higher ???? but improves lesion detectability and aids in lesion characterization.
  - Biopsy clips and microcalcifications may appear dark or light on CEM due to image processing effects.

IV. IMAGE QUALITY AND DOSE

A. Mammography Quality Standards Act

- **Mammography Quality Standards Act (MQSA)** requires mammography facilities in the United States to be **certified** every 3 years.
  - **U.S. Food and Drug Administration (FDA)** is responsible for enforcing MQSA but often subcontract this task to the American College of Radiology (ACR) and state regulatory agencies.
- ACR provides explicit accreditation guidelines for radiologist, technologist, and medical physicist practice and training.
  - **MQSA** requires that the "lead **interpreting physician**" (i.e., radiologist) be ultimately **responsible** for all aspects of clinical mammography.
- The **ACR phantom** or MQSA phantom contains **fibers (i.e., architectural distortion), speck groups (i.e., microcalcifications)**, and **masses.**
- To **pass**, the phantom image must show a minimum number of **fibers, speck groups,** and **masses** specified by the ACR or vendor.
  - Image **artifacts** must also be **minimal.**
  - Simulates a breast **4.2 cm compressed and 50% glandularity.**
- **Glandular tissue** is the radiosensitive tissue in the breast.
- **Average glandular dose (AGD)** for a single view of the **phantom** must be below **3 mGy.**
- Images for interpretation cannot have any lossy compression.
- Patient images must be held onto for 10 years if they are the only images of the patient or 5 years if other images exist.

B. Spatial Resolution

- The use of very **small focal spots, 0.3 mm** in contact mammography, **minimizes focal spot blur.**
  - In magnification mammography, the focal spot is reduced to only 0.1 mm, which maintains the resolution of contact mammography.
- Breast **compression immobilizes** the **breast**, which helps to **minimize motion blur.**
- **Scintillators** in digital mammography are **thin** and may be made of **columns** to minimize detector blur.
- **Photoconductors** in digital mammography have **minimal blurring** because the charge liberated by incident x-rays does not diffuse as does light in scintillators.
- The **pixel size** is usually the limiting factor in **digital mammography** and is typically **70 µm** in size (i.e., 14 pixels per mm).
  - **MQSA** requires each facility to achieve the **vendor specifications** in digital mammography, which are typically **7 lp/mm.**

C. Contrast-to-Noise Ratio

- **Contrast** is controlled by the **beam quality**, which may be varied by the operator.
- **Mottle (noise)** is **determined** by the value of K_{air} at the image receptor, which is normally fixed (e.g., **100 µGy**).
- **Increasing beam quality** with an AEC system **reduces patient dose and subject contrast,** as depicted in Table 8.4.
- Higher beam qualities also reduce exposure times, minimizing motion blur.
  - Higher energy **contrast reductions** can be **offset** by **image processing.**
- **Beam qualities** are selected by **radiologists** on image **quality** and patient **dose considerations.**
- Tungsten targets, which result in higher beam qualities, are replacing molybdenum targets (Table 8.2).
  - Use of **higher beam qualities** has resulted in **lower patient radiation doses,** while maintaining image quality and diagnostic performance.

TABLE 8.4	Effects of Beam Quality on Digital Mammography Performed Using an Automatic Exposure Control System		
X-Ray Beam Quality	**Exposure Time**	**Subject Contrast**	**Patient Dose**
Low	Long	High	High
High	Short	Low	Low

D. Patient Doses

- **AGDs** are determined by medical physicists who take into account x-ray techniques (i.e., entrance K_{air} and **HVL**).
  - **Breast doses** also depend on patient breast characteristics (i.e., **thickness** and **glandularity**).
- **The AGD** for the phantom is ~**1.2 mGy per view.**
- For a two-view screening mammogram, the AGD would be ~2.5 mGy.
  - **Left** and **right glandular doses** are *never* **added** together.
- At a constant beam quality and using AEC, **increasing** the **compressed thickness** by **10 mm** would likely **double** the **AGD.**
  - The tissue HVL at the low photon energies encountered in mammography is typically 1 cm (Table 8.1).
- Beam quality, however, generally increases with large increases in compressed breast thickness (Table 8.2), which limits dose increases in thicker breasts.
  - Use of **increased beam quality** nonetheless **increases AGD** as breast **thickness** and **density increase.**
- **The AGD** for an **80 mm dense breast,** imaged at the highest beam quality, most likely **exceeds 3 mGy** per view.
- **The effective dose** for a screening mammogram is ~0.4 mSv.
- Fetal doses from screening mammography are negligible.

E. Benefits and Risks

- **One million 50-year-old** women receiving a glandular dose of 3 mGy theoretically corresponds to a risk of **6 fatal breast cancers.**
  - Radiation risks have only been demonstrated at doses of a few Gy, a thousand times higher than current doses in mammography.
- Screening one million women is expected to identify between 4,000 and 6,000 cases of breast cancer, with a quarter being fatal.
- **Screening programs** should reduce the (average) fatality rate between 20% and 50% saving 200 to 500 lives.
  - Screening benefits have been demonstrated in epidemiological studies.
- The **benefit-to-risk** ratio of **screening mammography** is greater than 30 (i.e., 200/6).
- **Radiation risks** in screening mammography, if any, are extremely low and should **not deter women** from having this **diagnostic test.**
  - Radiation risks from **screening mammograms** are equivalent to the risk of **dying** in an **accident** when traveling ~**1,000 miles** by **car.**
- Patients should be encouraged to consider whether any **mammographic examination** would result in a net benefit (i.e., be **worthwhile**).

Chapter 8 (Mammography) Questions

8.1 How many cancers are most likely detected per 1000 screening mammography examinations?
A. 1
B. 4
C. 16
D. 64

8.2 What is the diameter (micron) of the smallest microcalcifications seen in mammograms?
A. 1
B. 10
C. 100
D. 1,000

8.3 What is the small focal spot size (μm) typically used in mammography?
A. 100
B. 300
C. 600
D. 1,200

8.4 Mammography x-ray tubes have windows that have x-ray attenuation properties that are _____ than those of conventional x-ray tubes.
A. greater than
B. comparable to
C. less than

8.5 What tube voltage (kV) is typically used in screening mammography?
A. 20
B. 30
C. 40
D. 50

8.6 What material is *never* used to filter x-ray beams on current clinical mammography imaging system?
A. Mo (Z = 42)
B. Rh (Z = 45)
C. Ag (Z = 47)
D. W (Z = 74)

8.7 A digital mammography x-ray beam most likely has a half-value layer of (mm Al).
A. 0.2
B. 0.5
C. 1.5
D. 3.0

8.8 Reducing the SID on a mammography imaging system would most likely increase:
A. Focal blur
B. Exposure time
C. Patient dose
D. Image scatter

8.9 In contact mammography performed with AEC, increasing the grid ratio would most likely _____ contrast and _____ patient doses.
A. increase; increase
B. increase; decrease
C. decrease; increase
D. decrease; decrease

8.10 What x-ray detector would likely offer the best characterization of microcalcifications in mammography imaging?
A. Scintillators (CsI)
B. Photostimulable phosphors (BaFBr)
C. Photoconductors (Se)

8.11 The number of pixels (million) in a mammogram is most likely:
A. 1
B. 4
C. 16
D. 64

8.12 What maximum luminance (cd/m^2) does the ACR recommend?
A. 6
B. 60
C. 600
D. 6,000

8.13 The optimal grid ratio in magnification mammography is most likely:
A. 2:1
B. 5:1
C. 10:1
D. No grids used

8.14 How does acquisition time for digital breast tomosynthesis compare to contact mammography?
A. Shorter
B. Comparable
C. Longer

8.15 How do patient doses in DBT compare to those in contact mammography?
   A. Half
   B. Comparable
   C. Double

8.16 MQSA requires the phantom dose (mGy) per view to be below what value?
   A. 1
   B. 2
   C. 3
   D. 5

8.17 What artifact causing a dark ring around highly attenuating objects is commonly seen in tomosynthesis and synthetic mammography images?
   A. Accordion
   B. Dead pixels
   C. Halo artifact
   D. Motion artifact

8.18 What measure of image quality is worse in mammography as compared to that in radiography?
   A. Spatial resolution
   B. Contrast
   C. Noise (mottle)
   D. Temporal resolution

8.19 The radiation dose (average glandular dose) of a 4-view screening tomosynthesis examination is most likely (mGy):
   A. 1.5
   B. 3
   C. 6
   D. 12

8.20 Screening a million 50-year-old women is expected to save 200 lives but might also result in an additional _____ fatal radiation-induced cancers.
   A. 1
   B. 10
   C. 100
   D. None

Answers and Explanations

8.1 B (4). In clinical practice, only 4 cancers are detected for every 1,000 examinations, which explains why doses need to be kept ALARA (i.e., >99% of patients are normal).

8.2 C (100 μm). The smallest microcalcifications seen in mammograms have sizes as small as about 0.1 mm. Malignant microcalcifications are typically 0.3 mm.

8.3 A (100 μm). Focal spot sizes of mammography x-ray tubes are 0.3 mm large and only 0.1 mm small (i.e., 100 μm).

8.4 C (Less than). Mammography uses low energies, so mammography x-ray tubes need to be used to reduce the loss of x-rays in the primary beam x-ray window.

8.5 B (30 kV). A representative x-ray tube voltages is 30 kV (20 and ≥40 kV are never used).

8.6 D (W). Tungsten is never used as an x-ray filter on any system, as its attenuation is very high and comparable to lead ($Z = 82$).

8.7 B (0.5 mm Al). A representative digital mammography x-ray beam HVL is 0.5 mm Al. Lower HVL would reduce breast penetration increasing doses, and higher HVLs would reduce contrast.

8.8 A (Focal blur). Short SIDs (<65 cm) are not used because of increased focal spot blur and image distortion.

8.9 A (increase; increase). Increasing the grid ratio will always increase both the image contrast and patient dose provided automatic exposure control is being used.

8.10 C (Selenium photoconductors). Best spatial resolution performance (i.e., MTF curves) are using photoconductors (e.g., amorphous selenium) which most likely deliver the sharpest images of microcalcifications.

8.11 C (16 million) A representative value of the number of pixels in a digital mammogram is 16 million, which is too many to be viewed on a 5-MP monitor.

8.12 C (600 cd/m²). A luminance of 600 cd/m² should be used in mammography diagnostic workstations.

8.13 D (No grids used). In magnification mammography, grids are removed because scatter is removed by the presence of an air gap.

8.14 C (Longer). X-ray tubes rotate to acquire about 15+ images so that the imaging time is likely 5 to 20 seconds, or several times longer than a typical contact mammogram.

8.15 B (Comparable). Patient doses are broadly comparable in DBT and contact mammography. Many expect DBT to replace contact mammography in the near future.

8.16 C (3 mGy). MQSA only pertains to the phantom (not patient) and requires the dose to be below 3 mGy.

8.17 C (Halo artifact). Photon starvation and beam hardening by highly attenuating objects will case a black "halo" to appear around the object.

8.18 D (Temporal resolution). Mammography requires a much longer time to acquire meaning is has reduced temporal resolution and is more susceptible to motion artifact.

8.19 B (3 mGy). Each breast likely gets 1.5 mGy in the CC view, and 1.5 mGy in the MLO view, so the overall *average breast tissue* dose is 3 mGy (i.e., both breasts get 3 mGy). Mammography has similar AGD.

8.20 B (10). Current radiation risks estimates, based on a linear no threshold extrapolation model, suggest about 10 fatal cancers in one million screened women (i.e., markedly fewer than the 200 lives expected to be saved but not negligible). This is most likely an overestimate of the risk.

CHAPTER 9

General Fluoroscopy

I. IMAGING CHAIN

A. X-Ray Beams

- X-ray tubes in general fluoroscopy are similar to those used in radiography but may have smaller focal spot options (0.3-1.2 mm).
- Fluoroscopy is normally performed at low x-ray tube currents (e.g. ~3-10 mA) and modest power (<0.5 kW), allowing use of smaller focal spots.
- Most fixed-room fluoroscopy systems have an additional 0.1 to 0.9 mm Cu filtration.
  - Cu filters reduce skin and pediatric doses up to 40%.
- Collimators can be adjusted by operators to limit the size of the x-ray beam, which is clinically required.
- Fluoroscopy systems generally use grids to remove scatter radiation.
  - Fluoroscopic grid ratios are similar to those in radiography (i.e., 10:1).
  - Grids may be removed for pediatric and small–body part imaging (<12 cm thickness) to reduce dose.

B. Image Intensifiers (Analog Fluoroscopy)

- Image intensifiers (II) convert incident x-rays into a bright light.
  - Light is amplified by flux gain and minification gain.
- The input phosphor (CsI) absorbs x-ray photons and reemits part of the absorbed energy as many light photons.
- Light photons emitted by the input phosphor are absorbed by a photocathode and results in the emission of low-energy electrons (photoelectrons).
- Low-energy electrons are accelerated to high energies across the image intensifier tube and focused onto the output phosphor, which is about one-tenth the diameter (Fig. 9.1).
- Flux gain is the increase in number of light photons due to electron energy gained during acceleration, typically ~50×.
- Minification gain is the increase in image brightness that results from reduction in image size from the input phosphor to the output phosphor, typically the ratio of areas ~100×.
- Energetic electrons are absorbed by the output phosphor and emit a large number of light photons.
  - Before image intensifiers, patient doses could be 1,000× larger to ensure a sufficiently bright image.

C. Digitized Analog Fluoroscopy

- Light is collected by a charge-coupled device (CCD) or specialized TV camera and is digitized in real time using an analog-to-digital converter (ADC).

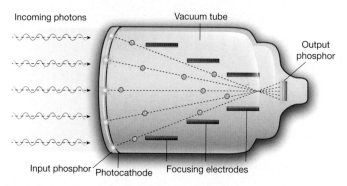

FIG 9.1 An image intensifier showing an incident x-ray pattern absorbed by the curved input phosphor (CsI scintillator) producing light that is then absorbed by a photocathode resulting in the emission of low-energy electrons. These electrons are accelerated to high energies using focusing electrodes, which are absorbed by the flat output phosphor (brightly) depicting the incident x-ray pattern. Distortions occur when a curved input image is viewed on a flat output phosphor.

- **Digitized TV image signals** are stored in a computer and can be **processed** or **displayed in real time.**
- **Last image hold (LIH)** displays a processed version of several recent fluoro frames combined into a still when the x-ray beam is switched off.
  - The image can be reviewed without dosing the patient.
  - A similar function (**last fluoro loop**) displays the last few seconds of fluoro repeatedly without dosing the patient.
- **Lower pulse rates** may improve LIH quality due to the tendency of machines to increase per-frame doses and thus decrease noise.
- **Digitization** also permits the use of temporal filtering to improve image quality.
- **Temporal filtering** (i.e., recursive frame averaging) is a technique of adding together and then averaging the pixel values in successive fluoro frames.
- **Temporal filtering** occurs in real time and **reduces** the effect of random **noise** and thus could **reduce patient dose** with parameter adjustments.
  - Too much temporal filtering will **increase motion blur.**

II. FLUOROSCOPIC IMAGING

A. What Is Fluoroscopy?

- **Fluoroscopy** involves viewing **dynamic images** in **real time** to assess motion.
- **Fluoroscopy images** are generally displayed at the rate of **30 to 60 frames per second** (33 ms per frame) on a monitor.
- Fluoroscopy **radiation pulse** rates are typically **lower** than the **image display** rates.
  - When 15 pulses per second are acquired, each frame is displayed twice on the monitor (filling 33 ms of TV time) to ensure a "flicker-free" display.
- **Tube currents** in fluoroscopy are a **hundred times lower** than that in **radiographic imaging.**
  - Because the number of x-ray photons used to create a **fluoroscopy frame** is very low, such images are not typically of **diagnostic image quality.**
- **Operators** are generally close to patients undergoing fluoroscopy and may be **exposed** to **scattered radiation.**
  - **Operators** have their exposures **monitored**, wear **lead aprons**, and utilize **pull-down shielding.**
  - **Operator dose** 1 m from the patient is 0.1% of patient dose not accounting for shielding.

B. Imaging System Variants

- Most radiology departments use **radiography/fluoroscopy (R/F)** units to perform **gastrointestinal (GI) studies** to visualize barium administered to patients.
  - **R/F units** can also be used to visualize iodine administered to patients undergoing **urological (genitourinary) examinations.**
- An R/F unit has the **x-ray tube under** the **table** and employs lead drapes hanging from the receptor to reduce operator scatter.
- **Tables** on **R/F** units can generally rotate **to help disperse barium.**
- R/F tables **attenuate** about **a third** of the incident **x-ray beam.**
- Dedicated systems for performing **urological** examinations are similar to R/F units except that the **x-ray** tube is located **above** the **patient.**
  - An **overhead x-ray tube minimizes magnification** of the kidneys but results in increased operator dose.
- To **reduce operator dose**, some units permit **remote control operation** where the operators can stand in the shielded area (i.e., not at the bedside).
  - Remotely controlled units also reduce operator fatigue because operators do not have to wear lead aprons and can work seated.
- **Portable fluoroscopy** systems are **C-arm** devices often used outside of radiology departments (e.g., operating rooms).
  - Mobile **C-arms** are frequently used by clinicians other than radiologists, but generally operated by **certified radiology technologists.**
  - Though inexpensive, they suffer from overheating for complex cases.
- **Mini C-arm** units produce very little radiation and are ideal for extremity procedures.
  - Minimal shielding is needed to operate these devices.

C. Fluoroscopy Techniques

- The patient should be placed as far from the x-ray tube as possible and the receptor should be as close to the patient as possible (see Table 9.1).
- **Iodinated contrast** requires the use of x-ray tube voltages of ~**70 kV**, where the average x-ray photon energy (i.e., 35 keV) is close to the iodine K-edge (33 keV).
- When the **average x-ray energy** is just above **33 keV, absorption** by **iodine** is maximized, and visibility of vasculature is maximized.
- Use of 70 kV in a barium meal study would result in negligible transmission through any part of the GI tract that contained any barium.
  - Unlike angiography, barium is readily visible in the GI tract because the mass of contrast material administered to patients is much higher.
- In **GI studies, high voltages (>100 kV)** are used to ensure some **penetration** of barium and easier visualization of bowel loops.

TABLE 9.1	Optimal Geometry		
Parameter	**Optimal Position**	**Effect**	**Comment**
Receptor	Close to the patient	Reduce patient and operator dose, reduce magnification	Limited independent motion available in some system types like C-arms
Patient	Close to the receptor and far from the x-ray tube	Reduce patient and operator dose, reduce magnification	Limited or not motion available in some systems like gastrointestinal units. Easier for taller operators.
X-ray tube	Far from the patient	Reduce patient, reduce magnification	Only able to change on overhead tube systems like urological units.

- Collimation is frequently used during fluoroscopy to restrict the x-ray beam to the specific area of interest.
  - **Collimation** reduces scatter, **improves contrast**, and **reduces** patient doses and **stochastic risks.**
- **High kV with low mA** can be used to **reduce dose** at the cost of **reduced image contrast.**
- **Removing the grid** and using **copper filtration** can **reduce dose** in pediatric exams.
- Modified barium swallows require smooth motion (30 pulses per second [pps]) to ensure accurate diagnosis, while procedures threading catheters/tubes can often use <15 pps.

D. **Radiography vs General Fluoroscopy**
- **Radiography** is **static**, whereas **fluoroscopy** is **dynamic.**
- Exposure times in radiography are typically very short (<0.1 seconds), whereas in fluoroscopy exposure times are generally measured in minutes.
- The number of **acquired images** in **radiography** is generally **low** and consists of a few images.
- In **fluoroscopy**, it is common to have thousands or **tens of thousands** of fluoroscopy images.
- Mottle in radiography is much lower than that in any single fluoroscopy frame.
  - Tube **currents** in **radiography** are **100 times higher** than **fluoroscopy**, resulting in **ten times less mottle.**
- Radiography is always of diagnostic quality, whereas fluoroscopy is generally not considered to be diagnostic unless **acquisition modes** are used.
- Although the patient dose per fluoroscopy frame is relatively low, the **large number** of **acquired frames** results in **patient doses that are ~10× that of radiography.**
- **Radiologists, technologists,** and **ancillary staff** are routinely **exposed** to radiation that is **scattered** from the **patient** during fluoroscopy.

E. **Acquisition Modes**
- **Acquisition modes** for fluoroscopy are **spot images, photospot images, and acquisition/cine loops.**
- **Spot films** are **conventional radiographs**, usually obtained by introducing an overhead x-ray tube to expose a digital detector.
- **Photospot images** are **diagnostic quality images** that are obtained through the **fluoroscopic imaging chain.**
  - **Photospot images** use x-ray **tube currents** that are increased from a **few mA** during **fluoroscopy** to **several hundred mA.**
- Increasing the number of x-ray photons hundredfold in a photospot image makes this diagnostic.
  - Inspection of *any* LIH with the corresponding photospot images sent to the PACS (picture archiving and communication system) illustrates the importance of mottle in x-ray imaging.
- **Photospot** imaging would always use a **large focal spot (1.2 mm).**
- **Photospot** imaging at **1,000 line TV mode** doubles the spatial resolution of fluoroscopy images acquired with 500 line TV mode.
- **Acquisition/cine loops** are high-dose (~8-15× fluoroscopy) images acquired in rapid succession for documentation purposes.

III. DOSE FACTORS

A. Electronic Magnification
- **Electronic magnification** irradiates a **smaller** diameter (**area**) of the image intensifier–scintillator device but maintains the same output image size as shown in Figure 9.2.
- Data in Table 9.2 show how **minification gain** is **reduced** with the application of **electronic magnification** modes (i.e., Mag 1, Mag 2, and Mag 3).

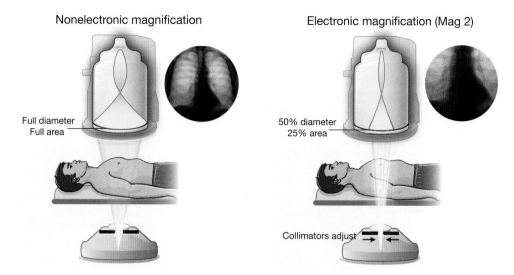

Nonelectronic magnification

Electronic magnification (Mag 2)

Full diameter
Full area

50% diameter
25% area

Collimators adjust

FIG 9.2 Normal image intensifier mode where the whole of the input phosphor is irradiated (left). Electronic magnification (Mag 2) irradiates only half the diameter of the input phosphor (25% of the area) that results in a magnified image with twice the limiting spatial resolution (right). To maintain the same brightness at the image intensifier output, the image intensifier automatic brightness control (ABC) quadruples K_{air} in Mag 2 mode, thereby quadrupling the patient peak skin dose. Kerma area product, however, is not affected because the irradiated area is reduced to a quarter.

- **Automatic brightness control (ABC) increases radiation** incident on the image intensifier in fluoroscopy to **maintain** a **constant brightness** at the image intensifier output.
- For a 36 cm image intensifier (Table 9.2), switching from Normal to **Mag 1** mode roughly **halves** the exposed image intensifier **area** which **halves** the **minification gain**.
- When **ABC mode** is operational, the radiation intensity (K_{air}) incident on the image intensifier (and patient) in **Mag 1** is roughly **doubled** compared to normal mode.
  - K_{air} roughly **quadruples** in **Mag 2** and so on.
- **Electronic magnification increases** patient **skin doses** (i.e., doubled in Mag 1).
  - Image mottle is reduced in mag mode due to the increased dose used.
- **Electronic magnification** does **not affect** the **kerma area product (KAP)**, because **increases** in entrance K_{air} are generally offset by **decreases** in **beam area**.
- With ABC, **KAP** is approximately the **same** in **normal** mode as in all three **electronic magnification modes** shown in Table 9.2.
  - **Patient stochastic risks are not increased** in **electronic magnification** because the total radiation incident on the patient is not changed.
- **Electronic magnification** has **no relationship** with **geometric magnification** used in mammography.

	Minification Gains for 36 cm Diameter Image Intensifier That Uses Three		
TABLE 9.2	**Electronic Magnification (Mag) Modes**		
Input Diameter cm (inches)	**Area cm² [Relative Area]**	**Minification Gain [Relative MG]**	**Name**
36 (14)	1000 [1.0]	320 [1.0]	Normal
25 (10)	500 [0.5]	160 [0.5]	Mag 1
18 (7)	250 [0.25]	80 [0.25]	Mag 2
13 (5)	130 [0.13]	40 [0.13]	Mag 3

B. Pulsed Fluoroscopy

- In **continuous mode fluoroscopy**, the **tube current flows continuously** (see Fig. 9.3) and any motion during the pulse (**33 ms**) results in a blurred image.
  - In 33 ms, the total x-ray production for a 3 mA tube current is approximately 0.1 mAs (i.e., 3 mA × 0.033 s).
- For **3.3 ms x-ray pulses,** and **30 mA tube currents** as depicted in Figure 9.3, the **total output (i.e., # of x-rays)** remains **the same (0.1 mAs).**
  - **Images created** at the image intensifier output in a **short time** still **require 33 ms** to be **read out** by the TV camera and displayed on a monitor.
- **Replacing continuous** by **pulsed fluoroscopy** (30 pulses per second) results in **improved temporal resolution** (i.e., reduced motion blur).
  - **Patient doses** are **unchanged** (i.e., same mAs per frame) (Fig. 9.3).
- **Pulsed fluoroscopy** only **reduces patient dose** when acquiring frames at **less than 30 frames per second** (e.g., 15 frames/s).
- Pulsed fluoroscopy with **reduced frame rates** uses a **higher dose per frame** to reduce the perceived level of random noise.

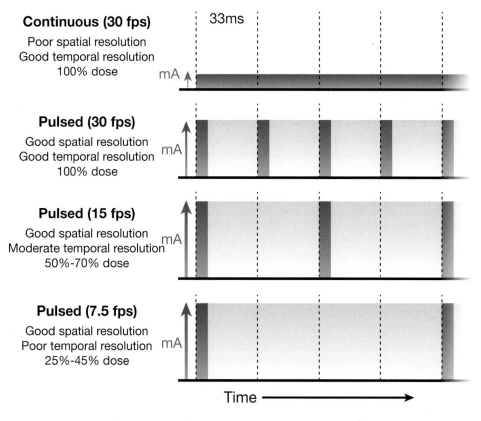

FIG 9.3 In continuous fluoroscopy (30 frames per second), the x-ray tube current is very low and always causes blur for fast-moving objects. In pulsed fluoroscopy (30 frames per second), the tube current is only on for a short time but increased to maintain the same mAs (and noise) for each frame as in continuous fluoroscopy. When the pulse rate is reduced to 15 frames per second, some systems will keep the mA constant, resulting in a 50% dose reduction as shown. Many systems will increase mA as pulse rate drops to keep noise "appearance" the same. This will result in a more modest reduction of ~30%. Further reducing the pulse rate will similarly reduce dose, at the cost of "choppy" motion.

- The human eye integrates frames together, resulting in lower perceived noise at higher acquired frames per second.
- Fluoroscopy performed at 15 acquired frames per second would likely increase the radiation per frame by about 30% (Fig. 9.3).
- Switching from **30 fps to 15 fps** would likely **reduce patient doses** by about **35%**, not the 50% expected at a constant radiation per frame.

C. Dose Settings and Collimation

- Fluoroscopy systems generally offer **choices** of **radiation intensities** to use during fluoroscopy.
  - Most systems permit use of "**low**," "**normal**," and "**high**" modes.
- Values of K_{air} at the image receptor in **low** mode are roughly **50%** of that offered in normal mode.
  - Low mode should be used when mottle is of less importance, such as a child who may have swallowed a coin (i.e., high-contrast lesion).
- Values of K_{air} at the image receptor in **high** mode are roughly **50% higher** than that in normal mode.
  - High mode should be selected when low-contrast lesions are being imaged, and mottle must be reduced to maintain diagnostic performance.
- When **collimation** is applied, the average image brightness is reduced as the outer regions that are no longer irradiated will be dark.
  - **Collimation** alone will demonstrate only a small increase in skin dose in the field of view, since minification gain is not altered.
- With **collimation**, there is **no change** in object **magnification** and thus no improvement in image spatial resolution.
- **Collimation reduces patient stochastic doses (risks)** and **improves image quality (contrast)** because of reduced scatter and improved image processing.
- Differences between collimation and electronic magnification are summarized in Table 9.3.

D. System Technique Curves

- **Imaging larger patients or body parts requires more radiation** incident on the patient to maintain a constant value of K_{air} at the image receptor.
- Increasing patient size results in the **system** increasing **tube voltage (kV)** and/or **current (mA).**
- **One option** to achieve more radiation incident on a larger patient would be to simply **increase** the **tube current (mA).**
  - Increasing the **tube current maintains image contrast** but results in **more patient dose than increasing kV.**
- **Another option** to achieve more radiation incident on a larger patient is to **increase** the **tube voltage (kV).**
  - Increasing the **tube voltage reduces image contrast but** will **give lower dose to the patient than increasing mA alone.**

Parameter	Comparison of the Effects of Electronic Magnification and Collimation for Image Intensifier–Based Fluoroscopy Systems	
TABLE 9.3		
Parameter	**Electronic Magnification**	**Collimation**
Radiation intensity[a] (K_{air})	Increased	Unchanged or small increase
Kerma area product (Gy-cm^2)	Unchanged[b]	Reduced
Resolution (detail visibility)	Increased	Unchanged

[a]Incident on both the patient and the image intensifier.
[b]Increase in $AK_{entrance}$ is canceled by the reduction in the exposed area.

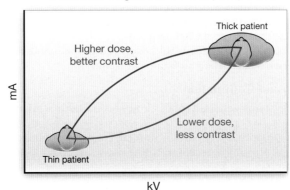

FIG 9.4 Imaging larger patients requires more radiation, which is normally achieved by increasing both tube voltage (kV) and tube current (mA). When the tube current is increased more than the voltage (red curve), patient dose and lesion contrast are higher than that when the voltage is increased more than the tube current (blue curve).

- **Larger patients** receive **lower doses** from an **increase in kV than** from a corresponding **increase in mA.**
- Most **fluoroscopy** systems modify both **kV** and **mA** when patient size changes, as depicted in Figure 9.4.
- In Figure 9.4, the red curve increases kV more than mA when imaging larger patients.
  - Using **the red curve** results in **lower doses** and **reduced contrast** *compared to* using **the blue curve** in the **same patient.**
- **Modern fluoroscopy systems** offer **several "ABC curves"** allowing operators to select optimal techniques.

E. **Regulatory**
- **US regulations limit fluoroscopy entrance K_{air} rates** to minimize skin doses, and the corresponding risks of skin burns.
  - US regulations (still) use a non-SI entrance exposure rate (i.e., **10 roentgens/min**), which corresponds to ~**87 mGy/min**
- **No regulatory limits** apply when **acquisition modes** are engaged **(i.e., photospot or acquisition/cine).**
- On **very large patients**, an entrance K_{air} rate of 100 mGy/min may still result in **inadequate image quality.**
- All modern fluoroscopy systems have a **high-level control (HLC) mode,** allowing the maximum entrance **K_{air} rate** to be increased to ~**200 mGy/min.**
  - Current US regulations for HLC use **20 roentgens/min** (~175 mGy/min).
- When the **HLC** is activated, **visible** and **audible indicators** indicate high-dose mode is being used.
  - **HLC** is only **used** in very **large patients** and has no relationship to the "high"-dose mode option in conventional fluoroscopy described previously.

IV. IMAGE QUALITY AND DOSE

A. **Contrast and Noise**
- **Contrast agents** added during fluoroscopy include **iodine, barium**, and **air.**
  - Barium and iodine are positive contrast agents (appear white), whereas air is a negative contrast agent (appears black).
- **Iodine contrast** is **maximized** using voltages of ~**70 kV.**

- **Contrast increases** with increased **collimation** because of reduced patient scatter and possibly improved image processing.
- **Fluoroscopy image noise (mottle)** is determined by the number of photons (i.e., K_{air}) at the image receptor.
- K_{air} at the image receptor is **low in fluoroscopy** imaging **(~0.02 µGy/frame).**
  - Fluoroscopy K_{air} at the image receptor **varies** markedly with **electronic magnification** and in acquisition modes.
- **Contrast-detail phantoms** are used to assess **fluoroscopic detection** of **lesions**, as depicted in Figure 9.5.
- **High-contrast** lesions of all sizes are **generally visible**, whereas **low-contrast** lesions are **invisible** because of **noise.**
- K_{air} at the image receptor is high in diagnostic imaging (**acquisition modes**) and in the range of **2 µGy/image.**

B. Resolution

- The **limiting resolution** of an **image intensifier** is **~5 lp/mm**, and viewing the output phosphor directly (i.e., removing TV) yields the full resolution.
  - Image intensifier resolution is determined by input phosphor (CsI) thickness, which is made of thin columns to limit the spread of light.
- When the **image intensifier** is **viewed** through a **TV camera/CCD**, the **limiting resolution** is **reduced.**
- **Limiting resolution** in modern image intensifier fluoroscopy is **typically 1 to 2 lp/mm.**
- **Fluoroscopy resolution** can be **improved** using **electronic magnification.**
  - **Halving** the **image intensifier field of view electronically** (i.e., Mag 2 in Table 9.2) **doubles spatial resolution.**
- **Resolution** in **photospot** imaging through an image intensifier is **2 lp/mm.**
  - Photospot images are acquired by digitizing more TV lines.
- **Resolution** in **spot imaging** is **3 to 4 lp/mm.**
  - Spot imaging is conventional radiographs acquired with an overhead x-ray tube and a digital image receptor in the table Bucky.

C. Artifacts

- Most artifacts in fluoroscopy require the vendor to service the system to correct them.
- The **image intensifier input** is **curved,** and projecting this surface onto a flat output phosphor results in **geometrical distortions** (Figure 9.1).

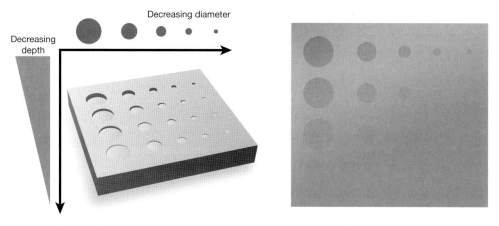

FIG 9.5 Contrast detail phantoms are used to assess lesion detection in images that have high noise levels such as a fluoroscopy. Holes of varying sizes and depth are drilled into an aluminum block (left). High-contrast lesions (deep holes) are generally visible, even when these are very small, whereas low-contrast lesions (shallow holes) are generally not seen, even when they are very large (right).

- A curved input permits the window to be thin (1.5 mm Al) despite the powerful vacuum, which minimizes the absorption of incident x-rays and improves patient dose.
- **Pincushion distortion** is produced by all image intensifiers, where straight lines appear curved toward the image center.
- **Vignetting** is a fall-off in brightness at the periphery of the image intensifier field.
  - Pincushion distortion and vignetting are of less concern with smaller field sizes (i.e., less minification).
- **S-distortion** is where straight lines appear wavy due to deflection of electrons in the image intensifier by **magnetic fields** (e.g., from the Earth).
  - S-distortions can vary as an image intensifier rotates due to changes in orientation with respect to the Earth's magnetic field.
- **Glare** occurs when there is a significant increase in x-ray transmission, as may occur at the interface of the heart and lung.
  - Visibility in the higher transmission area is reduced because of light scattering in the image intensifier's output phosphor (**veiling glare**).
- **Saturation** occurs when the image intensifier response has reached its peak value and appears as a uniform white intensity in the image (no contrast).
- **Lag** occurs when there is a persistence of any moving object (i.e., appears smeared out).
  - Averaging many fames using recursive filtration will result in increased lag.

D. Incident Patient Radiation

- **Entrance K_{air}** in a typical-sized adult is about **10 to 20 mGy/min.**
- In normal-sized patients, **entrance K_{air}** for diagnostic images is between **1 mGy and 3 mGy** per **photospot image.**
  - **One minute of standard fluoroscopy** most likely results in the same patient dose as **10 photospot images.**
- Patient fluoroscopy entrance K_{air} rates **increase** with **increasing patient size.**
  - **Tube voltage (kV)** also **increases** to **improve penetration** through the **largest patients,** which is generally automated (not manual).
- At the same beam quality, **increasing** the **patient** thickness by **3 cm** could roughly **double** the incident (entrance) K_{air} **rate.**
  - **Reducing** the **patient** thickness by **3 cm** would roughly **halve** the incident (entrance) K_{air} **rate** if beam quality is kept constant.
- Table 9.4 shows **representative** values of **KAP** in **fluoroscopy examinations.**
  - **Average KAP** is **20 Gy-cm²,** with all examinations within a factor of two of this benchmark value.
- **Fluoroscopy examinations** use **KAP** values that are about **20 times higher** than the corresponding value in **radiography.**

TABLE 9.4	Representative Values of Kerma Area Product (KAP; Gy-cm²) Encountered in Fluoroscopy-Guided Gastrointestinal and Urological Examinations			
Examination	Fluoroscopy KAP	Photo Spot Images KAP	Spot Images (Radiographs) KAP	Total Examination KAP
Video fluoroscopic swallow study	5	5	0	10
Upper gastrointestinal	7.5	7.5	0	15
Ba enema	8	8	24	40

E. **Patient Doses and Risks**

- In fluoroscopy-guided **GI** and **urological** exams, **skin doses** are always expected to be **below 500 mGy.**
  - **Skin burns** are **not expected** to occur in these types of fluoroscopy-guided examinations.
- An average **patient effective dose** in **general fluoroscopy is a few mSv** (e.g., 4 mSv for small bowel follow-through).
  - **Modified barium swallow** is <1 mSv.
- Ba swallows, upper GI studies have lower doses, as do most urological examinations, whereas barium enemas have higher doses.
  - Most **GI studies** would be considered **moderate-dose examinations.**
- A **25-year-old** exposed to an effective dose of **4 mSv** could increase their **cancer risk** by about 4 in 10,000 **(i.e., 0.04%) above** the base line of **40%.**
  - **Radiologists** need to ensure that the **patient benefit** is expected to be **greater** than this **estimated increase** in **patient cancer risk.**

Chapter 9 (Fluoroscopy) Questions

9.1 What is the likely power loading on the x-ray tube during fluoroscopy?
A. <1 kW
B. 1 kW
C. 10 kW
D. 100 kW

9.2 What focal spot size is typical during abdominal fluoroscopy?
A. 0.01 mm
B. 0.1 mm
C. 0.6 mm
D. 6.0 mm

9.3 What image intensifier component absorbs light and emits low-energy electrons?
A. Input window (Al)
B. Input phosphor
C. Photocathode
D. Output phosphor

9.4 The patient should be _____ the x-ray tube and _____ the image receptor.
A. close to; close to
B. close to; far from
C. far from; close to
D. far from; far from

9.5 Increasing recursive filtering will degrade which image property?
A. Spatial resolution
B. Temporal resolution
C. Noise
D. Contrast

9.6 What is the most likely tube current used during continuous fluoroscopy?
A. 0.3 mA
B. 3 mA
C. 30 mA
D. 300 mA

9.7 R/F units (i.e., x-ray tube under table) attenuate about _____% of the x-ray beam by the table prior to being incident on the patient.
A. 1
B. 3
C. 10
D. 30

9.8 How do grid ratios used in fluoroscopy compare to those used in radiography?
A. Greater
B. Comparable
C. Lower

9.9 What tube voltage is ideally used when iodine is administered to a patient to visualize the vasculature?
A. 30 kV
B. 70 kV
C. 110 kV
D. 130 kV

9.10 What tube voltage is ideally used when barium is administered to a patient to visualize the lower GI tract?
A. 30 kV
B. 70 kV
C. 110 kV
D. 130 kV

9.11 What is the percentage reduction in area when switching from normal mode to Mag 1 (electronic magnification)?
A. 90%
B. 50%
C. 25%
D. 10%

9.12 How do patient dose rate in pulsed fluoroscopy (30 pulses per second) compare to those in continuous fluoroscopy?
A. Higher
B. Comparable
C. Lower

9.13 How will dose per frame typically change when dose rate is reduced in pulsed fluoroscopy?
A. Increased
B. Maintained
C. Reduced

9.14 Collimation improves what image property?
A. Spatial resolution
B. Temporal resolution
C. Mottle
D. Contrast

9.15 As a patient gets bigger how does ABC alter tube output?
A. Increase
B. No Change
C. Decrease

9.16 Increasing kV as opposed to mA when imaging a larger patient most likely improves:
A. Dose
B. Contrast
C. Resolution
D. CNR

9.17 What is the maximum regulatory entrance K_{air} rate incident on a patient undergoing standard fluoroscopy?
A. 10 mGy/min
B. 50 mGy/min
C. 100 mGy/min
D. 200 mGy/min

9.18 One minute of standard fluoroscopy most likely delivers the same patient dose as how many photospot images?
A. <1
B. 1
C. 3
D. 10

9.19 Which image intensifier artifact is most likely observed when a mobile C-arm is moved close to an MR scanner?
A. Pincushion distortion
B. Vignetting
C. Lag
D. S-distortion

9.20 What is the effective dose of abdominopelvic barium studies?
A. Very low (<0.1 mSv)
B. Low (0.1-1 mSv)
C. Moderate (1-10 mSv)
D. High (>10 mSv)

Answers and Explanations

9.1   **A**   (<1 kW). The tube voltage (80 kV) with a tube current of 2 to 3 mA corresponds to a power loading of only 160 to 240 W.

9.2   **C**   (0.6 mm). The small x-ray tube focal spot (i.e., 0.6 mm) is used during fluoroscopy because this tolerates the extremely low power loading (e.g., <1 kW).

9.3   **C**   (Photocathodes). It is the photocathode that absorbs light and emits low-energy electrons that are subsequently accelerated to high energy to create a visible image when absorbed by the output phosphor.

9.4   **C**   (far from; close to). Bringing the patient far from the tube and bringing the receptor close to the patient reduces patient dose, operator dose, and magnification.

9.5   **B**   (Temporal resolution). Recursive frame averaging (recursive temporal filtering) averages several frames together to improve noise but decreases temporal resolution (more motion blur).

9.6   **B**   (3 mA). Continuous fluoroscopy tube currents are a few mA, and increased by about 100 when photospot images are being acquired.

9.7   **D**   (30%). Tables are required by the FDA to be no more than 2 mm Al equivalent, and this thickness attenuates about 30% of the incident beam. Fluoroscopy HVLs are about 3 mm Al equivalent, so 3 mm Al equivalent attenuates 50%.

9.8   **B**   (Comparable). Grid ratios in radiography and fluoroscopy are essentially the same because the amount of scatter is determined by the amount of scatter from the patient. Scatter-to-primary ratios are identical in fluoroscopy (low mA) and radiography (high mA).

9.9   **B**   (70 kV). With a tube voltage of 70 kV, the average x-ray beam energy (~35 keV) is very close to the iodine K-edge (33 keV), which maximizes x-ray absorption by the iodine and improves visibility of vasculature that contains this contrast agent.

9.10   **C**   (110 kV). A tube voltage of 110 kV is required to penetrate the barium contrast in the GI; at low tube voltages, any part of the GI that had any barium would simply appear white, offering poor GI tract visualization.

9.11   **B**   (50%). Normal mode normally exposes 100% of the image intensifier's phosphor area, Mag 1 exposes 50%, and Mag 2 exposes 25%.

9.12   **B**   (Comparable). Switching from continuous to 30 pulses per second results in the acquisition of exactly the same number of frames in each second (30), so the dose will not change. Pulsed fluoroscopy will result in sharper images because of reduced motion blur.

9.13   **A**   (Increased). At reduced acquisition frame rates in pulsed fluoroscopy, the dose per frame is increased to maintain the same perception image quality (signal to noise ratio).

9.14   **D**   (Contrast). A reduced x-ray beam area means less scatter and thereby higher lesion contrast. It also allows the image processing to better distribute gray levels, further improving contrast.

9.15   **A**   (Increase). as the patient anatomy becomes thicker and more attenuating the ABC increases tube output to maintain the same video brightness.

9.16 A (Dose). Radiation doses will be lower (i.e., improved) in this larger patient as compared to imaging the same patient with increased mA.

9.17 C (100 mGy/min). Current US regulations require the maximum entrance K_{air} rate in standard fluoroscopy to be ~100 Gy/min (actually 10 R/min, which translates to 87.6 mGy/min).

9.18 D (10). A good rule of thumb is that 1 minute of fluoroscopy (10 mGy/min) most likely delivers the same patient dose as 10 photospot images (10 × 1 mGy/photospot image).

9.19 D (S-distortion). When electrons are affected by stray magnetic fields (e.g., adjacent to an MR scanner), S-distortion occurs.

9.20 C (Moderate). Abdominopelvic barium studies will generally have effective doses in the range of 1 to 10 mSv. Modified swallows are <1 mSv.

CHAPTER 10 Interventional Radiology

I. IR IMAGING

A. Interventional Radiology

- **Interventional radiology (IR)**, aka **vascular and interventional radiology**, is a procedural subspecialty of radiology.
  - IR procedures utilize a variety of modalities, but this chapter will focus only on fluoroscopy.
  - Examples of IR procedures include **stenting**, **vertebroplasty**, **angioplasty**, and **chemoembolization.**
- Interventional radiologists **use images to direct needles** and **catheters** throughout the body, which **avoids making large incisions** as in traditional surgery.
- Minimally invasive procedures often have lower complication rates and decreased recovery time compared with surgery.
- IR imaging chains use fixed-room C-arms that can be easily maneuvered and high-quality x-ray generators and x-ray tubes.
  - IR facilities use **flat-panel detectors (FPDs),** whereas GI/GU facilities may use image intensifiers or flat-panel imaging systems.
- An **IR imaging chain** costs more than **$1,250k**, compared to **$350k** for an **R/F** systems.

B. Flat-Panel Detectors

- **FPDs** used in IR are conceptually **similar** to those used in **digital radiography.**
  - FPDs for general fluoroscopy also exist but still are typically only for upper end systems.
- FPDs in IR typically use 40 × 40 cm square **scintillators (CsI)**, which is larger than the round image intensifier (II) detectors used in general fluoroscopy.
  - Other fields of view (FOVs) are available as preset values (e.g., 32, 20, 16 cm).
- **FPD pixels** are ~175 μm, offering good resolution (detail) in **photospot imaging.**
- **FPDs** do not use TV or charge-coupled device system and are **read out electronically** for **real-time processing** and/or **display.**
- **FPD** have a **linear response** over a very **wide dynamic range** like their radiography counterparts.
  - **Saturation artifacts** occur much less often in FPDs.
- When FPDs are used for fluoroscopy, it is essential that electronic noise is minimized because the detected signals are a hundred times lower than in radiography.

C. FPD Operation

- **FPDs do not employ electronic magnification** used in image intensifiers.
- When the **FPD FOV** is **reduced** (e.g., 40 to 32 cm), there is no technical reason why the AK_{image} must increase (i.e., **no loss of minification gain**).

- In practice, when **FPD FOV** is **reduced (i.e., zoom), AK$_{image}$ increases** to **improve image quality** to reduce the perceived mottle by radiologists.
- A **40 cm FOV** (normal mode) would likely have **similar AK$_{image}$** rates for fluoroscopy performed with **FPD** and **IIs.**
- **Halving** the **FOV** would likely result **quadruple** the II **AK$_{image}$** in **Mag 2** mode but only **double** the corresponding FPD **AK$_{image}$.**
- **FPD fluoroscopy** performed with **larger FOVs** would likely **add four pixels together (aka binning)** to **reduce mottle** and the amount of **data** generated.
  - **Binning** also **halves** the **resolution**, which is clinically acceptable in fluoroscopy when using large FOVs.

D. FPD vs II Image Quality

- **Contrast** in fluoroscopy and photospot imaging is determined by the choice of x-ray **tube voltage (kV)** and is identical for both II detectors and FPD.
- **Noise** is determined by the **number** of **photons** captured by the **image receptor.**
- II detectors and FPDs are similar (400 μm CsI), but **FPDs have a carbon** cover that transmits more x-rays than the **1.5 mm Al** used in **image intensifiers.**
- FPDs offer a **fixed limiting resolution** of **3 lp/mm**, determined by the (fixed) pixel size, and is half of this value with binning.
  - General fluoroscopy resolution using an II is 1 to 2 lp/mm.
- Significant **differences** between **II detectors** and **FPDs** relate to **artifacts** and **distortions.**
- II detectors exhibit pin cushion distortion, s-distortion, vignetting, and glare.
  - **The fidelity** of **FPDs** used in IR is **excellent**, with none of the problems associated with image intensifiers.
- FPDs may exhibit **dead pixels and poor uniformity** correction similar to digital radiography.

E. Diagnostic Imaging

- **IR equipment** has more **sophisticated hardware** including more **powerful x-ray tubes**, added **copper filtration, automatic exposure rate control (AERC)**, and **equalization filters.**
- **AERC** is designed to keep **consistent noise or contrast-to-noise** in the image.
  - AERC systems may automatically alter kV, mA, filtration, and pulse width.
- **Equalization filters (aka soft collimators)** use **Pb/plastic mixtures** to reduce transmission of x-rays to peripheral regions used as anatomical landmarks.
- In **digital subtraction angiography (DSA)**, a **mask image** without contrast is subtracted from the corresponding image with contrast to show contrast-containing structures (like **vasculature**) with **no background anatomy.**
  - DSA improves vasculature visibility by the removal of "anatomical background," which is of greater importance than quantum mottle.
- **Road mapping** permits an image to be captured and displayed on a monitor, while a second monitor shows live images.
- **Road mapping** may also be used to capture images with contrast material that can be **overlaid** onto a **live fluoroscopy image.**
- **Tube voltages** in angiography and **DSA imaging** are roughly **70 kV,** to match the average photon energy to the K-edge of iodine (33 keV).
- **Tube currents** are typically **400 mA, exposure times** are **50 ms**, resulting in a total technique of **20 mAs.**
- A typical **matrix size** is **1k^2**, resulting in a data content of **2 MB**, with **frame rates** in angiography and DSA up to **8 frames/s** (though **DSA typically uses 3 fps to reduce patient dose).**
- The receptor air kerma (i.e., **AK$_{image}$**) in **angiography** and **DSA** is **similar** to that of **radiographic imaging** (i.e, **3 μGy/image**).

⬛ **II.** **IR SKIN DOSES**

A. Irradiation Geometry

- The **source-to-image receptor distance (SID)** is roughly **100 cm.**
  - A typical-sized adult patient has an abdominal anteroposterior (AP) dimension of 23 cm with a **source-to-skin distance (SSD)** of **75 cm.**
- **Shorter SIDs increase skin doses** and image distortion resulting from variable magnification.
  - Shorter SIDs may arise when the table is lowered for shorter personnel and can be obviated by having operators use a raised platform to stand on.
- **Longer SIDs** require **increased x-ray tube output** (inverse square law).
  - Larger SIDs result in longer image exposure times, increasing motion blur.
- **Geometric magnification** introduces **focal spot blurring, increased skin doses,** and an **air gap** permits **scatter** exiting the patient to **irradiate nearby operators.**
  - **Geometric magnification** in IR imaging is **minimized** by **reducing** the **gap** between the **patient** and the **image receptor.**
- All fluoroscopy equipment in the United States has a **spacer** to limit how close the patient's skin can get to the x-ray tube focal spot.
  - The **minimum focus-to-skin distance** is **38 cm** for **fixed systems,** and **30 cm** for **mobile units** (e.g., C-arms in operating rooms).
- **Entrance skin surface** of the patient should be at or above (i.e., toward the receptor) the interventional reference point discussed later in this chapter (Fig. 10.1).

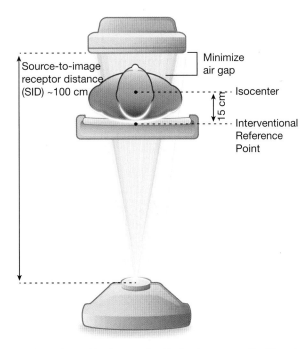

FIG 10.1 Ideal geometry to reduce skin dose and optimize image quality. Dose is reduced with the patient far from the source and close to the detector due to the inverse square law. Moving the detector away from the patient causes magnification and dose increase due to AERC. The entrance skin surface should be at the interventional reference point or more away from the source so that skin air kerma reported on the monitor is similar to or greater than the actual skin dose. AERC, automatic exposure rate control.

B. Dose Rates in IR

- **Entrance doses** are generally **100 times** higher than **exit doses**, with half of the dose deposited in the first 3 to 5 cm of tissue.
- **Skin dose rates** in a normal-sized adult (23 cm tissue) are **~15 mGy/min** during **fluoroscopy**, and **~3 mGy/image** in **angiography.**
  - About 30% of skin dose in the abdomen is due to backscatter from deeper in the patient.
- Dose rates can be **much higher** in very **large patients**, and the x-ray tube voltages raised to **>100 kV** to ensure adequate **penetration and acceptable mottle at the cost of lower contrast.**
- Dose rates can be **much lower** in **smaller patients** and voltages reduced to **60 kV** in **infants** and thin body parts (e.g., popliteal artery).
- Table 10.1 shows how skin dose rates vary with patient size.
- **Grids** are **optional** in IR procedures performed in **infants** and **knees**, where **removing the grid (with AEC)** will **halve** all **patient doses** (Table 10.1).
- **Skin dose rates** in **lateral body projections** are about **double** those of **AP projections.**
  - Operators should use a lateral projection when clinically appropriate, reverting to lower dose projections when clinically indicated.

C. IRP Doses

- The **interventional reference point (IRP)** (aka patient entrance reference point) is an imaginary point, **15 cm closer** to the **focal spot** than the system isocenter (Fig. 10.1).
  - **IR gantries rotate** around the **isocenter**, located close to the center of the patient.
- Manufacturers display **IRP air kerma** values to the operator on monitors, and provide a summary at the end of the procedure.
  - Manufacturers compute air kerma based on selected techniques (kV and mA) combined with the assumed irradiation geometry.
- **IRP air kerma** values are referred to as **cumulative doses** and include contributions from both **fluoroscopy** and **photospot imaging.**
  - Since the IRP travels with the gantry, **cumulative doses add up dose even if the beam hits different pieces of skin.**
- Cumulative doses pertaining to practice in academic medical centers (AMCs) are shown in Table 10.2.
  - Patient doses at AMCs are likely higher than average because they perform relatively complex IR procedures and use trainees.

TABLE 10.1	Examples of How Fluoroscopy K_{air} Rates and Selected X-Ray Tube Voltage (kV) Vary With Patient Size in Interventional Radiology			
Patient[a]	AP Dimension	Lateral Dimension (cm)	Tube Voltage (kV)	Relative Entrance K_{air} Rate
Neonate (no grid)	10	10	60	0.1
Neonate (grid)	10	10	60	0.2
Pediatric patient	15	20	65	0.4
Small adult	20	30	70	0.7
Average adult	23	30	75	1.0
Large adult	30	40	85	3.0
Obese patient	40	50	100	7.0
Obese patient (lateral)	40	50	120	10.0

Entrance K_{air} rate for a 23 cm patient is roughly 10 to 15 mGy/min.
AP, anteroposterior.
[a]AP projection unless otherwise indicated.

TABLE 10.2	Typical Number (%) of Patients Who Might Exceed a Specified IRP K$_{air}$ and Peak Skin Doses (PSD) for Cases Performed at US Academic Medical Centers	
Specified IRP K$_{air}$ or PSD (Gy)	% of Patients Exceeding Specified IRP K$_{air}$	% of Patients Exceeding Specified Peak Skin Dose
1	50	40
2	30	25
3	20	10
5	5	2

IRP, interventional reference point.

- **AK$_{entrance}$** specified by vendors is always **measured free in air** (not tissue) and **excludes patient backscatter.**
  - Tissue doses are **higher** than AK$_{entrance}$ because of differences between **air** and **tissue** (e.g., **+10%**), and the presence of **backscatter** (e.g., **+30%**).

D. Peak Skin Doses

- Converting a **cumulative dose** into the patient **PSD** is **difficult** and will depend on the irradiation geometry as shown in Figures 10.1 and 10.2.
  - Overlap of multiple beams will markedly influence PSDs.
- **Skin dose estimates** require knowledge of the **actual patient skin location**, which is unlikely to be at the assumed IRP location.
  - **Uncertainties** in the **location** of skin introduce dose **errors of ±50%.**
- Account must be taken whether the x-ray beam passes through the table before being incident on the patient.
  - **There is no table attenuation** in **lateral projections**, but ~30% loss for posteroanterior (**PA**) projections.
- Measured or calculated PSD values can be compared with the IRP cumulative dose, and a **dose index (DI)** computed **(PSD/IRP dose).**

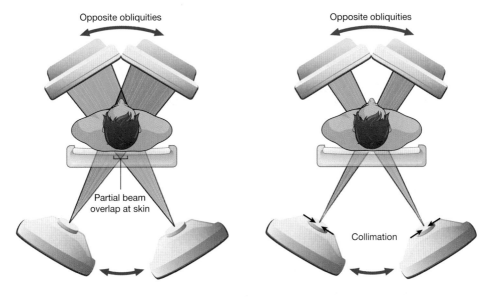

FIG 10.2 Performing opposite oblique views without collimation (left) may result in overlapping x-ray beams and a high peak skin dose that could result in a skin burn. Use of tight collimation (right) reduces the likelihood of x-ray beam overlap, and the corresponding risk of a patient skin burn. Collimation also reduces the total amount of radiation incident on the patient (KAP), and the corresponding patient carcinogenic radiation risk, as well as the scatter radiation incident on operators. KAP, kerma-area product.

- Scientific studies for procedures performed at AMCs have shown that most **dose index** values encountered in **clinical practice** lie **between 0.5 and 0.8.**
- Table 10.2 shows the percentages of procedures at AMC exceeding specified PSDs.
- **PSDs** in **nephrostomy, inferior vena cava filter placements,** and **pulmonary angiography rarely exceed 2 Gy.**
  - **TIPS (transjugular intrahepatic portosystemic shunt)** and **embolization** procedures have the **highest PSDs.**
- Up to **20%** of **spine neuroembolization** procedures to treat **arteriovenous malformation** and **tumors** may result in **PSDs exceeding 5 Gy.**

E. **Skin Dose Policy**
- All **IR sections** need a formal **policy** for **informing patients** about **potential radiation skin burns.**
  - When **high doses** are expected, the possibility of radiation burns should be included in the **informed consent** process.
- For current equipment, the **cumulative dose** provided by the vendor may be taken to be the **(nominal) PSD.**
  - In most cases, this will **likely** be **conservative.**
- For doses **below 2 Gy,** no action is required, as **tissue damage is not expected.**
- **Between 2 and 5 Gy,** it is prudent to **inform** the **patient** of the dose, **where/when a burn might occur.**
  - The patient should be provided with explicit medical advice as the action to be taken if any damage appears.
  - At these doses, damage will be temporary if it occurs at all.
- For **doses exceeding 5 Gy,** a **review** by a **medical physicist** should assess the validity of the IRP dose as the PSD, and recommend any modifications.
  - **Patients** should be **contacted 1 to 2 weeks after** the **procedure** to inquire about possible radiation burns.
- The **Joint Commission (JC)** defines a fluoroscopy **sentinel event** as permanent damage caused by radiation when clinical and technical optimization were not implemented and/or recognized practice parameters were not followed.
  - A sentinel event requires a full root cause analysis and a visit by a JC inspector.
- It is estimated that only **1 in 10,000 IR procedures** result in a **serious tissue damage requiring major clinical intervention** (e.g., skin grafts).

III. IR PATIENT AND OPERATOR EFFECTIVE DOSES

A. **KAP and Organ Doses**
- **Kerma-area product (KAP)** values are computed as $AK_{entrance}$ times the corresponding x-ray **beam areas** in fluoroscopy and photospot imaging and have the unit **Gy-cm^2.**
- **Mean KAP** in an **AMC** is about **200 Gy-cm^2.**
  - IR procedures have KAP values an order of magnitude higher than that in fluoroscopy-guided procedures, two orders of magnitude higher than that in radiography.
- **Half** the **procedures** in an **AMC** would likely fall in the range of **100 to 300 Gy-cm^2.**
- **Nephrostomy** placement has a KAP of ~**25 Gy-cm^2.**
- **Average** values for **spine arteriovenous malformation embolization** can be higher than **500 Gy-cm^2.**
- **KAP,** when combined with **beam quality** information, can be used to estimate **doses to all organs** in the patient.
  - **Converting KAP** into **organ doses** needs to account for exposed body **region, projection,** as well as **patient physical characteristics (size).**
- Patient **organ doses** are used to estimate **organ risks** which can be **summed** to provide an estimate of the **patient cancer risk.**
  - Patient cancer risk is the only radiation risk when skin doses do not exceed the threshold for tissue damage.
- Figure 10.3 shows how KAP correlates with cumulative doses in IR procedures.

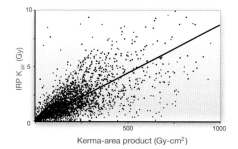

FIG 10.3 There is a modest correlation between IRP K_{air} and kerma-area product (KAP) for most IR procedures. IRP K_{air} is related to the patient peak skin dose, and corresponding likelihood of a radiation burn. KAP is a measure of the total radiation incident on the patient, and used to estimate the patient stochastic risk, primarily carcinogenesis. IRP, interventional reference point.

B. Patient Effective Doses

- **Patient effective doses** are **computed** from **organ doses** estimated from the KAP incident on patients undergoing IR procedures.
- Table 10.3 shows nominal conversion factors that may be used for normal sized adults.
  - **Increased patient size** in body examinations **reduces conversion factors.**
- E/KAP conversion factors for pediatric patients markedly increase as patient age/size is reduced.
  - **Body E/KAP conversion factors** are about **ten times higher** in **7 kg patients** than in normal-sized adults (70 kg).
- Table 10.4 shows typical imaging characteristics of common IR procedures, and the corresponding effective doses that are mainly "high dose" (>10 mSv).
- The **median patient effective dose** at AMCs is **30 mSv.**
- Approximately **half** the **patients undergoing IR** procedures in an AMC would be expected to have effective doses **between 10 and 50 mSv.**

TABLE 10.3	Nominal Effective Dose per Unit Kerma-Area Product (KAP; mSv/Gy-cm²) Conversion Factors Used to Estimate Patient Effective Doses for Normal-Sized Adults	
Body Region	**Projection**	**Nominal E/KAP mSv/Gy-cm²**
Head	All	0.03
Body	Anteroposterior	0.25
	Posteroanterior	0.15
	Lateral	0.10

TABLE 10.4	Representative Imaging Values Encountered in IR Procedures, With the Corresponding Kerma-Area Products and Effective Doses			
Procedure	**Fluoroscopy Time (min)**	**Number of Images**	**KAP (Gy-cm²)**	**Effective Dose (mSv)**
Nephrostomy (stone access)	15	10	40	6
Pulmonary angiography (IVC filter)	10	150	100	15
Renal angioplasty (stent)	20	150	200	30
Transjugular intrahepatic portosystemic shunt (TIPS)	40	250	400	60
Spine embolization (AVM)	75	1,300	600	90

AVM, arteriovenous malformation; IR, interventional radiology; IRP, interventional reference point; IVC, inferior vena cava.

C. Scatter Radiation

- **Operators** performing **IR procedures** are **exposed** to **radiation scattered** from **patients.**
- Operator doses **1 m from the patient** (scatter) is about **0.1%** of the **patient dose.**
- **One meter** from a 23 cm thick patient undergoing **fluoroscopy**, the scatter intensity will be **15 μGy/min (i.e., 1 mGy/h).**
  - At the same distance from this patient, the **scatter** is **3 μGy/image** during **photospot** imaging (0.3 mGy per 100 photospot images).
- The principal source of scatter in IR is the area where the x-ray beams enter into a patient.
- Under-the-table x-ray tubes thereby have low operator doses, whereas over-the-table x-ray tubes result in high eye doses.
- For lateral projections, **operators** need to **stand** at the **image receptor side**, not at the x-ray tube side, as depicted in Figure 10.4A.
- **Large patients** require **higher AK$_{entrance}$** values, which also **increases operator doses** as shown in Figure 10.4B.
- Table 10.5 shows how patient and operator doses are affected by changes in fluoroscopy operation.

D. Operator Effective Doses

- **IR** and **cardiology** have **high occupational effective doses.**
- **Operator effective doses** are about **5 μSv** for an IR procedure performed with a **KAP** of **~200 Gy-cm²**.

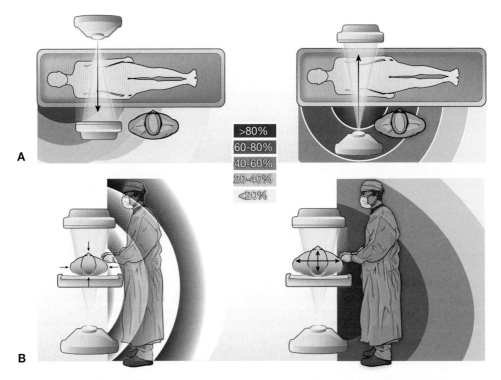

FIG 10.4 A: Virtually all of the scatter radiation in interventional radiology originates where the x-ray beam enters the patient. Operator doses are thus much lower when the radiologist stands on the image receptor size (left) as opposed to standing next to the x-ray tube (right) because the radiation incident on a patient is generally 100 times more intense than the radiation exiting a patient. **B:** Operator doses are generally directly proportional to the patient dose, and will be much lower with a small patient (left) than with a larger patient (right) because larger patients require much more radiation (see Table 10.1).

TABLE 10.5	Effects of Changes in a Flat-Panel Detector Imaging Parameters on Patient and Operator Doses in Interventional Radiology		
Change	**Patient**		**Operator Effective Dose**
	Skin Dose	**Effective Dose**	
Field of view area halved	+50%	−25%	−25%
0.2 mm Cu added	Halved	Halved	Halved
Switch from antero-posterior to lateral projection	Doubled	Doubled	Doubled

- For a **workload** of **1,000** procedures, **annual effective doses** will be about **5 mSv.**
- Operator effective doses vary markedly depending on procedure complexity.
- **Operator effective doses** in **IR** and **cardiology** are generally between **1 and 10 mSv.**
- An **IR fellow** can expect to receive an annual effective dose of about **5 mSv.**
- **Technologists** record doses **between 1 and 2 mSv,** with lower doses to ancillary staff.

E. **Operator Extremity/Lens Doses**
- Dosimeters worn above a lead apron at the level of the collar likely **overestimate eye lens doses.**
- **IR operator eye lens doses** are generally **below** the current US regulatory eye lens dose limit of **150 mSv per year.**
- IR personnel do not routinely monitor extremity doses as is done in nuclear medicine and radiopharmacies.
  - **IR extremity doses** are **much lower** than the regulatory limit (i.e., **500 mSv/y**).

IV. IR RADIATION PROTECTION

A. **Dose Monitoring**
- **Personnel working** in IR **wear dosimeters** to assess their **occupational doses** and ensure that these are below regulatory limits.
- Typically, a single **dosimeter** is worn **outside** the **lead apron** at the collar level.
  - This **overestimates effective doses.**
- Operators may instead wear **two dosimeters (double badge)** to get a better dose estimate.
  - One is worn under the lead apron at the waist and the other above the apron at the collar.
- **Dosimeter** can be used to **estimate** the **eye lens dose**, which is becoming a matter of concern to operators working in IR.
  - There is increased **clinical evidence** of **biological effects** in **eyes** of **staff** working in **IR.**
- **Pregnant workers can work** in an IR environment and, if they declare their pregnancy, will need to wear an extra dosimeter under their lead apron to ensure the **fetal dose** does **not exceed 5 mSv for the duration of the pregnancy (a regulatory limit).**
- Badge readings do not typically account for lead aprons, thyroid shields, or leaded glasses.

B. **Operational Factors**
- **Operators** can **reduce** their **exposures** by **limiting** the amount of radiation used to perform IR procedures, namely, the **KAP.**
- **Collimating** x-ray beams to the anatomy of interest not only **reduces** patient and operator **doses** but also reduces scatter and **increases image contrast.**

Chapter 10 (Interventional Radiology) Questions

10.1 The AERC in FPD systems typically keeps what image property consistent as the beam is moved to thinner and thicker body parts?
A. Contrast
B. Noise
C. Brightness
D. Resolution

10.2 What is the shape of the response curve of FPDs to radiation?
A. Sigmoidal
B. Exponential
C. Logarithmic
D. Linear

10.3 How do patient doses using FPDs with large fields of view compare to doses using image intensifiers?
A. Higher than
B. Comparable to
C. Lower than

10.4 How do patient doses using FPDs with small fields of view compare to those using image intensifiers?
A. Higher than
B. Comparable to
C. Lower than

10.5 What type of detectors employ pixel binning during fluoroscopy?
A. Only flat-panel detectors (FPD)
B. Only image intensifiers (II)
C. FPD or IIs
D. Neither FPDs nor IIs

10.6 How does spatial resolution change when one pixel is unbinned to four pixels during zoom?
A. Double
B. No change
C. Half
D. Quarter

10.7 Which parameter is least likely to be used in a digital subtraction angiography acquisition?
A. 75 kV
B. 500 mA
C. 25 mAs
D. 4:1 grid

10.8 The minimum focus to patient distance is _____ cm for fixed systems and _____ cm for mobile units.
A. 30 for both
B. 30; 38

C. 38; 30
D. 38 for both

10.9 In IR imaging, as patient size increases from infants to obese adults, x-ray tube voltages most likely increase from _____ to _____ kV.
A. 60; 60
B. 60; 120
C. 120; 60
D. 120; 120

10.10 In normal-sized adults, skin doses for lateral projections of the abdomen are what percentage higher than those of PA projections?
A. 10%
B. 30%
C. 50%
D. 100%

10.11 Where is the interventional reference point (IRP) is located for a C-arm?
A. At isocenter
B. Patient skin (entrance)
C. 15 cm from isocenter (toward focus)
D. 15 cm from isocenter (toward detector)

10.12 What percentage of IR patients likely exceeds a cumulative (IRP) dose of 2 Gy?
A. 10%
B. 30%
C. 50%
D. >50%

10.13 What percentage of IR patients likely exceeds a peak skin dose of 5 Gy?
A. <5
B. 5
C. 10
D. 20

10.14 Automatic exposure rate control may alter all system parameters below except what?
A. kV
B. mA
C. Filtration
D. Pulse rate

10.15 What is the frequency of IR procedures that would require major clinical intervention (e.g., skin graft)?
A. 1 per 100
B. 1 per 1,000
C. 1 per 10,000
D. 1 per 100,000

10.16 What shielding is likely accounted for in the operator badge reading?
A. Ceiling shield
B. Thyroid shield
C. Lead apron
D. Lead glasses

10.17 The average patient effective dose for IR procedures performed at AMC is most likely:
A. 3 mSv
B. 30 mSv
C. 300 mSv
D. >300 mSv

10.18 Patient scatter radiation results in doses at 1 m what percentage of radiation intensity incident on the patient?
A. 10%
B. 1%
C. 0.1%
D. 0.01%

10.19 What is the primary source of dose to the operator?
A. Tube housing leakage
B. Primary beam
C. Tube filter scatter
D. Patient scatter

10.20 Increasing which factor is most likely to increase operator doses in IR?
A. Distance from source
B. Lead shielding
C. Exposure time
D. A, B, and C

10.21 Wearing leaded glasses is most likely to reduce eye lens doses by what percentage?
A. 30%
B. 65%
C. 90%
D. >95%

Answers and Explanations

10.1 **B** (Noise). FPD systems use AERC, which attempts to keep image noise or, less commonly, contrast-to-noise constant as the anatomy thickness changes. This is similar to ABC keeping image brightness consistent for image intensified systems.

10.2 **D** (Linear). Digital x-ray detectors (e.g., CsI) have a linear response over a very wide range of radiation intensities, which is why they are superior to the sigmoidal response of both film and image intensifiers.

10.3 **B** (Comparable to). For large fields of view, doses are very similar for both FPDs and IIs, because these both use essentially the same detectors (CsI scintillators).

10.4 **C** (Lower than). For small fields of view, doses are lower for FPDs, because application of electronic magnification with IIs *requires* substantially increased doses for smaller areas.

10.5 **A** (Only flat-panel detectors (FPD)). Pixel binning (combining multiple pixels to make one) is only done with flat-panel detectors, usually for fluoroscopy performed using the larger fields of view.

10.6 **A** (Double). As FOV is reduced during zoom the binned pixels will eventually unbin. If the pixel size halves during unbinning, then the resolution will roughly double.

10.7 **D** (4:1 grid). DSA imaging typically uses the same grids as in most of radiography and fluoroscopy of the body (i.e., 10:1 grid ratio).

10.8 **C** (38; 30). The FDA requires a minimum focus-to-patient distance of 38 cm for fixed systems, and 30 cm for mobile units, to minimize the risk of skin burns.

10.9 **B** (60; 120). 60 kV would most likely be used to image a neonate, whereas 120 kV would likely be used to image obese adults.

10.10 **D** (100%). A good rule of thumb is to assume that lateral projection skin dose is twice the PA skin dose in normal-sized adults undergoing body imaging.

10.11 **C** (15 cm from isocenter (toward focus)). The interventional reference point (IRP) is located 15 cm from isocenter as one moves toward focus, and is an estimate of the location of the point where the x-ray beam enters the patient and delivers the highest (skin) dose.

10.12 **B** (30%). About 30% of IR patients are likely to have an IRP dose (cumulative dose) higher than 2 Gy.

10.13 **A** (<5%). Only about 2 % of IR patients are likely to receive a peak skin dose higher than 5 Gy.

10.14 **D** (Pulse rate). AERC can typically alter kV, mA, filtration, and pulse width. Pulse rate selection is left to the operator.

10.15 **C** (1 per 10,000). Frequency of IR procedures requiring major clinical intervention has been estimated at about 1 in 10,000.

10.16 **A** (ceiling shield). The ceiling shield keeps radiation from hitting the badge and so the badge reading accounts for ceiling shield usage. None of the other shields block radiation from hitting the badge.

10.17 **B** (30 mSv). 30 mSv is the average patient effective dose for IR procedures performed at academic medical centers in the United States.

10.18 **C** (0.1%). Patient scatter radiation results in doses at 1 meter that are about 0.1 % of the radiation intensity incident on the patient.

10.19 **D** (patient scatter). The primary source of patient dose is scatter from the entrance surface of the patient.

10.21 C (Exposure time). Increasing exposure time increases operator doses, whereas increasing shielding and distance from the source will reduce operator doses.

10.21 B (65%). Wearing leaded glasses reduce eye lens doses only by about 65%, with the eye lens doses mainly due to "scatter" from radiation incident on face skin around the glasses.

Computed Tomography I

I. IMAGING CHAIN

A. X-Ray Tubes

- Figure 11.1 shows the essential components of the x-ray imaging chain.
- **Power** to the x-ray tube is **supplied** to the tube by **slip ring** technology with high voltages delivered through contact rings in the gantry.
- Tube **voltages** range from **70 to 150 kV**, but the user can only select from 4 or 5 specified values in that range (e.g., 70, 100, 120, 150 kV).
  - Lower voltages (70 kV) are utilized for pediatric imaging and higher voltages (150 kV) to improve penetration in obese patients.

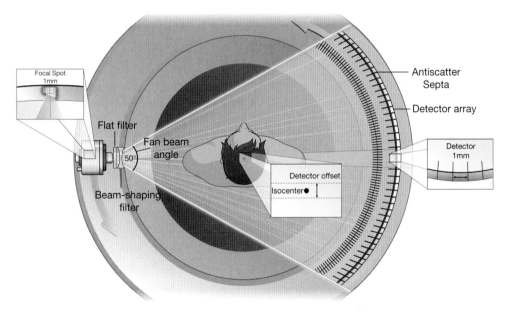

FIG 11.1 Schematic of the x-ray tube and detector array in a third-generation scanner where both the x-ray tube and detector array rotate around the patient (isocenter). The key components include the x-ray tube focus, flat filter, beam-shaping filters, antiscatter septa/grid, and detector array (scintillators). Quarter detector offset eliminates data redundancies when the same anatomy is imaged at opposing angles and improves radial sampling that helps to minimize in-plane aliasing and improve spatial resolution. The size of the focal spot and detector are generally the key determinants of the best achievable resolution performance.

- **Tube currents** can reach **1,000 mA.**
- The shortest **rotation time** for a **360°** rotation of the x-ray tube is about **0.2 seconds.**
  - Rotation times were ~3 seconds in the 1980s and ~1 s in the 1990s.
  - Short rotation times limit the maximum mA available due to heating concerns.
- At a given tube voltage (kV), x-ray output is the product of the tube current (mA) and the x-ray tube rotation time (s)—mAs.
  - Selected **mAs** is only a *relative* indicator of **CT radiation**, since the absolute **radiation output** depends on **tube design** and **voltage (kV).**
- CT scanners generally have a **large focal spot** (**1.2 mm**) and a **small focal spot** (**0.6 mm**).
  - New scanners may have a third extrasmall size for musculoskeletal imaging **(0.4 mm).**
- The x-ray tube **anode-cathode axis** is positioned **perpendicular** to the **imaging plane** to **reduce** the **heel effect.**
  - The heel effect is prominent in cone beam systems and requires extra mitigation from image processing.

B. Filtration

- **Filtration** on computed tomography (CT) x-ray tubes is **generally higher** than that in radiography and general fluoroscopy.
  - **Heavy filtration reduces** x-ray **beam hardening effects.**
  - **Special filters** (e.g., tin) may also be used to better separate high and low energies needed for **dual-energy scanning.**
- **Bow tie filters** are used in CT imaging and attenuate little along the central ray.
- In a bow tie filter, beam attenuation increases with increasing distance from this central ray, as shown in Figure 11.2.
- As attenuation is reduced at the patient periphery, filtration increases to compensate.
  - **Bow tie filters** are made of a **low–atomic number (Z) material** such as Teflon to **minimize beam hardening differences** with tissues.
- Use of **bow tie filters** results in all detectors receiving similar exposures (**reduced dynamic range**).
  - Without bow tie filters, transmission through thinner body regions results in higher detector signals and beam hardening artifacts would increase.
- **Bow tie filters** also help to **reduce scatter** and **patient dose.**
  - CT scanners normally have different **bow tie filters** for scanning an adult **head**, adult **body**, and **pediatric patients** and for **cardiac** imaging.
- Effective use of bow tie filters requires the patient to be **accurately centered** in the CT gantry **isocenter.**
  - **Incorrect centering** results in **poor image** quality (noise) and may result in **unnecessary radiation** dose to the patient.

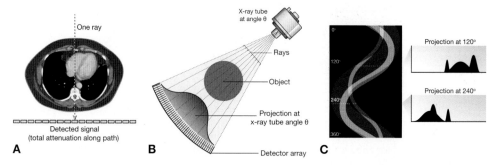

FIG 11.2 A: A ray measures the total attenuation along the x-ray beam path length that corresponds to one detector at a given x-ray tube angle; **B:** A projection is all the rays at a single x-ray tube projection angle; **C:** A sinogram is a plot of all the projections versus x-ray tube angle.

C. **Scatter Removal and Detectors**

- Scanners have **antiscatter collimation** in the form of **thin lamellae** (Fig. 11.1) or 2D cross-hatched collimators.
- **Antiscatter collimation** is located **between** the **detector elements** oriented along the long patient axis and aligned with the x-ray focus.
- CT scanners use **scintillators** that produce light when x-ray photons are absorbed with **low afterglow characteristics.**
  - **Scintillation detectors** are **coupled** to **light detectors.**
- **Detectors** absorb most of the incident x-ray photon energy (i.e., high **quantum detection efficiency**).
  - CT scintillators generally have **detection efficiencies higher** than **90%.**
- In CT detectors, an electric signal is produced that is proportional to the incident radiation intensity.
  - **Multislice** scanners and short gantry rotation times result in extremely **high data output rates (bandwidth)** from the CT detectors.
- A small (or zero) number of **photons reaching** the **detector** is referred to as **photon starvation.**
- **Obese patients** cause very **low detector signals.**
  - When x-ray **signals** are **low, electronic noise** can become significant, and x-ray detection is **no longer quantum mottle limited.**

D. **CT Geometry**

- A **third-generation** scanner (i.e., **tube and detector both rotate**) is shown in Figure 11.1.
  - Virtually **all current clinical** CT systems use **third-generation acquisition geometry.**
- **CT scanners** have a distance from the x-ray tube focus to the isocenter of about 60 cm, and a **magnification 1.5×–2×.**
  - Detector dimensions in CT are their size projected to the isocenter (i.e., actual physical sizes are 1.5×–2× the quoted values).
- A **fan beam angle** (Fig. 11.1) of **50°** corresponds to a **field of view** (FOV) with a **50 cm diameter.**
  - Larger fan angles with more detectors are needed to produce larger FOVs.
- There will be roughly **1,000 individual detectors** in an arc with dimensions as small as 0.5 mm measured at isocenter.
- CT scanners are designed so that the central rays of projections acquired at **0° and 180° do not overlap** but are **offset** by **half a detector width** (Fig. 11.1).
  - A quarter detector **offset improves data sampling** and the corresponding spatial resolution performance.
- Midrange scanners generate **64 to 128 axial slices** in a **single rotation.**
  - **Craniocaudal coverage in a single rotation would be 40 mm (64 detectors × 0.625 mm per detector).**
  - Some 128-slice scanners still have 40 mm coverage, since they use two slightly offset focal spots (i.e., **flying focal spot**) to improve through-plane resolution.

II. THEORY

A. **Axial (Step and Shoot) Acquisitions**

- In **axial scanning,** the table and **patient** remain **stationary** while the x-ray tube rotates through 360° and acquires the necessary projection data (Fig. 11.1).
- At a given location of the x-ray tube, **each individual detector measures** the **x-ray transmission** through the patient, referred to as a **ray.**
- Each ray measures the total attenuation in the patient along a line in one detector (Fig. 11.2A).
  - **CT images** are two-dimensional **patterns** of **x-ray attenuation coefficients.**

- The **collection of rays** for all the detectors in each slice at a **given tube angular position** is called a **projection** (Fig. 11.2B).
- **Each projection** has about **1,000 individual data points** corresponding to the 1,000 individual detectors (rays) in a single detector array.
- **Projection data sets** are **acquired** at **different angles around** the **patient**.
- A CT image generally requires **1,000 projections** for a **single rotation** of the x-ray tube.
- A graphical plot of **projection** versus **x-ray tube angle** is called a **sinogram** (Fig. 11.2C).
  - **Each** reconstructed **slice** always requires a complete **sinogram**.
- **Axial scanning** is much **slower than helical scanning** and is typically used only with cone beam detectors and special protocols.

B. Helical Acquisitions

- In **helical scanning**, the **patient moves** through the CT gantry at the same time **as the x-ray tube rotates**.
  - **Helical scanning** is primarily used to **reduce** the total CT **scan time**.
  - A 40 mm coverage scanner will take **one-fifth the time to perform a brain scan in helical mode** compared to axial mode.
- **CT pitch** is the **table increment distance during a 360° rotation of the x-ray tube divided by** the **nominal x-ray beam width**.
- If a **table moves 40 mm per 360°** rotation of the x-ray tube on a 64 multidetector computed tomography (MDCT) scanner (i.e., **beam width 40 mm**), the **pitch is 1**.
  - A table movement of **20 mm** corresponds to a **pitch of 0.5** and table movement of **80 mm** corresponds to a **pitch of 2**.
- At any given long patient axis (z-axis) position, **helical CT** scanning **provides one** of the **1,000 projections** that are **required** (see sinogram in Fig. 11.2C).
- There are **999 lines "missing,"** which are **obtained** using **interpolation algorithms**.
  - At each x-ray tube angle location, use is made of projections available "upstream" and "downstream" of the z-axis location of interest.
- **After interpolation** has been performed, a **sinogram** is **generated at each z-axis location** where image reconstruction is to be performed.
- In helical scanning, **effective mAs** is the **(true) mAs divided** by the **CT pitch**.
- **Effective mAs** is helpful to **predict dose** and **image quality** in **helical CT**.
  - **Increasing effective mAs** always **increases** patient **dose** and always **reduces** image **mottle**.

C. Filtered Back Projection

- Generating an image from the acquired data involves determining the linear attenuation coefficients of the individual image pixel.
- Data in **sinograms** are the **essential prerequisite** to **reconstruct** a **CT slice**.
- **Filtered back projection (FBP)** image reconstruction algorithms multiply projection data by a **mathematical reconstruction filter/kernel**.
  - This is **a computer algorithm, not a physical filter** like the bow tie.
- These **filtered projections** subsequently **undergo** a process of **back projection**.
  - **Back projection smears each projection back across the whole image at the angle it was acquired**.
- FBP is computationally inexpensive but has given way in recent years to advanced reconstruction methods that improve image quality.
- The **same sinogram data can be reconstructed changing kernel, FOV, thickness, and orientation** without the need to dose the patient multiple times.

D. Reconstruction Filters/Kernels

- Many **different reconstruction kernels can be chosen,** and each gives a slightly different image quality.
- There is always a **trade-off between spatial resolution and noise** when selecting a reconstruction kernel.

	Relative Image Noise Values, and the Corresponding Image Sharpness, a Range of Reconstruction Kernel Used in Filtered Back Projection (FBP) Image Reconstruction		
TABLE 11.1			
FBP Reconstruction Kernel	**Relative Noise**	**Qualitative Image Sharpness**	
Smooth	1	Blurred	
Standard (soft tissue)	1.5	Average	
Bone	3	Sharp	
Bone plus (edge)	5	Very sharp	

- Some vendors use application-specific names (bone or soft tissue kernel), whereas others use names such as H40 (head) or B70 (body).
- Some **kernels (e.g., bone) increase** both **resolution and noise**, whereas others (e.g., **soft tissue) reduce noise** and **resolution.**
  - Some may also alter Hounsfield unit (HU) values (especially for high HU materials).
- Table 11.1 shows how the amount of noise, and the corresponding image sharpness, in reconstructed CT images depends on the choice of kernel.
- Detection of large **low-contrast liver lesions** would use a **kernel** that **reduces noise.**
- Imaging an **inner ear** would use **a kernel** that offers the **best resolution.**
  - With high intrinsic contrast (i.e., bone vs air), increased noise is of little importance.
- **Each sinogram** can be **reconstructed** using any **number** of **kernels**, but this requires **viewing multiple image series.**

E. **Advanced Reconstruction**
  - **Iterative reconstruction (IR)** algorithms approach the correct solution using multiple iteration steps.
  - Each IR algorithm starts with an **assumed image** and then **computes projections** from the image.
    - **Computed projections** are then **compared** with the actual **acquired projections** from the patient.
  - **Improvements** in the image are based upon **difference** between a **calculated projection** and an **acquired (patient) projection.**
  - The process is **repeated (iterated) several times until** the **agreement** between a **calculated projection** and an **acquired (patient) projection** is **satisfactory.**
  - **IR algorithms** generally offer **better reconstruction** at the cost of a much **higher computation time.**
    - **Statistical iterative reconstruction** algorithms generally **reduce noise** and **some artifacts (e.g., streak).**
  - **Model-based IR algorithms** offer amazing quality by accounting for scanner degradations (e.g., focal spot size) but **require exceptionally long computation times** (e.g., 1 h per series).
  - **Deep-learning algorithms** are typically trained on model-based IR algorithms to give a similar quality but perform much faster.

III. IMAGES

A. **Hounsfield Units**
  - **CT images** are **maps** of the **relative linear attenuation values** of tissues.
  - Relative **attenuation coefficients (μ)** are expressed as **CT numbers** or **HU.**
    - **Godfrey Hounsfield** was one of the pioneers of clinical CT in the early **1970s.**
  - **HU** of a material is the **attenuation** of the **material relative** to the corresponding **attenuation** by **water.**
    - **Positive HU** values indicate attenuation **greater** than that of **water,** and **negative HU** values indicate attenuation **less** than that of **water.**

- By definition, the **HU value** for **water** is **always 0 HU**, and the **HU value** for **air** is calibrated to **−1,000 HU**.
- At **120 kV**, the HU for **fat** is approximately **−100 HU**, for soft **tissues** approximately **50 HU**, and for compact **bone > 1,000 HU**.
- Lesions with an **HU value** of **10 attenuate 1% more than water**, and an **HU value** of **−10 attenuate 1% less than water**.
- **HU values may differ** across scanners or even from one visit to another due to machine and patient setup variations.

B. HU and X-Ray Energy

- **Attenuation coefficients** are generally **dependent** on **photon energy (keV)**.
  - HU values will change with **kV** and **filtration**.
- Table 11.2 lists typical HU values for a range of tissues as a function of photon energy.
  - **Positive HU values increase** as **photon energy decreases**, and vice versa.
- The **energy dependenc**e of material's **HU** also depends on the **material atomic number** relative to that of water (7.5).
- **Changes** in **HU** with energy are **large** for **high Z** materials such as **iodine (Z = 53).**
  - Diluted iodine with an HU of **400** at 80 kV would likely have an HU of only **100** at 140 kV.
- Tissues with **atomic numbers close** to **water (e.g., brain)** show modest **changes in HU** with **photon energy** that are of **little clinical importance.**
  - Soft tissue HU values drop from **60** to **50 HU** as tube **voltage increases** from 80 to 140 kV.

C. Pixels and Voxels

- The display or reconstruction **field of view (dFOV)** is the **diameter** of image being reconstructed.
  - It is smaller than the scan field of view (sFOV) which is the largest diameter image that could be faithfully reconstructed.
- A **head CT** may have an **FOV** of **250 mm** and a **body CT** an FOV of **400 mm.**
- Image **matrix sizes** in **CT** are generally **512 × 512** except in very special circumstances where high spatial resolution is required.
- **Pixel sizes** are **~0.5 mm** for a **head** scan (i.e., 250/512 mm) and **0.8 mm** for a **body** scan (i.e., 400/512 mm).
- **Smaller pixels** do **not improve resolution** once the **inherent limits** have been **reached.**
  - Fundamental factors that **limit CT resolution** are **sizes** of the **focal spot** and **detector element.**
- For MDCT, the acquired **slice thickness** is generally **~0.6 mm, but the slices are reconstructed thicker.**
- **Display 0.6 mm thick slices** would result in **too many images** (1,000 for a 60 cm long scan)
  - **Thin slices** would also appear **very noisy** because of the limited number of photons making each image.
- **CT images** are normally reconstructed with a **3 or 5 mm slice thickness,** unless high resolution is required.

TABLE 11.2	Hounsfield Unit (HU) Values Computed at Different Photon Energies			
Photon Energy	Photon Energy (keV)			
	40	50	60[a]	80
Fat	−150	−110	−90	−70
Soft tissue	62	58	54	52
Dilute iodine	410	270	180	90

Dilute iodine HU factor is obtained by dividing the computed iodine HU by 1,000.
[a]Average energy expected for CT spectra obtained at 120 kV.

D. CT Image Data

- **CT image** contains a **quarter of a million pixels (i.e., 512 × 512).**
- **Each pixel** is coded using **12 bits**, which requires 2 bytes of computer memory.
  - Only 12 of the available 16 bits in 2 bytes are used.
- Using **12 bits** enables **4,096 shades** of **gray** to be generated (i.e., 2^{12}).
- Each **CT image** thus has a computer storage requirement of **0.5 MB** (quarter of a million pixels × 2 bytes per pixel).
  - A complete **chest/abdomen/pelvis CT** series with 100 images would require storage of **50 MB.**
- Acquired (raw) data have a higher storage requirement, because **each sinogram** requires up to **2 MB** of data per slice.
  - There may also be **ten times more acquired (thin) slices than displayed (thick) slices.**
- **Acquired data** are required to **modify** the **dFOV**, slice thickness, or **kernel without dosing the patient.**
  - **Acquired data** are **not sent** to **PACS (picture archiving and communication system)** because of extra storage.

E. Image Display

- **CT** examinations are viewed on **3 megapixel monitors.**
- The **monitor brightness** of each CT pixel is related to the **pixel HU value.**
  - Higher HU values by convention appear brighter, reflecting their increased x-ray attenuation.
- The HU values of any pixel **never changes**, but its **brightness** can be **modified** by adjusting **window** and **level settings.**
- Choice of **level (center) value** affects the **brightness** of a given pixel.
  - As level increases, lesion brightness is reduced, and vice versa.
- Choice of **window value** affects the **contrast** of a pixel relative to its neighbors.
  - As **window width increas**es, displayed **image contrast is reduced**, and vice versa.
- Figure 11.3A shows how the **window and level settings** act to **map pixel values** (horizontal axis) **to monitor brightness** (vertical axis).
- Figure 11.3A (**window width 100 HU** and **window level 50 HU**) has all HU **less than 0 HU appearing black**, and all HU **greater than 100 HU appearing white.**
  - In Figure 11.3A, the **HU of 50 appears midgray**, but changing the level to 100 makes it appear black, while a level of 0 makes it appear white.
- Figure 11.3B shows **lung** and **mediastinal** displays in **chest CT.**

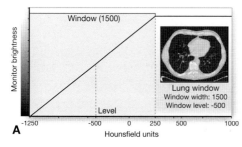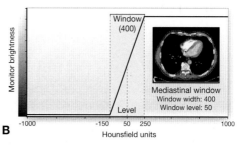

FIG 11.3 Graphical depiction how the choice of a window width, and corresponding window level, map the pixel HU values (horizontal axis), which are fixed, into monitor brightness (vertical axis), which is adjustable. **A:** A typical CT lung display uses a level of −500 HU and a window width of 1,500 HU. **B:** A typical CT mediastinum display uses a level of 50 HU and a window width of 450 HU. A typical head display uses a level of 40 HU and a window width of 80 HU. A typical liver display uses level of 60 HU and a window width of 150 HU. HU, Hounsfield unit.

IV. CT OUTPUT

A. Quantity

- Vendors specify the **output of CT scanners** by measuring energy deposition (**dose**) in **acrylic cylinders.**
- Phantom measurements are expressed as **volume computed tomography dose index (CTDI$_{vol}$) in mGy.**
  - CTDI$_{vol}$ **better reflects CT output than mAs,** as shown in Figure 11.4A.
- For a given set of techniques (kV, mA, rotation time, and pitch), **CTDI$_{vol}$** can be made in a **small (16 cm diameter)** phantom—CTDI$_{vol}$(S), or a **large (32 cm diameter)** phantom—CTDI$_{vol}$(L).
- Using identical techniques (kV and mAs) a **small phantom records twice the phantom dose as a large phantom.**
  - CTDI$_{vol}$**(S) of 10 mGy and CTDI$_{vol}$(L) of 5 mGy** indicate the **same CT output** (Fig. 11.4B).
- For a given patient examination, an **increase in CTDI$_{vol}$** simply indicates that **more radiation** is being **used** to perform the **CT examination.**
  - For a given patient, **using more radiation reduces** image **mottle** and also **increases patient dose.**
- At constant kV, **CTDI$_{vol}$** is directly **proportional to mAs,** and at constant mAs, directly **proportional to kV$^{2.6}$.**
  - Increasing the **x-ray tube from 80 to 140 kV**, with no adjustment to the mAs, increases CT output by a factor of 5 (i.e., **500%).**
- **Dose-length product (DLP)** is the **product** of **CTDI$_{vol}$** and **scan length**, which is expressed in **mGy-cm.**
  - Since DLP is based on CTID$_{vol}$, it will also depend on small or large phantom use.
- **DLP measures** the **total amount** of **radiation (energy) incident** on a **patient.**
  - **DLP** will be approximately proportional to the **total energy imparted** to the patient, and the corresponding **patient stochastic radiation risk.**

B. Effective mAs

- In planar x-ray imaging (e.g., radiography), **increasing mAs will increase dose and reduce noise.**
  - This is true in step-and-shoot CT scanning as well.
- Helical scanning introduces pitch as a factor.
- Two scans with the same mAs but different pitch will deliver different dose and different noise.
  - **High pitch will reduce dose and increase noise** for the same mAs.

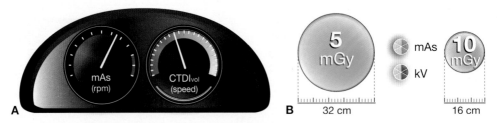

FIG 11.4 A: Car tachometers do not quantify speed (left), and x-ray tube output is not quantified by the mAs alone because it neglects tube voltage, beam filtration, and x-ray tube design. Computed tomography dose index (CTDI) is an absolute measure of x-ray tube output, analogous to the speed-ometer on any automobile (right). **B:** For fixed techniques (kV, mAs) with a constant CT output, CTDI measurements made on small (16 cm diameter) phantoms will be twice those made in large (32 cm diameter) phantoms. Vendors specify CT output for a pediatric abdomen using the 32 cm or 16 cm phantom, so phantom size must always be provided. CT, computed tomography.

- **Effective mAs is the mAs/pitch** and preserves the idea that higher effective mAs gives more dose and less noise for helical scanning.
- If **tube current modulation (TCM)** is used, the mA will increase as pitch increases to **keep dose and noise constant.**

C. Quality

- **X-ray beam qualities in CT (i.e., half-value layer [HVL])** are **relatively high** because the beams use **heavy filtration.**
- X-ray beam **quality** is primarily **controlled by** the choice of x-ray **tube voltage.**
  - Increasing the kV will result in higher average photon energies.
- Table 11.3 shows values of typical x-ray tube voltages, average photon energies, and the resultant HVLs normally encountered in CT.
- **Higher** x-ray beam **qualities increase patient penetration** but **reduce** image **contrast.**
  - High kV is used to ensure enough radiation penetrates the patient to hit the detector.
- **Increasing CT beam quality** *only* **reduces patient doses** when **tube output (mAs)** is **adjusted** so that **intensity K_{air}** at the CT detectors is kept constant.

D. Patient Transmission

- **Patient transmission** is determined by **beam quality** as well as **tissue atomic number (Z), density (ρ),** and **thickness.**
- Most patients are considered to be soft tissue with an atomic number of 7.5 and a density of about 1 g/cm^3.
- For soft tissues, and the high beam qualities used in most **CT**, the **tissue HVL** is about **4 cm.**
- Patient thickness for a neonate body is about 10 cm, but this can increase to 50 cm for the largest obese adults.
  - This **increase** in **thickness** for **patients** (i.e., **40 cm**) corresponds to **10 tissue HVLs.**
- At constant beam quality, an **obese adult transmits 1,000× less radiation** than a **neonate** (i.e., 2^{10}, or 1024).
  - CT images of **large patients** are likely **unsatisfactory (i.e., noisy/mottled)** because so **little radiation** reaches the **CT detectors.**
- Table 11.4 shows how x-ray beam transmission varies with beam quality and patient size.

TABLE 11.3	Nominal Values Effective Photon Energies, and the Corresponding Half-Value Layers for the X-Ray Tube Voltages Commonly Used in CT Imaging	
X-Ray Tube Voltage (kV)	Effective Photon Energy (keV)	Half-Value Layer (mm Al)
80	40	4.5
100	50	7
120	60	9
140	70	11

CT, computed tomography

TABLE 11.4	Transmission of CT X-Ray Beams (80 and 120 kV) Through Soft Tissue	
Tissue Thickness (cm)	Transmission at 80 kV (%)	Transmission at 120 kV (%)
10	8.6	12
15	3.0	4.5
20	1.0	1.8
30	0.12	0.26
40	0.015	0.040

CT, computed tomography.

- **Beam quality** must be **increased** in **larger patients** to improve **penetration.**
  - When **patient penetration** is **inadequate** (i.e., negligible), **adjusting** the **mA** does **not improve image quality.**

E. **Automatic Exposure Control**
  - **Radiography, mammography,** and **fluoroscopy** all use a **radiation detector** at the **image receptor,** whereas **CT does not.**
  - CT automatic exposure control (**AEC$_{CT}$**) typically **requires** operators to **manually set a reference kV, reference mA or noise index, pitch,** and **rotation time (s)** for an **average patient.**
  - **AEC$_{CT}$ TCM increases** the **mA** when patient **attenuation increases,** and **reduces** the **mA** when patient **attenuation** is **reduced (Fig. 11.5).**
    - Commercial systems may have an operator-selected **maximum** and **minimum mA** that can be used.
  - **Tube currents** are **modulated** as the **x-ray tube rotates** around the patient (**angular modulation**).
  - **Tube currents** are **modulated** as the **patient moves** through the CT gantry (**longitudinal modulation**).
  - Changes in **patient size** (i.e., attenuation) will require **CT tube currents** to be **adjusted,** with **smaller patients requiring less radiation,** and vice versa.
  - The scanner knows the attenuation based on the **prescan localizer radiograph (some systems also use projection data).**
  - **AEC$_{CT}$ automated kV selection** selects a low kV when the patient is small and high-Z materials are the object of interest.
    - Operators select a "strength" indicating how aggressive the system is at reducing kV.
    - Strength is typically set **high for angiography and low for noncontrast adult studies.**
  - Low kV allows for **higher contrast in iodine and bone and lower doses for small patients** but may cause an **increase in noise** due to low penetration.

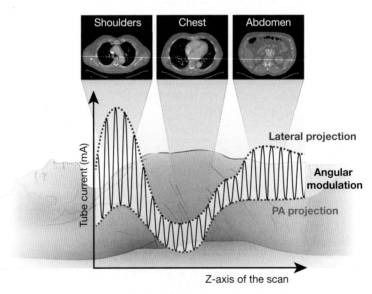

FIG 11.5 Tube current modulation is a type of automatic exposure control where the mA is reduced when patient attenuation is low. Tube current is high in the shoulder region, drops in the chest (low attenuating air in lung), and increases in the thicker pelvic region. As the tube revolves around the patient more mA is used in lateral projections (red line) since the patient is more attenuating (thicker) than in AP-PA projections (blue line). AP, anteroposterior; PA, posteroanterior.

Chapter 11 (Computed Tomography I) Questions

11.1 What modality has the highest filtration?
A. Mammography
B. Radiography
C. General fluoroscopy
D. Computed tomography

11.2 How do focal spot sizes for CT compare to radiography?
A. Much larger
B. Similar
C. Much smaller

11.3 What factor is considered by the machine when selecting the beam-shaping filter (i.e., bow tie)?
A. kV
B. mAs
C. Scan type (helical vs axial)
D. Protocol body part

11.4 Removing the lamellae/grid would likely make what image quality property worse?
A. Contrast
B. Resolution
C. Mottle
D. Artifacts

11.5 What percentage of incident x-rays (120 kV) is typically absorbed by a CT detector?
A. ≤10%
B. 30%
C. 70%
D. ≥90%

11.6 What is the geometric magnification at bore isocenter?
A. 0.5
B. 1.0
C. 2.0
D. 4.0

11.7 What is the pitch for a CT scan with x-ray tube rotation time of 0.5 s, beam width of 40 mm, and table speed of 160 mm/s?
A. 0.5
B. 1
C. 1.5
D. 2

11.8 How does patient dose change if both CT pitch and effective mAs are doubled and tube current modulation is not used?
A. Doubles
B. Not affected
C. Halved
D. Quatruple

11.9 How does image noise change if receptor dose quadruples in CT?
A. 1/4×
B. 1/2×
C. 2×
D. 4×

11.10 Which reconstruction kernel will have the lowest level of image noise (mottle)?
A. Ramp
B. Bone
C. Edge
D. Smooth

11.11 Which reconstruction method is most likely to result in the "best" CT images?
A. Back projection
B. Filtered back projection
C. Iterative reconstruction (statistical)
D. Iterative reconstruction (model based)

11.12 What do CT images depict?
A. X-ray attenuation
B. X-ray transmission
C. Pixel mass
D. Voxel density

11.13 What is the difference in x-ray attenuation coefficient between gray (40 HU) and white matter (34 HU)?
A. 0.2%
B. 0.6%
C. 2%
D. 6%

11.14 When x-ray tube voltage decreases from 140 to 80 kV, what tissue will show the highest increase in HU?
A. CSF
B. Gray matter
C. Fat
D. Bone

11.15 What is the typical in-plane pixel dimension for a head CT?
  A. 0.1 mm
  B. 0.2 mm
  C. 0.5 mm
  D. 1.0 mm

11.16 How much storage space is needed for a head CT examination with 20 images?
  A. 1 MB
  B. 10 MB
  C. 100 MB
  D. >100 MB

11.17 Which CT image most likely uses the greatest display window width?
  A. Head (tissue)
  B. Chest (mediastinum)
  C. Chest (lung)
  D. Abdomen (liver)

11.18 How does AEC for CT impact tube voltage?
  A. Modulates the voltage based only on patient thickness in a slice
  B. Selects the voltage based on user settings and patient attenuation
  C. Modulates the voltage based on user settings and patient attenuation
  D. Selects the voltage for the scan based on patient thickness

11.19 Low kV increases HU of iodine in abdominal angiography but makes what image property worse?
  A. Contrast
  B. Noise
  C. Temporal resolution
  D. Spatial resolution

11.20 What percentage of the incident CT x-ray beam intensity is most likely transmitted through 45 cm of soft tissue?
  A. 1
  B. 0.3
  C. 0.1
  D. <0.1

Answers and Explanations

11.1 **D** (Computed tomography). CT has extensive filtration to reduce beam hardening and the artifacts that it causes.

11.2 **B** (Similar). For CT x-ray tubes, the small focal spot is ~0.6 mm and large focal spot ~1.2 mm. CT resolution is lower than that of radiography due to other factors (e.g., reconstruction).

11.3 **D** (Protocol body part). The filter compensates for the changing thickness of the body part being imaged. Choosing a cardiac or head protocol will impact the filter used during scanning.

11.4 **A** (Contrast). Removing lamellae/grid will allow more scatter to hit the receptor and thereby decrease image contrast.

11.5 **D** ($\geq$90%). CT detectors are usually thick scintillators with high Z that have excellent x-ray attenuation properties and absorb most of incident x-ray photons (i.e., $\geq$90%).

11.6 **C** (2.0). Geometric magnification is 1.5$\times$ – 2$\times$, with a typical focus to the isocenter distance of about 60 cm, and double this distance between the focus and CT detector array.

11.7 **D** (2). In one x-ray tube rotation (0.5 s), the table moves 80 mm, which is twice the x-ray beam width (40 mm), so the pitch is 2.

11.8 **A** (Double). Patient dose is directly proportional to effective mAs. Since effective mAs is the mAs divided by pitch, doubling effective mAs at twice the pitch value requires that the mAs be quadrupled (i.e., patient dose doubles).

11.9 **B** (1/2$\times$). Noise will roughly go as the square root of dose and thus will double if dose is quadrupled.

11.10 **D** (Smooth). Using a smooth kernel minimizes noise (as suggested by the name) but also provides the blurriest images.

11.11 **D** (IR model based). Model-based iterative reconstruction techniques offer improved image quality but are computationally intensive. Scientists hope deep learning will allow similar quality increases with reduced computation cost.

11.12 **A** (x-ray ray attenuation). CT images are two-dimensional patterns of x-ray linear attenuation coefficients.

11.13 **B** (0.6%). HU of gray matter is about 6 HU higher than that of white matter. Each increase of 1 HU corresponds to an increase of about 0.1% in attenuation.

11.14 **D** (Bone). Bone shows (by far) the largest increase in HU when kV decreases, because its atomic number (Z = 14) is furthest away from that of water (Z = 7.5).

11.15 **C** (0.5 mm). A head is about 250 mm, and a CT image is typically a matrix size of 512 $\times$ 512, so the pixel dimension is 0.5 mm (i.e., 250 mm divided by 512).

11.16 **B** (10 MB). One CT image has 250,000 pixels (500 $\times$ 500) and requires 2 bytes for each pixel. One CT image is thus 0.5 megabytes (250,000 pixels $\times$ 2 bytes/pixel) so 20 CT images requires 10 MB.

11.17 **C** (Lung window). Displaying the lung in chest CT images use very wide windows (e.g., 1,500), whereas all the other displays would use narrower windows (e.g., <500).

11.18 B (Selects the voltage based on user settings and patient attenuation). The user will select reference voltage and a setting for aggressiveness, then the system will select a single voltage for the scan based on those settings and patient attenuation.

11.19 B (Noise). Low kV will increase iodine HU and thus increase contrast, but the lower penetration means there will be more noise in the image, unless dose is increased using other parameters like mA.

11.20 D (<0.1%). Much less than 0.1% of the incident x-ray beam is likely to reach the CT detector after passing through 45 cm of soft tissue, which explains why CT images of obese patients are generally of such poor quality (i.e., mottled or noisy).

CHAPTER 12
Computed Tomography II

I. CLINICAL IMAGING

A. Adult Head

- X-ray tube **voltages** in **head computed tomography (CT)** are typically **120 kV**.
- Increased tube voltages (e.g., **140 kV**) may be used in the **posterior fossa** to **minimize beam hardening artifacts.**
- Lower tube **voltages (e.g., 100 kV)** may be used in small pediatric and **angiographic imaging** where it maximizes the visibility of iodinated contrast media.
- The x-ray beam intensities in **head CT** are relatively high, using a **CTDI$_{vol}$(S) of 60 mGy.**
  - High intensities are required to **reduce mottle** and visualize subtle soft tissue structures (e.g., gray vs white matter).
- Table 12.1 shows the ACR (American College of Radiology) CT Accreditation reference doses for adult head CT examinations.
  - Typical site dose cannot exceed these falues for ACR accredited sites.
- Use of image processing (e.g., **iterative reconstruction**) has **reduced radiation (CTDI$_{vol}$)** used in head CT.
- **CTDI$_{vol}$** can be **reduced** when imaging **airways** and **bony structures** (i.e., high-contrast objects) because noise has less impact on visibility.
- **Dose-length product in the small ACR phantom (DLP(S))** for a routine head CT examination is roughly **1,000 mGy-cm** (i.e., 16 cm scan length).

B. Adult Body

- Tube **voltages** in **abdominal** and **pelvic CT** scanning are typically **100 to 120 kV**.
  - Lowering tube voltage reduces penetration in adult patients.
- An average-sized adult undergoing a routine **abdominal** and/or **pelvic CT** scan would use a **CTDI$_{vol}$(L) of 15 mGy.**
  - For the specific task of **detecting soft tissue lesions** (e.g., liver scan), the **CTDI$_{vol}$(L)** might be **increased** to **20 mGy.**

TABLE 12.1	Values of CTDI$_{vol}$ Associated With the ACR CT Accreditation Program			
Patient	Body Region	Phantom Size	Clinical CTDI$_{vol}$ (mGy)	"Failing" CTDI$_{vol}$ (mGy)
Adult	Head	Small	60	>80
	Abdomen	Large	15-20	>30
Pediatric	1-y-old head	Small	25	>40
	5-y-old abdomen	Small	5	>20

ACR, American College of Radiology; CT, computed tomography; CTDI$_{vol}$, volumetric computed tomography dose index.

- Table 12.1 shows the ACR CT Accreditation reference doses for adult abdominal CT examinations.
- Total **dose-length product in the large ACR phantom (DLP(L))** for an **abdominal** or **pelvic CT** (not both combined) scan is roughly **300 mGy-cm.**
  - An **abdominal/pelvic CT** scan would have a **DLP(L)** of about **500 mGy-cm.**
- **Chests** are less than attenuating than abdomens, and in chest CT, the **CTDI$_{vol}$(L)** is likely reduced (e.g., around **10 mGy**).
- For **contrast studies**, tube voltages for average and small patients are typically **100 kV** to increase the visibility (contrast-to-noise ratio [CNR]) of the iodinated material.
- **DLP(L)** for a typical **chest CT** examination is about **300 mGy-cm** (i.e., scan length of 30 cm).

C. Cardiac Imaging

- A CT coronary angiogram is acquired when the heart has its least motion: end diastole at <70 bpm and end systole at >70 bpm.
- **64-Slice (or greater)** CT is **essential** for cardiac scanning, to ensure both good **spatial** and **temporal resolution performance.**
  - With 4 cm of coverage, gating is needed to allow the scanner to acquire data at the same cardiac phase for different cardiac slices on successive RR intervals.
  - **Iodinated contrast** is administered, which is best imaged at the lowest possible x-ray tube **voltage (80 or 100 kV).**
- **Retrospective gating** studies acquire the necessary projections throughout the heart at all phases of the cardiac cycle.
  - Retrospective gating uses **low pitch (0.2-0.3),** which results in relatively **high patient doses (700 mGy-cm DLP; 10 mSv effective dose),** because the x-ray tube is kept on continuously.
- **Prospective gating** studies **minimize** patient **exposure (200 mGy-cm DLP; 3 mSv effective dose),** because the x-ray tube is **switched off** in most phases of the **cardiac cycle.**
  - Only one cardiac phase can be acquired in this technique.
- **Volume/wide-array CT scanners** have **beam widths** that are sufficiently wide to **capture** the **heart** in a **single rotation** of the x-ray tube (12-16 cm).
  - **Dual-source CT** scanners can operate at very **high pitch values (>2.0)** and may also be used to acquire the **complete cardiac data** in a **single heartbeat.**
- **Cardiac calcium scoring** studies can quantify calcium-only burden and is typically used for older patients.
  - A lower technique can be used due to the high Hounsfield unit (HU) of calcium (DLP 70 mGy-cm; 1 mSv effective dose).

D. Adults and Size

- An **adult head** can be modeled as a water cylinder with a diameter of **18 cm of water.**
  - Head size does not generally change much with adult patient size, age, or sex.
- **"Average-sized" adult abdomens** can be modeled as **water cylinders** with diameters of **28 cm,** and **chests** with diameters of **24 cm.**
- When **patient size changes** in body CT, it is essential to **modify** the **radiation output** so that acceptable amounts of radiation hit the **detectors.**
  - X-ray tube **voltage** (penetration) should to be **increased** in **larger patients** and may be **reduced** when scanning **infants** and young children and in angiographic studies.
- Figure 12.1 shows how the tube current needs to be adjusted for different-sized patients and varying x-ray tube voltages to keep **detector K$_{air}$ constant.**
  - In practice, detector K$_{air}$ is increased but not kept constant in bariatric patients, since visibility of their larger structure is less impacted by noise.
- At **120 kV,** reducing patient size from **24 to 18 cm** would require a **fivefold reduction in mAs.**
  - Increasing patient size from **24 to 42 cm** would require a **20-fold increase in mAs (not typically possible due to heating so kV is also increased).**

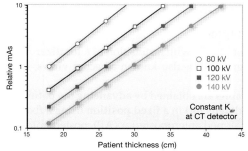

FIG 12.1 How mAs needs to be adjusted to maintain a constant K_{air} at the CT detectors when patient size changes at a given tube voltage. Data were normalized to unity at 120 kV for a 26 cm patient, and account for changes in patient transmission as well as x-ray tube output at each tube voltage (kV). Also shown is how mAs needs to be adjusted for a given patient size when x-ray tube voltage is modified (fixed detector K_{air}). CT, computed tomography.

- For a 26 cm patient, reducing the tube voltage from **120 to 80 kV** would require a **five-fold increase** in **mAs**.
  - Increasing tube voltage from **120 to 140 kV** would require **mAs** to be **halved**.
- Data in Figure 12.1 show that **maintaining** a constant amount of radiation at the image receptor (K_{air}) is **challenging**, even when kV is adjusted.

E. Pediatric

- **Noncontrast studies** in **infants** use roughly **80 kV**.
  - As patient size increases, x-ray tube voltage increases, and **large children** use **adult voltages (i.e., 120 kV)**.
- **Angiographic examinations** typically use the **low tube voltages (i.e., 80 kV)**.
  - When patient **penetration** at **80 kV** is **inadequate (i.e., too much noise)**, **100 kV** would be used.
- Tube current and rotation time (i.e., $CTDI_{vol}$) should be adjusted to ensure radiation intensity at the CT detector (K_{air}) and resultant image mottle are satisfactory.
- Pediatric CT typically requires lower **levels of mottle** than that in **adult CT due to less visceral fat, bone calcification, and smaller structures.**
- **Short rotation times** are used to **minimize motion blur** in young pediatric patients.
- Limiting the **scan length** and eliminating **unnecessary contrast phases** will substantially lower pediatric radiation dose.
- Going from adult to neonate $CTDI_{vol}$ and DLP drops 60% for the head and 90% for chest and abdomen/pelvis scans.
- Table 12.2 shows **kV and dose values** for performing abdominal CT scans of children as a function of **pediatric size**.
  - Data in Table 12.1 show the current **ACR CT Accreditation reference dose** for a **5-year-old abdomen** CT (20 kg).

TABLE 12.2	Typical Values for Abdominal Imaging in Infants and Small Children				
Weight (kg)	AP (cm)	Lateral (cm)	Tube Voltage (kV)	$CTDI_{vol}$(L) (mGy)	SSDE (mGy)[a]
<10	<13	<17	80	0.5-2	1-5
10-20	13-14	17-19.5	100	2-3	5-6
20-30	14-15.5	19.5-22	100-120	3-4	6-7
30-40	15.5-17	22-24.5	120	4-5	7-8
40-50	17-19	24.5-27	120	5-6	8-9

AP, anteroposterior; $CTDI_{vol}$(L), volumetric computed tomography dose index in the large phantom; SSDE, size-specific dose estimate.
[a]Size-Specific Dose Estimate.

- **Iodine maps** are not true iodine concentrations and should be considered semiquantitative.
- **Iodine removal** from contrast-enhanced scans generates a **virtual noncontrast (VNC) image** (Fig. 12.3).
  - VNC images often contain **more noise** and slightly **altered HU (e.g., in fat)** compared to true noncontrast images.
- **Dual-energy CT radiation dose is similar to a typical single-phase scan** and can be lower than a dual-phase scan if VNC is utilized.
- **Virtual monoenergetic** images at specific keV are created by processing the low- and high-voltage images.
  - **140 keV images mitigate metal artifact,** and **low-keV images (e.g., 50 keV) enhance iodine contrast.**
  - **Low-keV images are relatively noisy,** since they rely more on the low-voltage acquisition data where the beam is less penetrating.

D. CT Fluoroscopy

- **CT fluoroscopy** is the display of **constantly updated images** produced by **continuous rotation** of the x-ray tube.
  - Reconstructions are **near real time but cannot use advanced techniques resulting in worse image quality.**
- In CT fluoroscopy, the CT image is constantly updated to include the latest projection data (e.g., **60° increments**).
- Images are typically **updated** at the rate of **6 per second**, which provides **moderate temporal resolution.**
  - Fluoroscopy and ultrasound update images at **30 frames per second** for **real-time** imaging.
- CT fluoroscopy facilitates **advancement** of a **needle** for **biopsies** or drainage procedures.
- Standard x-ray **tube voltages (e.g., 120 kV)** are used in CT fluoroscopy.
- **Lower tube currents (20-50 mA)** are used compared to conventional CT (200-300 mA).
  - **Reducing** the **tube current** helps to **minimize radiation doses but increases noise.**
- Tube currents and radiation **dose** may be **further reduced** for diagnostic tasks such as tracking a **biopsy needle** where increased mottle does not affect performance.

III. IMAGE QUALITY

A. Contrast

- By definition, the **Hounsfield unit (HU)** of a **tissue** is the **contrast between** the **tissue and water** (HU = 0).
- **Changes** in **lesion contrast** most strongly **depend** on lesion **atomic number Z.**
- The **further away** the **lesion atomic number** is to that of **water (soft tissue),** the **more** the **change** in **lesion contrast** when **photon energy** is **adjusted.**
  - Large differences between lesion atomic number and that of water (soft tissue) result in big changes in lesion contrast when photon energy is adjusted.
- **CT subject contrast** is the **difference** in **intensity (HU value)** of a **lesion relative** to the **background tissues.**
- A **fat nodule** (HU of −90) in **soft tissue** (HU of 50), when imaged at 120 kV, **differs** by about **140 HU.**
  - **Fat attenuates** about **14% less** than **soft tissues.**
- A blood vessel that contains **dilute iodine (HU of 180)** will have a **contrast** of **130 HU compared** to **soft tissues (HU 50).**
- **Special reconstruction kernels, reconstruction methods, and dual-energy reconstructions** may alter contrast.
- AEC may select lower tube kV automatically to improve iodine contrast.

B. Noise

- **Mottle** in CT represents **random fluctuations** in **attenuation coefficient.**
- An image of a uniform water phantom with a **noise of ±3 HU** has **68%** of the **pixels** with HU values at **0 ± 3 HU.**
  - Ninety-five percent of pixels are at ±6 HU and 99% at ±9 HU.
- **CT mottle** depends primarily on the **number** of **x-ray photons** used to **make** the **image.**
- The number of **photons** composing a **CT image** is directly **proportional** to the **effective mA**, x-ray tube **rotation time (s),** and reconstructed **slice thickness.**
- **Quadrupling** the CT **tube current (mA)** will **halve** the resultant **mottle** because four times more photons were used to create the CT image.
  - **Quadrupling scan time, or slice thickness**, also **halves** image **mottle.**
- **Tube current modulation (TCM)** will produce more **consistent noise** over the entire scan by raising and lowering mA as needed.
- Use of reconstruction kernels producing **high spatial resolution** will **increase mottle.**
- Use of **iterative reconstruction** generally **reduces** that amount of **mottle** but **also changes noise texture.**
  - Simple **noise measures (e.g., standard deviation)** cannot assess performances of filtered back projection (FBP) versus iterative reconstruction methods because of **differences** in **noise texture.**

C. Temporal Resolution

- The **shortest time** that a **standard CT** imaging can acquire 1,000 projections during a **360° x-ray tube** rotation is currently close to **0.3 seconds.**
  - Some vendors claim rotations times as low as 0.2 seconds.
- **Temporal resolution** in standard CT, the time required to produce an image, is thus close to 250 ms.
- After an x-ray tube has **rotated** from **0° to 180°** plus the fan beam angle, it is possible to synthesize a set of projections pertaining to x-ray tube angles 180° to 360° (**rebinning**).
- **Image quality** of a **180° (i.e., half-scan reconstruction)** is **inferior** because of **reduced spatial sampling** and the use of about half the photons of a full 360° rotation.
- The **best achievable temporal resolution** on a standard CT scanner is approximately **half** the x-ray **tube rotation time** (i.e., **~150 ms**).
- **Dual-source CT** scanners acquire image data (projections) at double the rate of single-source scanners, offering better **temporal resolution** performance.
  - **Temporal resolution** of current **dual-source CT** scanners is about **75 ms,** one quarter of the x-ray tube rotation time.

D. Spatial Resolution

- **Focal spot size** and **detector element size** are hardware that **determine the in-plane spatial resolution.**
  - This is at **least 0.6 line pairs per mm (lp/mm) for a large FOV** and can exceed 1.5 lp/mm using a smaller FOV.
  - **Spatial resolution is worse for CT than planar x-ray modalities** (e.g., radiography at 4 lp/mm).
- Spatial resolution may be **worse than hardware limits** depending on **reconstructed pixel size, reconstruction kernel, and reconstruction type (e.g., FBP).**
- **Detector element size determines the maximum resolution** in the **longitudinal direction** (along the long patient axis).
  - Longitudinal spatial resolution will be **worse if thick slices** are reconstructed.
- For **musculoskeletal and inner ear** exam, resolution is maximized using the **smallest focal spot, sharp reconstruction kernel, and large matrix size (giving small pixels).**
- **Reducing x-ray tube rotation times** will help to **minimize motion blur.**
- **Detail (bone) reconstruction kernels** are used to achieve **the best possible resolution.**

- **Reconstructing** a smaller FOV than that of the acquired data means smaller pixel sizes to **improve resolution.**
- Once the **limits imposed** by **focal spot blur** and **detector blur** have been **reached, larger matrix sizes** (i.e., smaller pixels) and small focal spots do **not improve CT resolution.**
  - **Large body parts have worse resolution** due to larger reconstructed pixel sizes, a large focal spot to account for heat, and typically smoother kernel use.

E. **Artifacts**

- **Partial volume** artifact is the result of averaging the linear attenuation coefficient in a voxel that contains more than one material (e.g., air and water give HU close to fat).
  - Smaller reconstructed pixel sizes help.
- **Random motion** (e.g., moving pediatric patient) produces streaks and blur in the image (Fig. 12.4).
  - **Restraining** the patient or **faster acquisition times** help.
- **Photon starvation** is a lack of sufficient photons hitting the detector along some rays that pass through high-density structures and results in a directional noise in the image.
  - **TCM** (or other things to increase dose) and **iterative reconstruction** mitigate this artifact.
  - Scanning a patient with their **arms above their head** reduces streak artifacts in the chest.
- **Beam hardening** artifacts is caused by **lower-energy photons** being **preferentially absorbed**, resulting in a more penetrating (**higher energy) beam.**
- This causes **artificially low HU** (darker pixels) **far from the attenuator** and **high HU** (lighter pixels) **adjacent to the attenuator.**
  - **Software algorithms** that incorporate prior knowledge of the patient (e.g., skull in head CT) have been developed to **reduce beam hardening artifacts in the head.**
  - **Higher kV (including virtual monoenergetic)** can mitigate this artifact.
- **Metal implants** can be considered a combination of **photon starvation** and **beam hardening** (Fig. 12.4).
- A **single ring artifact** may arise when a **single detector** is **faulty.**
  - **Multiple ring artifacts** appear when a scanner is **not properly calibrated.**
  - Ring artifact may also occur if **so few photons hit the detector that electronic noise is large enough to be seen in the image.**
  - A ring artifact example is shown in Figure 12.4.
- **Truncation** artifact occurs when the patient exceeds the FOV and attenuation cannot be accounted for in the image (Fig. 12.4).
  - This often appears with a bright area at the edge of the image where unaccounted-for attenuation is piled up.
- **Aliasing artifacts** can occur when **edges** are image because of **inadequate data sampling** (i.e., too few detectors in each centimeter of the detector arc).
- **Cone beam artifacts** occur with large detectors due to **inadequate anatomical coverage** related to undersampling in the cone beam direction.

IV. DOSIMETRY

A. **Organ Doses**

- Key determinants of **organ doses** in CT are the amount of **radiation used** (i.e., $CTDI_{vol}$), **scan length**, and **patient size** (see Fig. 12.5).
- An **adult head and neck CT**, performed at a **$CTDI_{vol}(S)$ of 60 mGy**, wholly irradiates the brain, thyroid, and the eye lens.
- Doses to the **eye lens** will be about **55 mGy**, and **brain doses** are about **50 mGy.**
  - **Thyroid doses** are **65 mGy** and are higher than brain doses because of the **smaller size of** the **neck**, and the **absence** of **attenuation** by the **skull.**
- A **whole-body scan** on an average-sized patient, performed at a $CTDI_{vol}(L)$ of **20 mGy,** wholly irradiates virtually all organs and tissues of clinical importance.

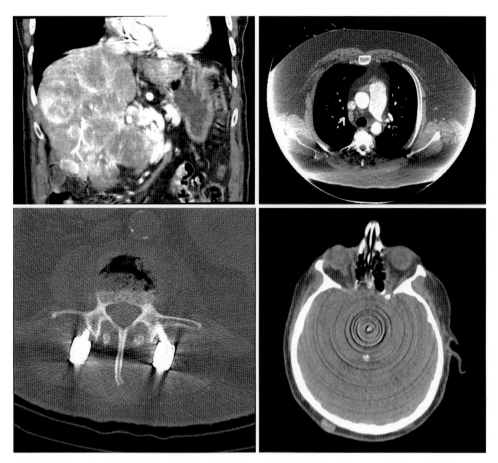

FIG 12.4 Top-Left: Motion artifact in a coronal abdomen reconstruction. The breathing motion causes duplicate surfaces at the lung interface and general blur throughout the image. Bottom-Right: Ring artifact can be seen in the axial head CT slice. This is likely due to poor detector calibration. Top-Right: Truncation artifact is visible in the chest CT of a bariatric patient. Note the brightness at the edge of the circular field of view. Beam hardening is also seen in the posterior portion of the image as a thick dark horizontal band across the patient. Bottom-Left: Metal artifact from fixation hardware is seen in the spine CT scan. Note the dark beam hardening bands between the metal. CT, computed tomography..

- Doses to the most sensitive organs doses are **red bone marrow (25 mGy)**, **lung (35 mGy), colon (30 mGy), stomach (30 mGy)**, and **breast (25 mGy)**.
  - Doses to moderately sensitive organs are the **bladder (35 mGy), liver (30 mGy), esophagus (40 mGy)**, and **thyroid (50 mGy)**.
- At **fixed CTDI$_{vol}$**, smaller patients (AP ~ 18 cm) have **organ doses** about **20% higher** than an average adult (AP ~ 23 cm).
  - **CTDI$_{vol}$** for the **small phantom** is **about double** CTDI$_{vol}$ for the **large phantom for the same exposure**.
- Absorbed doses in body **regions** that only **receive scattered radiation** are **very low compared to** organ doses in the directly irradiated volume.
- **Size-specific dose estimate (SSDE)** is CTDI$_{vol}$ times a correction factor based on patient size.
  - SSDE gives a better estimate of **average absorbed dose in a slice** than CTDI$_{vol}$ alone (Table 12.2).

B. Cancer Risks in CT

- For **chest CT** scans in **men, lung cancer** accounts for about **70%** of the **total cancer risks,** and **leukemia** for about **20%** of the total risk.
  - For **chest CT** scans in **20-year-old women, breast cancer** can contributes up to **45%** of the **total risk,** similar to the risk from lung cancer.
- For **abdomen scans** in **male individuals,** the most important organs contributing to the total **patient risk** are the **colon (~40%)** and the **stomach (~20%).**
  - For **abdomen scans** in **female individuals,** the principal contributors to **risk** are **stomach (25%), colon (25%),** and **lung (25%).**
- For **pelvic scans** in **male individuals,** the **bladder (40%), colon (30%),** and **prostate (20%)** are principal contributors to **patient cancer risk.**
  - In **female individuals** undergoing **pelvic scans, bladder (50%)** and **colon (20%)** are major contributors to **cancer risk.**
- **Average risks** from body CT scans (effective dose 5 mSv) are **0.06%** in a **25-year-old woman,** and **0.04%** in a **25-year-old man.**
  - These risks estimates are similar the **average risk of 0.1%** for a uniform whole-body dose **10 mSv** in a **25-year-old** used in radiation protection practice.

C. Adult Effective Doses

- For a given DLP, **CT organ doses** may be **combined into effective dose (E),** thereby providing **E/DLP conversion factors (k-factors).**
  - **E/DLP conversion factors** depend on the scanned **anatomy,** patient **age** and **size** but are generally **independent** of **tube voltage (kV).**
- **E/DLP factors** also depend on the **size** of **phantom** in which $CTDI_{vol}$ is measured.
  - When a **large phantom replaces** a **small phantom,** values of $CTDI_{vol}$ **and DLP** are **halved,** and **E/DLP** conversion factors are **doubled.**
- Table 12.3 shows E/DLP conversion factors for normal-sized adult patients undergoing a range of CT examinations.
  - **Effective doses,** which are always based on organ doses, will **change** with **patient size** in the **same manner** as **organ doses** (Fig. 12.5).
- Table 12.4 summarizes representative techniques, and the corresponding effective doses, for a normal-sized adult patient.

D. Pediatric Doses

- At **constant output, organ** and **effective dose** for **CT** examinations in infants and young children **increase** as **patient age** is **reduced.**
  - Table 12.5 shows how pediatric E/DLP conversion factors increase with decreasing age.
- When a **newborn** undergoes a **head CT** scan, the **E/DLP** conversion factor is about 12 μSv/mGy-cm, or **five times higher** than that for **adults** (2.4 μSv/mGy-cm).
- At a fixed x-ray tube output, **organ doses** generally **increase** as patient **size** is **reduced.**

TABLE 12.3	**E/DLP Conversion Factors for Normal-Sized Adult Patients**	
Scan Region	**E/DLP (μSv/mGy-cm) With CTDI$_{vol}$ Measured in:**	
	16 cm Diameter Phantom [S]	**32 cm Diameter Phantom [L]**
Head	2.4	4.9
Neck	5.3	11
Chest	10	20
Abdomen	8.2	16
Pelvis	7.1	14
Whole body	7.7	15

CTDI$_{vol}$, volumetric computed tomography dose index.

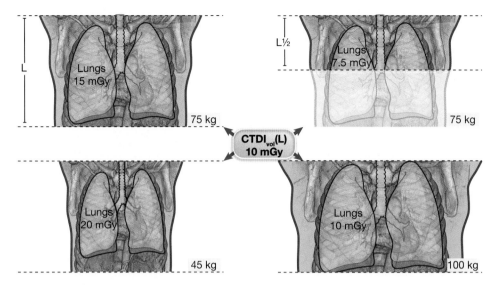

FIG 12.5 Organ doses depend primarily on the intensity used (CTDI$_{vol}$), scan length, and patient size. A chest CT performed at a CTDI$_{vol}$ of 10 mGy will result in a lung dose of about 15 mGy (upper left), but reducing the scan length to a half will also halve the resultant average lung dose (upper right). Reducing the patient size from 75 to 45 kg increases the lung dose for a complete chest CT to about 20 mGy (lower left), whereas increasing the patient size to 100 kg reduces the lung dose to about 10 mGy. CT, computed tomography; CTDI$_{vol}$, volumetric computed tomography dose index; CTDI$_{vol}$(L), volumetric computed tomography dose index in the large phantom.

- **- Smaller patients attenuate** the primary beam **less** than larger patients.
- Doses adjacent to the directly irradiated region increase because adjacent organs are much closer and have lower masses.
- A **1-year-old child** undergoing a **head CT** scan (CTDI$_{vol}$(S) 30 mGy and DLP(S) 480 mGy-cm) would have an effective dose of nearly **4 mSv.**
  - **- Infant effective doses** in head CT are nearly **twice** those of **adults,** despite **using** only **half** the **radiation.**
- A **1-year-old** child undergoing a **chest CT** scan (CTDI$_{vol}$(L) 2.5 mGy and DLP(L) 30 mGy-cm) would have an effective dose of nearly **2 mSv.**
  - **- A 1-year-old** has an **effective dose** a **third** of that of **adults** in chest CT, despite using **ten times less radiation.**

E. **Embryo/Fetal Doses**

- **Embryo** and **fetal doses** are very low to negligible if not directly in the x-ray beam.

TABLE 12.4	Adult Patient (70 kg) Effective Doses		
Body Region	**Head[a]**	**Chest[b]**	**Abdomen or Pelvis[b]**
CTDI$_{vol}$ (mGy)	60	10	15
Scan length (cm)	15	30	20
DLP (mGy-cm)	900	300	300
E/DLP (μSv/mGy-cm)	2.4	20	15
Effective dose (mSv)	2	6	4.5

CTDI$_{vol}$, volumetric computed tomography dose index; DLP, dose-length product; E, effective dose.
[a]Small phantom data.
[b]Large phantom data.

	E/DLP Conversion Factors for Children, Relative to Those of Normal-Sized	
TABLE 12.5	Adults, Undergoing CT Examinations	
Age (y)	$(E/DLP_{child})/(E/DLP_{adult})$	
10	1.6	
5	2.2	
1	3.3	
0 (newborn)	5.0	

CT, computed tomography, DLP, dose-length product; E, effective dose.

- Because this low dose is primarily due to internal scatter, **placing** a **lead apron** on the patient's abdomen would have **negligible effect** on **embryo doses.**
- **Doses** to the embryo/fetus are directly **proportional** to the total radiation (i.e., **CTDI$_{vol}$**).
- They also depend on **maternal size, gestational age, and scan length** (see Fig. 12.5).
- **Pulmonary embolism** is **most frequent CT indication** in pregnant patients (40% of all scans and 85% of chest scans).
  - Fetal dose typically ranges from **0.01 to 0.07 mSv** and increases with gestational age.
- **Appendicitis** is the most frequent indication for CT scan with the fetus in the FOV (30% of all scans and 58% of abdominopelvic scans).
  - **Mean fetal dose is 20 mSv** and only rises above 50 mSv with multiple phases.
  - **Fetal shielding** cannot be used, since it would **interfere the imaging.**
- A **qualified medical physicist** should be consulted if fetal dose may rise above **50 mSv,** and a **formal dose estimation** should be performed if dose could be **above 100 mSv (the threshold for tissue effects).**
- Technique (dose) typically should **NOT be decreased** for a pregnant patient compared to a same-sized nonpregnant patient, since it could result in **substandard image quality.**

Chapter 12 (Computed Tomography II) Questions

12.1 CTDI$_{vol}$(S) for a routine adult head CT examination would most likely be:
A. 15 mGy
B. 30 mGy
C. 60 mGy
D. 120 mGy

12.2 How does tube voltage for a routine head CT compare to voltage for a CTA?
A. CTA higher
B. Both about the same
C. CTA lower

12.3 What is a typical DLP for a routine adult chest CT?
A. 3 mGy-cm
B. 30 mGy-cm
C. 300 mGy-cm
D. 3,000 mGy-cm

12.4 CT scans of bariatric patients most likely use _____ mAs and _____ kV.
A. increased; increased
B. increased; decreased
C. decreased; increased
D. decreased; decreased

12.5 How is tissue characterization affected as the difference between voltages used in dual-energy CT decreases?
A. Gets better
B. No change
C. Gets worse

12.6 What is the ACR CT Accreditation reference dose limit for CTDI$_{vol}$(S) in pediatric abdominal CT?
A. 5 mGy
B. 10 mGy
C. 20 mGy
D. 60 mGy

12.7 Radiation doses associated with a projection radiograph are what percentage of the dose of an adult chest CT examination?
A. <5%
B. 10%
C. 25%
D. 50%

12.8 What monoenergetic reconstruction likely has the worst noise?
A. 140 keV
B. 80 keV
C. 60 keV
D. 40 keV

12.9 What is the HU difference between fat and soft tissues?
A. 1,500 HU
B. 150 HU
C. 1.5 HU
D. 0.15 HU

12.10 How does contrast change when effective mAs increases?
A. Increases
B. Unchanged
C. Decreases

12.11 How dose noise (mottle) change when mAs quadruples?
A. Quadruples
B. Doubles
C. Halves
D. Quarters

12.12 Increasing the CT x-ray tube voltage at constant mAs most likely _____ contrast and _____ image noise.
A. increases; increases
B. increases; decreases
C. decreases; increases
D. decreases; decreases

12.13 What is the best temporal resolution typically seen on a dual-source CT scanner using half-scan reconstruction with an x-ray tube rotation time of 300 ms?
A. 30 ms
B. 75 ms
C. 150 ms
D. 300 ms

12.14 What is the typical spatial resolution in CT?
A. 0.7 lp/mm
B. 4 lp/mm
C. 7.8 lp/mm
D. 14 lp/mm

12.15 When should patient shielding be utilized during CT scanning?
A. Protect adult eyes during head CT
B. Female breast dose reduction during chest CT
C. When a pregnant patient needs an abdominopelvic CT
D. Patient shielding should not typically be used

12.16 Tube current modulation is effective in mitigating what artifact?
A. Beam hardening
B. Motion
C. Photon starvation
D. Ring

12.17 150 keV virtual monoenergetic reconstructions can mitigate what artifact?
A. Ring
B. Metal
C. Partial volume
D. Truncation

12.18 What is the effective dose to a typical adult undergoing a routine single-phase chest CT scan?
A. 0.5 mSv
B. 5 mSv
C. 50 mSv
D. >50 mSv

12.19 How does the effective dose for a child compare to that for an adult if the same DLP was delivered to both?
A. Pediatric dose higher than that of adult
B. Pediatric dose comparable to that of adult
C. Pediatric dose lower than that of adult

12.20 What is the typical embryo dose from a chest CT examination?
A. <0.1 mGy
B. 1 mGy
C. 10 mGy
D. >10 mGy

Answers and Explanations

12.1 **C** (60 mGy). Most routine head CT examinations are performed at 120 kV and a CTDIvol(S) of 60 mGy, and the ACR limits routine head CT to be below 80 mGy for an adult.

12.2 **C** (CTA lower). CT angiography requires a lower tube voltage (e.g., 100 kV) to increase the visibility of iodine contrast, which absorbs more x-rays as the beam energy is reduced.

12.3 **C** (300 mGy-cm). The exam would use a CTDIvol(L) of 10 mGy and a scan length of 30 cm, which multiplied together results in about 300 mGy-cm.

12.4 **A** (increased; increased). Both CT voltage and tube output (mAs) need to be increased when performing CT scans of bariatric patients.

12.5 **C** (Gets worse). As the low and high kV used in dual energy scanning get closer the HU of different tissues become more similar and tissue characterization gets worse.

12.6 **C** (20 mGy). For a 5 year old child undergoing an abdominal CT examinations, the ACR CT Accreditation program expects CTDIvol(S) to be below 20 mGy, and will fail applicants who submit values higher than 25 mGy (NB: CTDIvol(S) of 20 mGy is the same CT output as CTDIvol(L) of 10 mGy).

12.7 **A** (<5%). Projection radiographs have very low patient doses, and are unlikely to exceed 5% of a typical routine head or body CT scan in adults.

12.8 **D** (40 keV). Low-energy monoenergetic reconstructions depend on the low-voltage image more. Since the low-voltage image is less penetrating, it is noisier. Some vendors increase mAs for the low-energy image to improve this at the cost of patient dose.

12.9 **B** (150 HU). Difference between fat (about −100 HU) and soft tissues (about 50 HU) is 150 HU.

12.10 **B** (Unchanged). Effective mAs changes impact noise but not contrast.

12.11 **C** (Halves). Quadrupling the mAs will quadruple the number of x-ray photons used to create a CT image, which halves the amount of noise (mottle).

12.12 **D** (decreases; decreases). Higher voltages (photon energies) reduce contrast, but high voltages increase x-ray tube output as well as patient penetration, so image mottle will be decreased as well. Patient dose will also increase.

12.13 **B** (75 ms). For dual-source CT, the best achievable temporal resolution is a quarter of the x-ray tube rotation time. For single-source CT scanners, the best achievable temporal resolution is half the rotation time (i.e., about 150 ms).

12.14 **A** (0.7 lp/mm). CT must be able to resolve at least 0.6 lp/mm for typical imaging and 0.8 lp/mm for high-resolution chest imaging according to the ACR Accreditation manual. 0.7 lp/mm is typical, and this can be doubled by using smaller FOV with same matrix size (i.e., using smaller pixel size). Cutting-edge systems such as photon counting and ultrahigh resolution will push this number higher in the future.

12.15 **D** (Patient shielding should typically not be used) Shielding should generally not be used due to the optimized doses delivered in modern scanners and because they may confuse the AEC and cause unintended dose increases.

12.16 **C** (Photon starvation). Photon starvation artifacts occur due to dose being too low in some projections. TCM will increase the dose to compensate and then patient attenuation increases.

12.17 B (Metal). Metal artifact is a combination of beam hardening and photon starvation. Increased penetration at high keV will reduce the artifact at the cost of lower image contrast.

12.18 B (5 mSv). A representative patient effective dose for a single-phase chest CT scan is a few mSv and would be classified as a moderate dose (1-10 mSv).

12.19 A (Pediatric dose higher than that of adult). For the same DLP, pediatric effective doses are about 3 to 5× higher than that in adults. Even when the amount of radiation used in children is reduced, their effective doses can still be higher than that in adults.

12.20 A (<0.1 mGy). A chest CT scan delivers organ doses of about 15 mGy in directly irradiated regions (lung and heart) but <0.1 mGy to the uterus (embryo) from internal scatter. Placing a lead apron on the patients abdomen will not significantly affect this very low embryo dose but might be used to reassure a concerned patient..

Advanced Modalities

Nuclear Medicine I

I. NUCLEI

A. Nuclei

- Atomic **nuclei** contain **protons** and **neutrons** (i.e., nucleons) held together by a strong force.
- **Atomic mass number (A)** is the sum of the number of **protons (Z)** and **neutrons (N)**, so A is equal to Z plus N.
  - **Iodine-127**, which can be written as ^{127}I, has an atomic number **(Z) of 53**, and **127 nucleons** (i.e., **N is 74**).
- Nuclides having the same mass number (A) are called **isobars** and those having the same atomic number (Z; protons) are called **isotopes**.
- **Stable low A nuclides** have approximately **equal numbers** of **neutrons** and **protons**, but stable high A nuclides have more neutrons than protons.
- **Unstable isotopes (i.e., radionuclides) emit radiation** in their attempt to attain stability.
- **Transformation** of an **unstable nuclide** is **radioactive decay.**
  - The original nuclide is called the **parent**, and nuclides resulting from the nuclear decay are called **daughters.**
- When decay involves a **change** in the number of **protons**, there is a change of element (e.g., fluorine to oxygen), termed a **transmutation.**
- Unstable nuclides undergo nuclear transformation as summarized in Table 13.1.

TABLE 13.1	Radioactive Decay Modes for Unstable Nuclei Containing Protons (Z), Neutrons (N), and Mass Number (A)			
	Daughter Nucleus Value			
Decay Mode	**Mass Number**	**Atomic Number**	**Neutron Number**	**Comments**
Isomeric transition	A	Z	N	Metastable if half-life is long
Beta minus (β^-)	A	Z + 1	N − 1	Nucleus emits electrons
Beta plus (β^+)	A	Z − 1	N + 1	Nucleus emits positrons
Electron capture	A	Z − 1	N + 1	Atoms emit characteristic x-rays[a]
Alpha decay	A − 4	Z − 2	N − 2	Only occurs with heavy nuclei (Z > 82)

[a]When inner shell vacancies are filled.

B. Isomeric Transitions

- **Ground states** are the nucleus's lowest energy state and are the most **stable.**
- **Higher energy levels** (i.e., excited states) are **isomeric states,** which are **unstable.**
- **Excited states** will transform into a lower energy level, **emitting gamma rays.**
  - **Gamma rays** are photons emitted by the nucleus during a decay and are used to create nuclear medicine images.
  - Isomeric transitions do not involve capture or emission of any particles.
- After an **isomeric transition,** both **parent** and **daughter** nuclei have the **same mass number** and **atomic number** (see Fig. 13.1).
- **^{99m}Tc** has an excited state at an energy level of **140 keV,** with transitions from this energy level to ground level resulting in emission of 140 keV gamma rays.
  - A 140 keV gamma ray is ideal for nuclear medicine (NM) because its **energy** is **high** enough to **escape** from a patient but **low** enough to be easily **detected.**
- **Isomeric states** with very **long lifetimes** (100×–1,000× longer than the shortest state) are called **metastable.**
  - A **metastable state** of an atom is denoted by a lowercase m following the mass number (e.g., ^{99m}Tc).

C. Beta Minus and Alpha Decay

- In **beta minus (β⁻)** decay, a **neutron** inside the nucleus is **converted** into a **proton** and emits a beta minus, as depicted schematically in Figure 13.1.
  - A beta minus is just an **electron emitted from the nucleus.**
  - One can think of the neutron (neutral) as breaking into a proton (+) and an electron (−) that is emitted.
- **Beta minus decay** occurs in **nuclei** with **too few protons** (i.e., excess of neutrons).
- Most **therapy radionuclides** (e.g., ^{90}Y and ^{131}I) are beta minus emitters, since electrons damage nearby tissue but are stopped before hitting other organs or leaving the body.
  - Beta minus particles from medical isotopes **travel a few millimeters in soft tissue** before losing all energy and stopping.
- **Beta particles** (i.e., electron or positron) **travel** a distance up to several millimeters in **soft tissue** (i.e., range).
  - **Beta** particle **range increases** with increasing beta particle **energy** and is also **increased** in low-density tissues such as the **lungs.**
- In **alpha decay,** a radionuclide emits an **alpha particle** consisting of **two neutrons** and **two protons (no electrons).**
  - ^{223}Ra is utilized for castrate-resistant prostate cancer bone metastases.
- **Alpha particles** pose a **high risk** if **ingested, inhaled,** or **injected.**

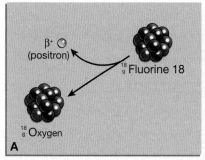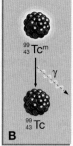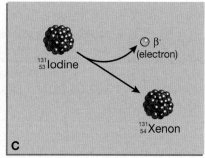

FIG 13.1 A: Proton-rich nuclei (e.g., ^{18}F) can emit positrons to reduce the positive charge in the daughter nucleus. **B:** Isomeric transition occurs when energetic nuclei (e.g., ^{99m}Tc) emit their excess energy as gamma rays with both the parent and daughter having the same atomic number. **C:** Nuclei with too little positive charge (e.g., ^{131}I) emit beta minus particles (i.e., electrons) to increase the positive charge in the daughter nucleus.

- **²²²Rn (Radon)** is a naturally occurring alpha-emitter gas that EPA has stated may be responsible for up to **15% of lung** cancers in the United States.
  - It is the **leading cause of lung cancer in nonsmokers** and second only to smoking for the entire US population.

D. Electron Capture and Beta Plus Decay

- In **electron capture (EC)**, a **proton** is **converted** into a **neutron** by **capturing** an **atomic electron**, usually in the K-shell (i.e., the closest one).
- EC and beta plus decay occur in **nuclei** with **too many protons** (i.e., neutrons deficient).
- In **EC, protons** inside the nucleus are **converted** into a **neutron** by **capturing** an **atomic electron.**
  - One can think of an electron (−) combining with a proton (+) to create a neutron (neutral).
- When the electron is captured from the K-shell, the resultant **K-shell vacancy** is filled by outer shell electrons, emitting **characteristic x-rays.**
- Important **electron capture radionuclides** used in nuclear medicine are ²⁰¹Tl, ⁶⁷Ga, ¹¹¹In, and ¹²³I.
- In **beta plus (β+)** decay (Fig. 13.1), a **proton** inside the nucleus is **converted** into a **neutron** with the emission of a beta plus particle (positron).
  - A positron is the **antimatter version of an electron** with the only difference being a positive charge instead of negative.
  - One can think of a proton (+) breaking into a neutron (neutral) and a positron (+) that is emitted.
- When the **positron loses** all of its **kinetic energy**, it undergoes an **annihilation reaction** with an **electron in the local environment (e.g., tissue).**
- The **mass** of the **positron and electron (511 keV** each) is converted into two **511 keV photons** that are **emitted** in **opposite directions** (i.e., 180° apart).
- All **PET (positron emission tomography) radionuclides** decay by positron emission, with the most popular being ¹⁸F.
- **EC competes** with **beta plus decay,** as both have too many protons (i.e., neutron deficient).
  - Positron emission is more likely as the **difference between parent and daughter energies (i.e., mass defect)** increases.
  - Positron emission is **impossible if the mass defect is below 1.022 MeV.**

E. Measuring Radioactivity

- **Activity** is the number of **decays per unit time.**
- The **SI unit** of **activity** is the **Becquerel (Bq),** where one Becquerel is **1 nuclear decay per second.**
  - The United States uses **non-SI** units of **millicuries (mCi),** where **1 mCi is 37 MBq.**
- **Radioactivity decays exponentially** and is characterized by the **decay constant λ.**
  - **Activity** is directly **proportional** to the **decay constant λ.**
- **Physical half-life ($T_{1/2}$)** is time for half of the radionuclides to transform (decay).
- After one half-life, half the initial activity remains; after two half-lives, a quarter remains; and after three half-lives, an eighth remains.
  - After **10 half-lives,** only **0.1%** of the initial activity remains, and most medical radionuclide emissions will **likely be at or below background levels.**
- Half-life and decay constant are **inversely proportional.**
  - Long-lived radionuclides have a very small value of λ, decay slowly, and hence little activity.
- **Effective half-life (T_e)** of a radionuclide in any organ encompasses both **physical half-life from decay (T_p)** and **biological clearance half-life (T_b).**
  - **Biological clearance** includes spit, defecation, and urination.
- **When T_p and T_b are the same,** T_e will be half of T_p, but **when one (e.g., T_p) is much shorter than the other (e.g., T_b),** then T_e will be just below the shorter half-life (e.g., T_p), as depicted in Figure 13.2.

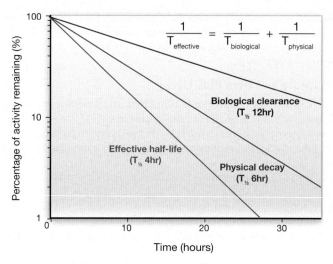

FIG 13.2 Effective half-life is 4 hours, shorter than the half-lives associated with both physical decay (6 hours) and biological clearance (12 hours).

■■ II. RADIOPHARMACEUTICALS

A. Producing Radioactivity

- **Radionuclides** (e.g., Lu-177) may be **produced** in a **nuclear reactor** by **adding neutrons** to a stable nuclide (**activation**).
- **Neutron activation products** cannot be chemically separated and are therefore **not carrier free.**
  - **Carrier-free** is when there are no other isotopes of an element except the desired one.
- **Reactor-produced neutron activation radionuclides** generally **decay** by a **beta minus** process.
- **Radionuclides** may be **produced** in **cyclotrons** where charged particles (e.g., **protons or deuterons**) are **added** to **stable nuclides.**
  - **Cyclotron-produced radionuclides** generally **decay** by a **beta plus** or by **electron capture.**
- **Cyclotron-produced isotopes** include ^{123}I, ^{18}F, ^{67}Ga, and ^{111}In.
- **Radionuclides** may also be obtained as **fission products** when heavy nuclides break up.
- Fission products include ^{131}I, ^{133}Xe, ^{90}Sr, and ^{99}Mo.
  - **Fission product radionuclides** generally **decay** by a **beta minus** process, similar to neutron activation.
- **Cyclotron** and **fission product** materials can be chemically separated and supplied as pure materials (i.e., are **carrier free**).
- Table 13.2 shows a summary of the most common gamma-emitting radionuclides.

TABLE 13.2	Key Characteristics of Common Gamma-Emitting Radionuclides			
Nuclide	**Photons (keV)**	**Production Mode**	**Decay Mode**	**Half-Life (T$_{1/2}$)**
^{67}Ga	93, 185, 300	Cyclotron	EC	78 h
^{99m}Tc	140	Generator	IT	6 h
^{111}In	173, 247	Cyclotron	EC	68 h
^{123}I	159	Cyclotron	EC	13 h
^{131}I	364	Fission product	β	8 d
^{133}Xe	80	Fission product	β	5.3 d

β, beta decay; EC, electron capture; IT, isomeric transition.

B. Generators

- In **generators**, a useful radionuclide (**daughter**) is **continuously produced** by radioactive decay of a longer-lived (**parent) radionuclide.**
- **Specific activity** refers to the **activity per unit mass** of material (i.e., Bq per gram).
  - For carrier-free radionuclides, **longer half-lives** have **lower specific activities.**
- **Technetium generators** consist of an alumina column loaded with ^{99}Mo, which **decays** to ^{99m}**Tc.**
  - **Saline** is passed through the column to **elute (wash off)** the ^{99m}Tc in the form of **sodium pertechnetate.**
- ^{99}Mo is not soluble in saline and remains in the column.
- ^{82}**Rb** is **obtained** from ^{82}**Sr** and is a positron emitter used in **cardiac imaging.**
- **The half-life** of ^{82}Rb is very short (**1.25 minutes**), which permits sequential studies every 5 minutes (see below).
- Isotopes available from **generators** for use in **NM** include gamma emitters (e.g., ^{113m}**In**) and positron emitters (e.g., ^{68}**Ga**).

C. Generator Equilibrium

- Consider a generator **initially** starting with ~**100 GBq** of ^{99}**Mo** and which has **no** ^{99m}**Tc** present.
- As ^{99}**Mo** decays, ^{99m}**Tc** activity is **produced.**
- Daughter activity (^{99m}Tc) increases until **equilibrium** is reached, which occurs after **four daughter half-lives.**
  - Because the half-life of ^{99m}Tc is 6 hours, a ^{99}**Mo generator** takes about **24 hours** to reach **equilibrium.**
- At **equilibrium,** the **activities** of **parent and daughter** are taken to be approximately **equal.**
  - In equilibrium, a 100 GBq ^{99}Mo generator also has about 100 GBq ^{99m}Tc.
- Because the **half-life** of ^{99}**Mo** is **66 hours**, generators remain **useful** for about **five working days** (i.e., ~**two parent half-lives**).
  - After 5 days, yield of a ^{99m}Tc generator is less than 25% of initial activity.
- **Transient equilibrium** is when the **parent radionuclide** is longer lived than the daughter (e.g., Mo-Tc generator).
- **Secular equilibrium** is when the parent is so long lived compared to the daughter that its half-life is essentially infinite (Sr-Rb generator).
  - **Both secular** and **transient equilibrium** occur after **four daughter half-lives**, and both have (approximately) **equal parent** and **daughter activities.**
- In **secular** equilibrium, **parent** and **daughter activities** are **exactly equal.**
  - In **transient** equilibrium, **parent** and **daughter activities** are only **approximately equal**, and directly proportional to each other.

D. Methods of Localization

- **Compartmental localization** looks for filling and leakage from anatomic compartments (e.g., Tc 99m red blood cells).
- **Phagocytosis** localization occurs when colloidal particles (e.g., Tc 99m sulfur colloid) are trapped (e.g., Kupffer cells).
- **Active transport** (e.g., I 131) and **passive diffusion** (e.g., Tc 99m hexamethylpropyleneamine oxime) utilize chemical gradients to move radioisotopes across cell membranes.
- **Facilitated diffusion** (e.g., F 18 fluorodeoxyglucose) utilizes energy to move radionuclides against the chemical gradient.
- **Embolization** utilized the large particle size to create microemboli in vessels (e.g., Tc 99m macroaggregated albumin or Y90 spheres).
- **Chemisorption** is when the radiochemical complex (e.g., phosphate from Tc 99m methylene diphosphonate) is incorporated into bone surface repair/building.
- **Receptor binding** utilizes the attachment sites for ligand molecules for localization (e.g., In-111 somatostatin or Ga-67 citrate transferrin).

- **Antigen binding** uses radiolabeled antibody binding to surface antigens (e.g., prostate-specific membrane antigen or Y-90 Zevalin).

E. **Generator and Pharmaceutical QC**
- Damaged generators may permit **parent isotopes (e.g., ^{99}Mo or ^{82}Sr) or contaminants (e.g., ^{85}Sr) to break into saline elute (breakthrough).**
  - **Molybdenum breakthrough** is kept below 1.5 μCi of ^{99}Mo per 1 mCi of ^{99m}Tc.
  - For each mCi of ^{82}Rb, **^{82}Sr breakthrough** is kept below 0.02 μCi and **^{85}Sr breakthrough** is kept below 0.2 μCi.
- **Dose calibrators** can determine the content of ^{99}Mo each time the generator is eluted using a **lead shield blocks** the ^{99m}Tc **gamma rays.**
- **Alumina** can also **break through** and cause unwanted precipitates and is tested using **colorimetric test paper.**
- **Radionuclide purity** (proportion of wanted to unwanted radioactive nuclides) is identified by their (distinctive) photopeak energies using gamma-ray spectroscopy (e.g., presence of ^{99}Mo in ^{99m}Tc).
- **Radiochemical purity** is the chemical purity of the isotope, checked using thin-layer chromatography (e.g., free **pertechnetate** in ^{99m}Tc**-labeled diethylenetriamine penta-acetate**).
- **Chemical purity** refers to the amount of unwanted **chemical contaminants** in the agent.
- **Sterility** and **pyrogen** testing should be performed before agents are administered to patients.
- **Severe adverse reactions** of **radiopharmaceuticals** are extremely **rare** (about **2 per 100,000**).

III. RADIATION DETECTORS

A. **Scintillators**
- When **gamma rays** are **absorbed** in a **scintillator** (e.g., **NaI**), the absorbed energy produces (a lot of) **light photons.**
  - The total amount of **light produced** is directly **proportional** to the **energy deposited** in the scintillator crystal.
- Light produced following the total or partial absorption of gamma ray energies is converted into electrons and amplified by a **light detector (photomultiplier tube [PMT]).**
- Scintillators display the resultant signals (pulses) that represent the total amount of light produced in the scintillator as an **energy spectrum.**
  - The **vertical axis** is the number of **counts** (photons) at a given energy, and the **horizontal axis** is the **photon energy** (Fig. 13.3).
- An **energy spectrum** from a **gamma emitter** usually contains a **photopeak** that corresponds to the full energy of the absorbed gamma ray.
  - The photopeak for ^{123}I is at **160 keV** (i.e., Fig. 13.3A) and for ^{99m}Tc is at **140 keV** (i.e., Fig. 13.3B).
- Gamma rays may undergo **Compton scatter,** so only part of the photon energy is deposited in the scintillator.
  - **Compton scatter** interactions **produce less light** than the corresponding photoelectric absorption events (^{99m}Tc scatter has energies <140 keV).
- Figure 13.3B shows the spectra obtained from ^{99m}Tc in a patient showing both the photopeak and Compton scatter photons incident on a scintillator.

B. **Detection Efficiency and Energy Resolution**
- **Detection efficiency** is the proportion of emitted source radiation into a detector signal.
  - The **intrinsic efficiency** is the **proportion** of **incident gamma rays incident** on the **detector absorbed** in the scintillator.
  - **Geometric efficiency** is the proportion of emitted photons that can hit the detector (this is highest when the source is surrounded by the detector).

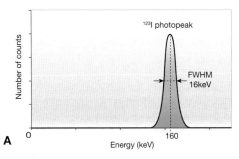
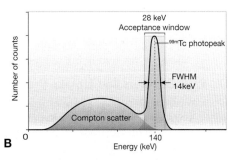

FIG 13.3 A: Gamma ray spectrum for ^{123}I showing an idealized spectrum (i.e., no scatter) with a photopeak at 160 keV, and a peak broadening of 16 keV (full width at half maximum) as 10% of the photopeak energy. **B:** Gamma ray spectrum for ^{99m}Tc which shows a photopeak at 140 keV, as well as scattered photons that "overlap" with the photopeak. Setting an acceptance window of 28 keV, twice the energy resolution of 14 keV (i.e., 10%), accepts most photopeak photons while excluding most scattered photons.

- **Increasing** the **photon energy** from **100 to 511 keV** reduces detection efficiency from **100% to 5%** (the photoelectric effect is proportional to $1/E^3$).
- When a **gamma ray photon** is **fully absorbed** (i.e., the photopeak) in a scintillator, the amount of **light produced** is directly **proportional** to **energy deposited (i.e., the gamma ray energy).**
  - Each absorbed gamma ray, however, generates a slightly different amount of light because of statistical fluctuations.
- After a large number of gamma rays are absorbed by a scintillator, there will be **distribution (spread)** of events **around** a **mean energy value.**
  - **Full width at half maximum (FWHM)** is the **width (spread)** of a **photopeak.**
- **Energy resolution** is the FWHM of the photopeak divided by the mean energy.
- The width of the ^{99m}Tc photopeak (140 keV) in a 10 mm NaI crystal is about 14 keV, so the energy resolution is 10%, **which is typical for most modern systems** (Fig. 13.3B).
  - A **10% energy resolution** for ^{123}I **(160 keV)** has an **FWHM energy** of **16 keV** (Fig. 13.3A).
  - Smaller energy resolution allows for **better scatter rejection** using energy windows.

C. Pulse Height Analysis

- A **pulse height analyzer (PHA)** is an electronic device used to determine which portion of the detected spectrum is used for subsequent analysis.
  - A PHA is used to **identify** which **gamma ray interactions** will be **used** to **create** a nuclear medicine **image.**
- **Pulse height analysis** involves setting of a **lower signal value (S_{low})** and an **upper signal value (S_{upper})** for the total light detected by the PMT from the scintillator.
- **Signals** that are **lower than S_{low}** or **higher than S_{upper}** will be **rejected** (excluded).
  - Pulse height analysis sets an accepted **energy window** for detections.
- **Lower-energy signals** (i.e., S_{low}) include **Compton scatter** events in a patient.
- **Higher-energy signals** (i.e., S_{high}) include **coincidence events** where light from two gamma rays overlap.
  - **Compton scatter** and **coincidence events** are **excluded** because they **degrade image quality.**
- **Signals** that **are between S_{low}** and **S_{high}** are **accepted** for subsequent analysis.
- Pulse Height Analysis **window width** (i.e., $S_{high} - S_{low}$) is about **twice** the **energy resolution.**
  - This **pulse height analysis window** width is expected to **accept most** of the **photopeak** events, and **rejects most** of the **scatter.**

- Figure 13.3B shows the **effect** of a **pulse height analysis window** on a **detected spectrum.**
  - Increasing the PHA window increases the number of photopeak events and also increases the number of scatter events, and vice versa.

D. Well Counters and Uptake Probes

- **Well counters** have samples inserted into a well within the crystal, which maximizes sensitivity by collecting most of the emitted gamma rays.
  - Their high sensitivity makes them useful for finding contamination during wipe tests.
- **Well counters identify radionuclides** from the **photopeak energy.**
  - A photopeak at **160 keV** identifies a radionuclide as ^{123}I, and a photopeak of **140 keV** identifies the radionuclide as ^{99m}Tc (Fig. 13.3).
- **Well counters** can also **quantify** the **amount (MBq)** of activity present by using an appropriate calibration factor.
  - A sample of **1 kBq** of activity could result up to **~1,000 detected counts per second.**
- **Uptake probes** quantify uptake of **radioiodine** in **patients** without imaging.
  - Measurement of **thyroid uptake** is usually performed **24 hours after administration** of the radioiodine.
- **Uptake** is usually measured at a **standard distance** (e.g., 30 cm) from a scintillator crystal (NaI).
- **Neck counts, corrected** for body **background counts**, are compared with a standard in a neck phantom to **estimate patient uptake** of activity.
- **Uptake probes** are also used to **monitor dose from liquid radioiodine** (^{123}I **and** ^{131}I) in **workers** who handle this volatile chemical.

E. Dose Calibrators

- A **dose calibrator** is an **ionization chamber** used to measure the activity of a radioisotope dose (MBq or mCi).
  - **Activity** is **measured** in a **syringe** but **prior** to **injection** into a patient.
- The response of a dose calibrator is dependent on the radionuclide, and each radionuclide has a user-selected unique setting.
  - **One MBq of** ^{18}F gives the same electronic output **as three MBq of** ^{99m}Tc.
- Custom-designed plastic sample holders and deep-well detectors are used to ensure consistent sample positioning in the well.
  - Current Nuclear Regulatory Commission **Regulations** require that the **administered dosage** be within **±20%** of the prescribed dose for both imaging and therapy radionuclides.
- **Dose calibrator constancy** is **checked daily** by measuring the same standard source, usually ^{137}Cs because it has a half-life of 30 years.
  - Day-to-day **measurement**s should **vary** by **less than 5%.**
- **Accuracy** is checked at installation and **annually** using commercially available **calibrated sources.**
- **Linearity** is **checked quarterly** by measuring the decay of ^{99m}Tc over 72 hours or more.
  - Linearity can also be checked by using a source placed into a calibrated cylinder of lead, which attenuates the source by a known amount.

IV. PLANAR IMAGING

A. Gamma Camera

- **Gamma cameras** produce **projection images** of the distribution of radioactivity in patients, built up **one gamma ray** (i.e., count) **at a time.**
- **Key components** of traditional gamma cameras are a **collimator, NaI scintillator** crystal, **PMT arrays**, and **processing** of the **PMT signals** (Fig. 13.4).

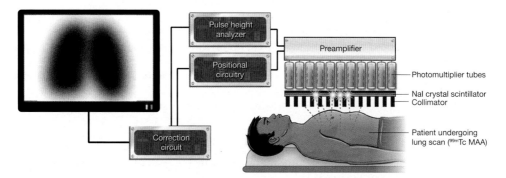

FIG 13.4 Only gamma rays that are traveling vertically out of the patient get transmitted through the parallel hole collimator. A fraction of the absorbed energy in the NaI detector is converted to light that is detected by a two-dimensional array of photomultiplier tubes. Total amount of light is processed by the pulse height analyzer to identify photopeak events, and the pattern of light provides positional information. After application of corrections to rectify nonrandom distortions, the resultant image is displayed as the number of detected photons in each pixel.

- Gamma rays emerging from the patient pass through a **lead collimator** that only allows photons traveling **parallel** to the **collimator holes** to **reach** the **scintillator.**
  - **Collimators provide spatial information** relating to the in-plane location of each single gamma ray interaction.
- Gamma rays that pass through the collimator are incident on a **NaI scintillator** crystal, typically **10 mm thick.**
  - **Scintillators** absorb incident gamma photons and produce many light photons.
- **Light output** from the scintillator is detected by an array of **PMTs** and converted to an **electrical signal.**
- **PHA accepts photopeak events** used to create an image and rejects scatter and coincidence (pile-up) events that degrade image quality.
  - Some radionuclides (e.g., ^{67}Ga and ^{111}In) use **multiple (PHA) energy windows** for **multiple gamma ray energies** (see Table 13.2).
- **Location** of the gamma ray **interaction** is determined by the relative strength of signals from each PMT (**Anger logic**).
- **Solid-state (digital) gamma cameras** may replace the PMT with a silicon photodiode and NaI detectors with cadmium-zinc-telluride.
  - Digital gamma cameras have improved energy resolution (~6%), spatial resolution, and sensitivity.

B. **Collimators**
- **Collimators** are typically made of **lead** and contain **multiple holes** (Fig. 13.5).
  - The **lead strips** between the holes are called **septa.**
- **Parallel-hole collimators** are the workhorse of nuclear medicine and do not magnify the patient—the **field of view (FOV)** does **not change** with **distance.**
- **Converging collimators** produce a **magnified image**, and **diverging collimators** project an **image size** that is **smaller** than the object size (for imaging anatomy larger than the detector).
- **Pinhole collimators** are cone shaped with a **single hole** at the apex, resulting in **images** that are normally **magnified** and **inverted.**
- **Low-energy collimators,** used with ^{99m}Tc and ^{123}I, have **thin septa.**
  - **Medium-energy collimators,** used with ^{67}Ga and ^{111}In, have **thick septa.**
- **Collimator sensitivity** is the **count rate per MBq** being imaged and is generally low (0.01% of incident photons).
  - Sensitivity is **constant with distance from the patient for parallel-hole collimators, increases** for converging collimators, and **decreases** for diverging and pinhole collimators.

- **Collimator resolution falls off rapidly** with **distance for all collimators.**
  - **System resolution** is **dominated** by **collimator resolution**, with the **blur** introduced by the **scintillator** being of **little clinical importance.**
- **General-purpose** collimators have **larger holes, thinner septa and transmit more** photons.
  - **High-resolution** collimators have **small holes, thicker septa and localize** the **activity better** (Fig. 13.5).
- Table 13.3 shows resolution and sensitivity performance of parallel-hole collimators.

C. Clinical NM Imaging

- Most **clinical NM imaging** is performed using ^{99m}Tc-labeled radiopharmaceuticals.
- [99m]Tc imaging typically uses a **20% energy window (i.e., ±10%)** accepting photon energies ranging from 126 to 154 keV.
  - **Applying a PHA (energy) window (peaking)** is done manually or automatically.
- A **count** refers to the registration of a single gamma ray by the detector, with about **500,000 counts** acquired for a typical **scintillation camera image.**
  - If the count rate is very high, the system fails to count some gamma rays that occur while the electronics register the current count (i.e., **dead time**).
- **Gamma cameras** have **corrections** made to the acquired image data that correct for system **spatial nonlinearity.**
- **Corrections** are made for **nonuniformities** in detector response (detection efficiency) at varying locations across the detector.
  - **Nonuniformity corrections** are computed from ^{99m}Tc or [57]Co flood (uniformity) images obtained with a high number of counts to minimize random noise (e.g., 200 million).
- **Corrections** are also applied to account for **differences** in the amount of **light generated** at **varying locations** across the detector by the scintillator.
- **NM image matrix** sizes generally range from **64 × 64 to 512 × 512.**
  - Recorded pixel values in an image reflect the counts detected and may be used to create activity maps.

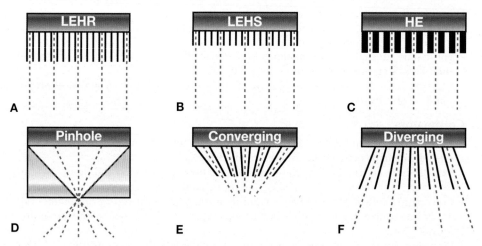

FIG 13.5 **A:** Parallel-hole low-energy high-resolution collimator, most commonly used with gamma cameras for planar imaging. **B:** Parallel-hole low-energy high-sensitivity collimator, which has increased transmission because it is thinner, but is therefore less able to localize the source of the photons (i.e., worse resolution). **C:** Parallel-hole high-energy collimator used to image ^{111}In and ^{67}Ga with much thicker septa. **D:** Pinhole collimator used to shallow objects with small fields of view (e.g., thyroid). **E:** Converging collimator used to image pediatrics (i.e., object is magnified). **F:** Diverging collimator used to image larger organs and patients (i.e., object is minified). HE, high-energy; LEHR, low-energy high-resolution; LEHS, low-energy high-sensitivity.

TABLE 13.3	Representative Full Width at Half Maximum (FWHM) Resolution		
Distance From Parallel-Hole Collimator (cm)	Collimator Spatial Resolution FWHM (mm) [Relative Sensitivity (%)]		
	High Resolution (HR)	All Purpose (AP)	High Sensitivity (HS)
0	2 [30]	3 [65]	5 [100]
5	5 [30]	7 [65]	10 [100]
10	8 [30]	10 [65]	15 [100]
15	12 [30]	14 [65]	20 [100]

- An average **count density** in NM images is **very low** (e.g., **100 counts per pixel**), resulting in very high levels of mottle (e.g., **10%**).

D. Image Quality

- **Contrast** is the **difference** in intensity (counts) in any **abnormality compared to** the intensity in the surrounding **normal anatomy** (background).
  - **Contrast** is **degraded** by **septal penetration** and **scatter.**
- Contrast in nuclear medicine images occurs when radiopharmaceuticals localize in the organ of interest **("hot spot").**
  - The absence of uptake **("cold spot")** also results in lesion contrast.
- Radioactivity is found in other tissues, which generates **undesirable background counts**, which degrades contrast (target-to-background ratio).
- **Gamma camera lung images** contain about **10 photons/mm²**, whereas **chest radiographs** have about **20,000 x-ray photons every mm².**
  - **A low** number of **counts** in NM images accounts for **their poor (i.e., mottled) appearance.**
- Ways of **increasing NM image counts** include **increasing** the **administered activity,** increasing **imaging time,** or using a **higher-sensitivity collimator.**
- **Gamma cameras** have an **FWHM** of **~8 mm,** with the **low-energy high-resolution (LEHR)** collimator most commonly used in clinical imaging.
  - **Intrinsic resolution,** performance of gamma camera without the collimator, is typically **3 mm** and negligible compared to the collimator.
- A **FWHM of 8 mm** corresponds to a **limiting spatial resolution** of roughly **0.06 lp/mm.**
  - Gamma camera resolution is nearly 10 times worse than that of computed tomography (0.7 lp/mm).
- The detector should be as close as possible to the radionuclide (i.e., brought close to patient skin line) to maximize resolution.
  - Bariatric patient scans have a reduced resolution due to patient thickness.

E. Artifacts

- **Patient motion** is a common artifact in all NM imaging (i.e., long imaging time).
- **Damaged collimators** can cause significant uniformity problems.
- **Septal penetration or star artifact** is exhibited when a low-energy collimator is used to image higher-energy photons (e.g., I 131) (hexagonal pattern).
- **Cracked crystals** produce defects in the image, reflecting the shape of crack(s).
  - Typically, defects include a void in the crack and a hot spot along the edge of the crystal to which light is displaced.
- **PMT failure or loose coupling to the scintillator** may produce a cold defect and shows up well on flood (uniformity) imaging.
- **Edge packing** refers to the increased brightness at the edge of the crystal due to internal reflection of light (like cracked crystal) and absence of PMTs.
  - **Crystals** are deliberately made **larger** than the imaged FOV to **minimize edge packing.**

- **Off-peak images (wrong energy window)** on the "low" side of the photopeak contain excessive Compton scatter.
  - When the **PHA window** is **not centered** on the photopeak (mistuned or detuned), the resultant image will **show** the location of **individual PMTs.**
- **Metal objects** worn by the patient produce **photopenic areas** that may mimic pathologic cold lesions.
  - Other high Z materials like jewelry or x-ray contrast material can cause similar artifacts.
- **Extravasation** of the administered radiopharmaceutical gives rise to a hot spot at the injection site, and **excessive scatter** from **adjacent tissues.**

F.   **Gamma Camera Quality Control**

- **Photopeak window** of the pulse height analysis is to ensure energy window accuracy.
- **Intrinsic floods (intrinsic uniformity)** are performed **without** the **collimator** using a **point source** (^{99m}Tc) and assess the performance of NaI crystal and associated light detectors.
- **Extrinsic flood** images are obtained **with** the **collimator** in place and assess the **system performance** including the collimator.
  - **Extrinsic uniformity** is **checked daily** by placing a large-area **disc** made of ^{57}Co ($T_{1/2}$ **270 days** and **120-keV gamma rays)** in front of the camera.
- **Uniformity** is the **standard deviation** expressed as **percentage** of **mean counts.**
  - **Nonuniformities** of **±5%** or more are **unacceptable** for clinical imaging, and modern cameras have a uniformity of 2 to 3%.
- **Quadrant bar phantoms** have four sets of parallel bars, with each rotated through 90°, with dimensions of 3.5, 3.0, 2.5, and 2.0 mm.
  - **Bar pattern phantoms** also check for **linearity** (i.e., the ability to image straight lines) and are **performed weekly** (Fig. 13.6).
- **High-count uniformity** acquisitions are performed **every month** for each camera head and collimator.
  - **High-count floods** are used to obtain **uniformity correction factors.**
- Common gamma camera quality control tests are given in Table 13.4.

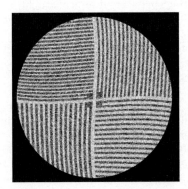 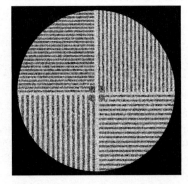

FIG 13.6 Gamma camera's employ data in the form of tables that contain position-specific correction factors. The acquired image (left) exhibits fixed (i.e., nonrandom) distortions that can be improved using correction circuits (see Fig. 13.4) that process acquired counts producing an improved image (right) with fewer distortions.

TABLE 13.4	Common Gamma Camera Quality Control Tests		
Test	**Frequency**	**Testing Isotopes**	**Reason**
Photopeak window (peaking)	Daily	Anything used that day	Ensure photons are counted only if at the correct energy
Extrinsic or intrinsic uniformity Low count rate	Daily	Co 57 or In 111	Ensure all areas of the image register the same output if hit with the same number of photons A few million counts needed
Extrinsic or intrinsic resolution	Weekly	Co 57 or Tc 99m	Determine image blur
Linearity	Weekly	Co 57 or Tc 99m	Detect geometric distortion
Intrinsic or extrinsic uniformity High count rate	Monthly	Co 57 or Tc 99m	Correct nonuniformities Tens to hundreds of millions of counts
Multiple window resolution	Annually	Ga 67 or In 111	Ensure different energies in a source all are correctly localized
Dead time/count rate	Annual	Tc 99m	Determine count rate losses that occur at high count rates

Chapter 13 (Nuclear Medicine I) Questions

13.1 What elemental property must change when transmutation occurs?
A. Atomic number (Z)
B. Proton number (N)
C. Mass number (A)
D. Total energy (E)

13.2 What nuclear change is characteristic of isomeric decay?
A. Atomic number (Z)
B. Proton number (N)
C. Mass number (A)
D. Total energy (E)

13.3 How does daughter atomic number change in β^- decay?
A. Increases by 2
B. Increases by 1
C. Decreases by 1
D. Decreases by 2

13.4 Which of the following radionuclides decays by electron capture?
A. ^{18}F
B. ^{99m}Tc
C. ^{123}I
D. ^{222}Rn

13.5 What is a typical adult dosage of ^{99m}Tc MDP?
A. 9 MBq
B. 90 MBq
C. 900 MBq
D. 9,000 MBq

13.6 Which radionuclide is least likely to be produced in a cyclotron?
A. ^{18}F
B. ^{67}Ga
C. ^{123}I
D. ^{99m}Tc

13.7 Which isotope (i.e., daughter) is unlikely to be obtained by eluting a radionuclide generator?
A. ^{99m}Tc
B. ^{82}Rb
C. ^{113m}In
D. ^{99}Mo

13.8 How does parent activity compare to daughter activity for a generator in secular equilibrium?
A. Parent greater than daughter
B. Parent equal to daughter
C. Parent less than daughter

13.9 What is the localization method for ^{99m}Tc macroaggregated albumin (MAA)?
A. Active transport
B. Capillary blockade
C. Compartmentalization
D. Simple diffusion

13.10 What is the output of a scintillator?
A. Visible light
B. Electron charge
C. Unscattered gamma rays
D. Electron-hole pairs

13.11 What percentage of ^{99m}Tc gamma rays incident on a NaI scintillator will be absorbed?
A. 15%
B. 33%
C. 67%
D. >85%

13.12 What is the half-life of ^{99m}Tc?
A. 1.25 min
B. 6 hours
C. 66 hours
D. 2.3 days

13.13 What is a reasonable energy window for ^{99m}Tc?
A. 30 to 120 keV
B. 80 to 140 keV
C. 126 to 154 keV
D. 140 to 511 keV

13.14 What is the decay rate expected from a 1 kBq sample of ^{99m}Tc?
A. <100
B. 100
C. 1,000
D. 10,000

13.15 Which is true of NM dose calibrator QC?
A. Constancy checked quarterly
B. Accuracy checked monthly
C. Geometric efficiency checked at installation
D. Linearity checked annually

13.16 What is the logically correct sequence of gamma camera components as one moves away from the patient to the detector?
A. Collimator, scintillator, PMTs
B. Collimator, PMTs, scintillator
C. Scintillator, PMTs, collimator
D. Scintillator, collimator, PMTs

13.17 Increasing collimator hole size likely _____ sensitivity and _____ spatial resolution.
A. improves; improves
B. improves; degrades
C. degrades; improves
D. degrades; degrades

13.18 What is the "tracer concept" in nuclear medicine imaging?
A. Small amounts of substance will not alter physiology.
B. Skin line is hot due to decreased attenuation.
C. Resolution is maximized by bringing the detector close to the patient.
D. Compton scatter reduces image spatial resolution.

13.19 Activity administered to an NM patient must be within what percentage of the prescribed dose according to NCR regulations?
A. ±1
B. ±5
C. ±20
D. ±50

13.20 How can the number of counts in an image be increased?
A. Decrease scan time
B. Decrease energy window width
C. Switch to a general-purpose collimator
D. Switch to filtered back projection reconstruction

Answers and Explanations

13.1 A (Atomic number (Z)). Nuclear transmutation requires a change in atomic number Z, where one element is transmuted into another element as happens in alpha and beta decay.

13.2 D (Total energy). In isomeric transitions, a higher (i.e., excited) nuclear energy level drops to a low energy level, thereby emitting the energy difference as a gamma ray (NB: A and Z remain exactly the same).

13.3 B (Increased by 1). In β- decay, the daughter atomic number is increased by 1, and in β+ decay, the daughter atomic number is decreased by 1.

13.4 C (^{123}I). The nuclide ^{123}I decays via electron capture (^{18}F is a positron emitter, ^{99m}Tc decays by isomeric transition, and ^{222}Rn is an alpha emitter).

13.5 C (900 MBq). A typical administered activity to a patient undergoing an NM imaging examination is 200 to 900 MBq (5-25 mCi) for ^{99m}Tc(though exceptions exist). 900 MBq is ~24 mCi.

13.6 D (^{99m}Tc). A ^{99}Mo generator produces ^{99m}Tc, which then decays by an isomeric transition, whereas all the other nuclei are positron emitters or decay by Electron Capture and are made using cyclotrons.

13.7 D (^{99m}Mo). Molybdenum 99 is a β- emitter that is produced in reactors or as a fission product and is used as the parent (not daughter) in ^{99m}Mo/^{99m}Tc generators.

13.8 B (Parent equal to daughter). Parent and daughter activities are equal in secular equilibrium so that 1 GBq of a long-lived parent produces 1 GBq of a short-lived daughter when it is eluted.

13.9 B (Capillary blockade). MAA lodges in a small number of capillary beds, causing microembolizations that are not dangerous to the patient.

13.10 A (Visible light). Scintillators emit visible light, and the signal representing total light detected (by PMTs) is plotted along the horizontal axis. A calibration system is used to determine the photon energy (keV) for a given amount of light (e.g., by using a ^{99m}Tc source, which produces 140 keV gamma rays).

13.11 D (>85%). NM NaI scintillators (e.g., gamma cameras and well counters) have excellent photoelectric absorption of low-energy photons (i.e., 140 keV).

13.12 B (6 h). Tc 99m is the most widely used radionuclide in nuclear medicine imaging, but its short half-life makes it difficult to store in bulk for use.

13.13 C (126-154 keV). Assuming a 10% energy window for a typical gamma camera, the energy window is set to double (20%), 10% below the 140 keV peak to 10% above the 140 keV peak.

13.14 D (10,000). 1 kBq emits approximately 1,000 gamma rays per second.

13.15 C (Geometric efficiency is assessed at installation). Constancy is checked daily. Linearity is checked quarterly, and accuracy is checked annually, whereas geometric efficiency is assessed at installation.

13.16 A (Collimator, scintillator, PMTs). Collimators occur first to select gamma rays that are traveling to pass through the holes, which are then absorbed in a scintillator that emits light detected by the photomultiplier tubes (PMTs).

13.17 B (improves; degrades). Increasing NM collimator hole size likely improves sensitivity and degrades spatial resolution performance.

13.18 A (Small amounts…). By using trace amounts of radioisotope, we can image physiology without disrupting it.

13.19 C (±20). NCR regulations require that activity administered to an NM patient be within ±20 % of the prescribed dose for both diagnostic and therapeutic agents.

13.20 C (Switch to a general-purpose collimator). High-resolution collimators decrease blur but block more "good" photons from being detected.

Nuclear Medicine II

I. SPECT AND SPECT/CT

A. Data Acquisition, Reconstruction, and Processing

- **Single-photon emission computed tomography (SPECT)** provides **tomographic views** of the **distribution** of **radioisotopes** in patients.
  - **SPECT** is to **gamma camera imaging** as **chest computed tomography (CT)** is to **chest radiographs.**
- **SPECT** uses **gamma cameras** to **acquire projection images (aka frames),** which are subsequently processed to generate tomographic images.
- **Parallel-hole collimators or fan-beam collimators** are commonly used for SPECT imaging.
  - **Fan-beam collimators** have a **limited field of view (FOV)** and are often used for **brain SPECT.**
- **Scintillation cameras** generally **rotate** around the patient, using **60 (or 120) frames** yields **60 (or 120) planar images** obtained at **6° (or 3°) intervals.**
  - When **each projection** image is obtained in **20 seconds (or 10 seconds),** the **scanning time** will be approximately **20 minutes.**
- In **cardiac** imaging, **180° rotations** are more common, and images make use of a **64 × 64 matrix size.**
- SPECT image reconstruction **seldom uses filtered back projection** due to the low number of projections which cause the appearance of **radial streaks due to undersampling.**
- **Iterative reconstruction** algorithms such as **ordered subset expectation maximization (OSEM)** are used to **reduce noise and artifacts.**
  - OSEM is a common iterative reconstruction algorithm used in SPECT.
- **Low-pass filters** (e.g., Butterworth) are often applied to further **smooth images (i.e. reduce noise)** but with reduced resolution as a detriment.

B. Attenuation Correction

- For ^{99m}Tc, **5 cm of tissue attenuates half** of the activity, and **10 cm reduces** the **detected activity** to about a **quarter** (Fig. 14.1).
- **Measured activity concentrations** in uncorrected **SPECT** images show **less activity** in the **patient center** than at the periphery.
- **CT** is typically used for attenuation correction in SPECT-capable systems.
  - Smaller SPECT systems (e.g., dedicated cardiac systems) may use a rod radionuclide source external to patient to create a **transmission image.**
  - **Coregistration** of **nuclear medicine (NM) images** with **CT** also **improves lesion localization.**

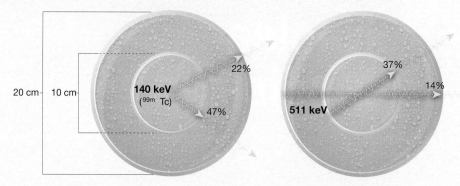

FIG 14.1 Attenuation of different energy photons. Left: roughly half of Tc-99m photons are attenuated in 5 cm of tissue and almost 80% are attenuated in 10 cm. Right: Approximately 60% of PET annihilation photons are attenuated in 10 cm and 85% are attenuated in 20 cm. Though the higher-energy photons of PET are more attenuating, two are always created by annihilation and both must escape, causing higher attenuation values compared to that of lower-energy Tc-99m. PET, positron emission tomography.

- **Correction factors** derived from CT (or rod-source) attenuation maps compensate for attenuation.
- Figure 14.2 shows how attenuation correction works.
- CT-scanners in SPECT are low cost because they typically have fewer slices and fewer cutting-edge add-ons.
- **Low-dose CT** scans performed for **attenuation correction and fusion-only purposes** likely use a $CTDI_{vol}$ **(L)** of **2 mGy** and would not be of diagnostic quality.
  - **High-dose CT** scans used to generate **diagnostic images** would likely use a $CTDI_{vol}$ **(L)** of **15 mGy.**
- **CT images** are obtained at **120 kV to 140 kV (~60 keV-70 keV),** lower than photon energies used in SPECT (e.g., **140 keV** for ^{99m}Tc), which requires transformation of attenuation data for correction factors.
- The magnitude of **SPECT attenuation correction factors** depends on **photon energy** and **thickness** of the **attenuator.**

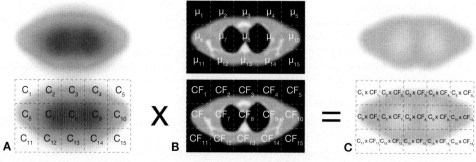

FIG 14.2 **A:** Apparent counts (C_1, C_2, etc.) in each pixel of a SPECT image are shown (left) which are low at the patient's center because of photon attenuation. **B:** The upper figure shows the attenuation coefficient for each patient pixel obtained from the CT image ($\mu1$, $\mu2$, etc.), which is used to generate a correction factor (CF) in each image pixel (CF_1, CF_2, etc.). **C:** Multiplication of the apparent counts in each pixel with the corresponding correction factors will result in the true activity distribution ($C_1 \times CF_1$, $C_2 \times CF_2$, etc.), eliminating the "cold" region in the patient center. SPECT, single-photon emission computed tomography.

- Scanners without a CT or external source may use **Chang's method,** which assumes the body has a uniform attenuation throughout.

C. Clinical Imaging

- **SPECT systems** generally use **two** or **three gamma cameras** to **reduce** the **time required** to acquire projection images.
- Use of **elliptical orbits** (i.e., **body contouring**) for scintillation camera traveling around the patient allows the distance to the patient to be minimized.
  - Keeping the **detector as close as possible to the patient** maximizes resolution.
- **Bone scans** generally use 900-MBq ^{99m}Tc-labeled **phosphonates** (e.g., methylene diphosphonate [MDP]).
  - A **360° rotation angle,** with **120 projections** (30 seconds per projection), and a **128 × 128 acquisition matrix.**
- **Cardiac SPECT** scan generally uses **900-MBq** ^{99m}Tc-labeled **tetrofosmin** or **sestamibi.**
  - A **180° rotation angle,** with **60 projections** (25 seconds per projection), and a **64 × 64 acquisition matrix.**
- **Neuroendocrine** or **neurologic tumor** scan generally uses **400 MBq** of ^{123}I-labeled **MIBG** (metaiodobenzylguanidine).
  - A **128 × 128 acquisition matrix,** 3° per rotation step, and 30 seconds per projection.
- A **white cell scan** generally uses leukocytes labeled in vivo with about **20 MBq** of ^{111}In.
  - A **360° rotation angle,** with **60 projections** (30 seconds per projection), and a **64 × 64 acquisition matrix.**

D. SPECT QC, Image Quality, and Artifacts

- Image **imperfections** that are tolerable in planar images are often unacceptable in reconstructed **SPECT images.**
- A ^{99m}Tc-filled **Jaszczak phantom** is the standard phantom used for SPECT quality control (QC) and has three sections.
  - **Uniformity section** to evaluate noise and artifacts.
  - **Spheres of acrylic (various sizes)** to evaluate partial volume and cold contrast detectability.
  - **Rods** of various sizes to evaluate resolution.
- **Continuous SPECT QC is performed by technologists.**
  - **Center of rotation** is performed using point sources or **line source monthly.**
  - **Jaszczak** phantom is imaged semiannually to semiquantitatively assess **spatial resolution, uniformity,** and **image contrast (quarterly).**
- **Quantum mottle** is a **major factor** in **SPECT** due to the **low number** of **photons** used to reconstruct each voxel.
- **Spatial resolution** of **SPECT** is **worse** than that for **planar imaging** because SPECT images are derived from planar images.
- The **major benefit** of **SPECT** is the **improved contrast** that results from the **elimination** of **overlapping structures.**
- **Ring or bull's eye artifact** occurs when detector uniformity is not properly corrected.
  - Nonuniformities appear as **rings due to detector rotation.**
  - It is **corrected by high-count flood (uniformity) image** to create new calibration coefficients.
- **Attenuation from a large breast or diaphragm** may create an artifact that simulates myocardial defects if not corrected.
- **CT artifacts** may impact attenuation-corrected images due to the incorrect attenuation and thus correction factors.
  - **High-Z materials** like metal and iodine **may cause artificial hotspots** due to their large attenuation correction factors—images without attenuation correction should be cross-referenced.

II. POSITRON EMISSION TOMOGRAPHY/COMPUTED TOMOGRAPHY I

A. Localization and Radiobiology

- Cancer cells are **"glucose hungry"** to support their rapid reproduction.
  - Warburg effect (aerobic glycolysis), upregulation of glucose transporters and hexokinase, activation of proliferation signals such as ras and myc, and downregulation of phosphatase (reverse hexokinase) all contribute to increased glucose use.
  - More avid cells use more glucose, allowing for **positron emission tomography (PET)-informed cancer staging.**
- **Fluorodeoxyglucose (FDG) is an analogue** of glucose utilizing F-18 in place of an OH group.
- **FDG is competitive with glucose** for facilitated diffusion/active transport uptake by the cell (reason for **patient fasting** before imaging).
  - Glucose transporters (**GLUTs**) facilitate **diffusion into cell** and are also responsible for **brown fat artifact** and crossing of the blood-brain barrier.
  - Sodium-coupled glucose transporters (**SGLTs**) are important for urinary excretion and kidney reabsorption of FDG.
- Glucose is phosphorylated by hexokinase and then the product (glucose-6-phosphate) goes through glycolysis.
  - FDG becomes FDG-6-phosphate and **cannot go through glycolysis, so it is stuck inside the cell.**
  - During radioactive decay, **F-18 becomes O-18 and it picks up a hydrogen** from the environment to become glucose again, allowing it to break down and be excreted by the cell.
- PET radioisotopes **emit a positron (beta plus),** which slows to a stop and interacts with a local electron (**annihilation interaction**).
  - The rest mass of the two particles turns into **two 511 keV photons emitted 180° from each other** (these are detected for PET imaging).

B. PET Scanner Hardware

- **Scintillators** are utilized to capture annihilation gamma rays.
  - Key **PET scintillator properties** are **photoelectric absorption efficiency, energy resolution,** and **light decay time.**

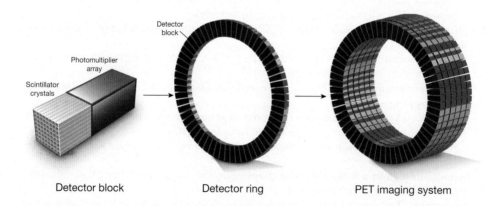

FIG 14.3 PET makes use of individual detector blocks (left) coupled to an array of light detectors (photomultiplier tubes or silicon photomultipliers). A large number of blocks are used to create a single detector ring (middle). Several detector rings are placed adjacent to each other to create a complete imaging system (right). PET, positron emission tomography.

- **Bismuth germanate scintillators** have the **best absorption** characteristics (high Z) but **worse energy resolution.**
- **Lutetium oxyorthosilicate (LSO) and lutetium-yttrium oxyorthosilicate (LYSO)** emit more light, thereby **improving** their **energy resolution,** and have **shorter light decay times (afterglow),** which offer **improved performance at high count rates.**
- **Crystals** are often arranged in **6 × 6 or 8 × 8 blocks,** resulting in 36 to 64 "crystals" per detector block, as depicted in Figure 14.3.
- Each **block** is **coupled** either to an array of traditional **photomultiplier tubes or digital silicon photomultipliers (SiPM),** which provide **positional information** and offer **pulse height analysis** capability.
  - SiPM generally offer 20% improvement in spatial resolution, improved energy resolution, and half the minimum coincidence time.
- **Detector blocks** are **arranged** in a **ring,** and **several rings** are **arranged concentrically** (Fig. 14.3).

C. Image Formation, Reconstruction, and Processing

- Commonly used **PET radionuclides** are summarized in Table 14.1.
- **PET** systems use fast electronics to **determine** whether **two detected 511-keV photons** were likely produced by a **single annihilation event.**
- **Two interactions** occurring within a specified **time interval** (coincidence timing window) are called a **true coincidence** event.
  - Only ~1% of **detected photons** are **accepted** by the **coincidence circuitry.**
- Simultaneous detection of two events (i.e., 511 photons) generates **line of response** (Fig. 14.4).
- **Line of response** data are used to generate projections and create a **sinogram** as shown in Figure 14.4 (i.e., **projections vs angle**), similar to those obtained in CT.
- Images are **reconstructed** using **iterative reconstruction** algorithms (e.g., **OSEM**).
- **Scatter coincidences** and **random (accidental) coincidences** degrade image quality and standardized uptake value (SUV) accuracy (Fig. 14.4).
  - **Scatter** and **random coincidences account for 30% to 70% of interactions each.**
  - **Scatter is worse with larger patients.**
  - **Random coincides are worse with higher dosages.**

D. Attenuation Correction

- **Sixteen-slice CT** scanners are **adequate** for most **PET/CT** applications, but **64-slice scanners** are required for **cardiac** applications.
- **Spiral CT** scanning (**eyes to upper thigh**) can be performed in less than **20s.**
- Average **photon energies** in CT images (**60-70 keV**) are nearly **10 times lower** than **photon energies** used in **PET** (i.e., **511 keV**) (Fig. 14.1).
- **The attenuation coefficient** at **PET energies** is estimated by **extrapolation** from the known attenuation properties of tissues.

TABLE 14.1	Positron-Emitting Nuclides for Positron Emission Tomography Imaging, With Average Positron Energy and the Corresponding Mean Range of Travel in Water			
Radionuclide	Atomic Number (Z)	Half-Life ($T_{1/2}$; minutes)	Average Positron Energy (MeV)	Mean Range in Water (mm)
Carbon 11	6	20	0.39	1.1
Nitrogen 13	7	10	0.49	1.4
Oxygen 15	8	2.1	0.74	1.5
Fluorine 18	9	110	0.25	1.0
Rubidium 82	32	1.25	1.4	5.9

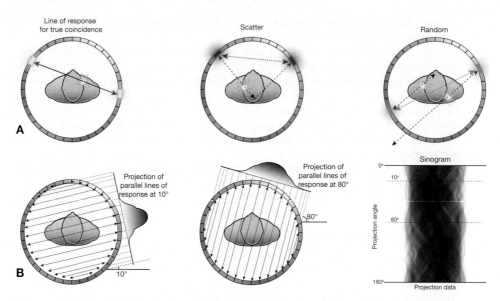

FIG 14.4 A: A line of response (LOR) is the solid line linking two detectors that captured 511 keV photons in coincidence (yellow detectors on left, solid black line). Scatter event (red detectors in middle, red dashed line) and random coincidence event (green detectors on right, green dashed line) also occur, as shown as erroneous dashed lines, and which will degrade image quality. **B:** Two projections containing all the detected LOR at 10° (left) and at 80° (middle) are shown in the complete sinogram (right) that shows acquired projections as a function of the projection angle.

- As in SPECT, attenuation coefficient **extrapolation** for **tissues** and **bone** is **straightforward** but causes **problems** for **metallic implants**.
- **Attenuation** in **PET** depends on the *total thickness* of the tissue (Fig. 14.5).
  - **Twenty centimeters** of **tissue only transmits 14%** of **511-keV photons** requiring an **attenuation correction factor** of about **7**.
  - **Attenuation correction factors** are **higher** in **PET** imaging than in SPECT, even though PET uses much higher energy photons.
- In a **large person,** the loss of counts because of **attenuation can exceed 95%**.

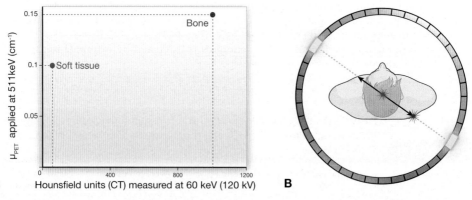

FIG 14.5 A: A CT scan is used to compute the attenuation coefficient (HU) of each pixel (i.e., Hounsfield unit), which is used to predict the attenuation of 511 keV photons (μ_{PET}). **B:** The red annihilation has no attenuation for the 511 keV photon traveling rightward and a maximum attenuation for the photon traveling leftward. The blue event in the center has equal attenuation for the two photons emitted. The attenuation correction factor takes *both photons* into account and turns out to be the same for *any* annihilation event along this line. In this example, the red and blue events would both use exactly the same correction factor determined by the total attenuation ($\mu_{PET1} + \mu_{PET2} + \dots$ etc) along the black path through the patient. CT, computed tomography; HU, Hounsfield unit.

E.   **Advanced PET Technology**
  - Measuring the difference in arrival times of the two annihilation photons from an annihilation event is used in **time-of-flight (TOF) PET.**
    - **TOF data** improve **signal-to-noise ratio (20%-100%)** and facilitates changes to improve **spatial resolution.**
    - **LSO or LYSO** have short light decay times and facilitate TOF imaging.
  - **Point spread function (PSF) recovery** models the interaction in the crystal and compensates for light spread as a function of angle and interaction depth.
    - Spatial resolution is improved in peripheral areas of the field of view.
  - TOF and PSF are often utilized together, and **care must be taken when comparing SUV or imaging characteristics over time.**
    - Best practice is to **use the same scanner** so that changes over time can be attributed to physiological changes and not difference in scanner technology.
  - **Whole-body PET** scanners utilize many more rings than does a typical scanner.
  - Added rings mean many **more coincidences detected between rings.**
    - Whole-body scanners have a **much better sensitivity,** which can be traded for improved spatial resolution or lower patient dosage.
    - Higher sensitivity can also be used to allow for **dynamic uptake studies** with reasonable amounts of noise.

III. POSITRON EMISSION TOMOGRAPHY/COMPUTED TOMOGRAPHY II

A.   **Standardized Uptake Value**
  - Defined as the **ratio of radionuclide concentration in a region of interest divided by injected concentration.**
    - Practically the denominator is determined by dividing injected activity by patient body mass (or lean body mass), which is really a volume using 1 mg/mL conversion for water.
  - More glucose-avid tissues (e.g., cancer) will accumulate a relatively larger amount of FDG, resulting in a higher SUV value.
  - **Increasing SUV** over time is a sign of **disease progression,** whereas decreasing SUV is a sign of therapeutic response.
  - It is important to **keep all factors as consistent as possible when scanning a patient serially** so that changes are attributable to physiology and not changing technical parameters
    - **Dosage** and **time between injection and scanning** can cause changes in SUV.
    - Reconstruction parameters, postprocessing filters, TOF, and PSF recovery can alter SUV values.
    - Small lesions will exhibit **artificially low SUV due to partial volume effects.**
  - SUV is **semiquantitative, allowing for comparison within the same patient for relative change** but not accurate enough for meaningful comparison across patients.

B.   **Clinical Imaging**
  - For adults, **500 MBq** (~3.7 MBq/kg pediatric) of ^{18}F is generally imaged within 40 minutes of injection.
  - **Axial coverage** in typical **PET** for a single detector position is about **20 to 25 cm.**
  - PET scans take **1 to 3 minutes** at **each bed position.**
  - Current clinical PET scans use about **five bed positions** to cover the body.
    - Up to **10 positions** are used for **head-to-toe PET** imaging of melanoma patients.
  - A **420 to 650 keV energy window** is often used to identify 511 keV annihilation photons.
    - This is narrowed to **440 to 580 keV for digital systems** due to improved energy resolution and sensitivity.
  - Adult patients fast 6 h (2-4 h pediatric) to **limit competitive glucose uptake.**
    - Glucose levels should be 80 to 120 mg/dL or 180 to 200 mg/dL for diabetic patients (muscle uptake)

- An intravenous line (22-24 gauge) is inserted **contralateral to the side of interest** when possible.
- The patient rests in a warm calm environment for biodistribution (45-60 min).
  - Warm room and blankets **limits brown fat activation.**
  - No motion, talking, eating, or other stimulation is advised to **limit nontarget uptake.**
- The patient should be placed in the **center of the bore to maximize spatial resolution.**

C. Quality Control

- **Image plane uniformity** is obtained with a cylinder filled with a positron emitter.
  - **Uniformity** is likely performed **every 2 weeks.**
- **Detector calibration** is performed with a positron source in FOV.
  - **Detector calibration frequency** is usually recommended by **vendor.**
- **PET sensitivity (counts per MBq)** is obtained using a sleeved rod source.
  - **Sensitivity** is likely performed **annually.**
- **Spatial resolution** is assessed by imaging of a point source 1 and 10 cm from the center of the bore.
  - Resolution is tested at acceptance and likely checked **annually.**
  - Resolution decreases 15% to 20% from bore center to 10 cm from bore center.
- Count rate **performance** and **scatter fraction** are assessed using a line source in polyethylene cylinder.
  - **Count rate** and **scatter fraction** tests require special software and are performed **annually.**
- **System performance,** including uniformity and hot contrast, is evaluated every **6 months** using a standardized QC phantom.

D. Artifacts and Image Quality

- **PET images** have **high counts** and much **lower** levels of **image mottle than gamma cameras.**
  - PET images use **several million counts, 10 times more** than **planar images.**
- The **ultimate limit** of **spatial resolution** is determined by the **range** of the **positron (1 mm for** ^{18}**F).**
  - ^{82}**Rb** has **worse resolution** than ^{18}F because of the much **longer distance traveled** by the **positrons** (Table 14.1).
- **Spatial resolution** of commercial **PET** systems is about **5-mm full width at half maximum (FWHM)** when imaging a line source of activity.
  - PET resolution is **worse** at the **edge** than at the center of the bore because 511-keV photons may be detected by adjacent detectors.
- Figure 14.6 shows examples of **partial volume artifacts,** which affect the counts in **small lesions.**
  - **Partial volume artifacts** occur for lesions **smaller** than **two to three times the FWHM spatial resolution (i.e., ~8-15 mm).**

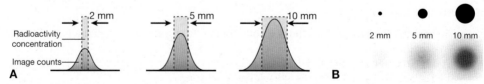

FIG 14.6 A: Three lesions with exactly the same radioactivity (i.e., MBq/mL). The small 2 mm lesion is blurred by the imaging system (FWHM 5 mm), markedly reducing the counts in the center. As the lesion size increases, the observed counts in the center of the lesion increases, and is maximized when the lesion diameter is two to three FWHM values (i.e., 10-15 mm). **B:** The upper image shows how lesions of varying size would appear with a perfect imaging system (i.e., no image blur), where all lesions show the true maximum intensity. The lower image shows the appearance of these same lesions in an image with 5 mm FWHM. FWHM, full width at half maximum.

- **A faulty detector** results in an **angled black line** in the **sinogram,** whereas a faulty block results in a thicker angled black strip in the sinogram.
- **Contrast material** (e.g., barium) and **metal implants** may **cause** "hot" **artifacts** in **attenuation-corrected PET** images (especially if there is patient motion).
- **Misregistration** is typically due to patient motion between the CT and PET scans.
  - Roughly 2% of lung base/liver dome lesions are incorrectly localized due to respiratory motion during PET.

IV. DOSIMETRY AND PROTECTION

A. Dose, Dosage, and Dosimetry

- Calculating **organ** and **effective dose** from administered radioactivity in NM is normally performed by **medical physicists.**
  - Organ doses require total number of decays in **source organs,** and published data on the **target organ** dose per decay in the source organ.
- **Organs** that **take up activity** generally receive the **highest doses.**
- **Reducing organ size** markedly **increases organ doses** (Table 14.2).
- ^{123}I or ^{131}I transported **across** the **placenta** after **12 weeks** can result in extremely **high fetal thyroid doses.**
- Highest **organ doses** from **diagnostic NM** procedures range between **10 and 50 mGy.**
- **Effective dose** for many of the ^{99m}Tc radiopharmaceuticals is **a few millisieverts.**
  - **Lung scans** have relatively low effective doses (**1.5 mSv**), whereas **stress cardiac** studies have higher effective doses (**10 mSv**).
- **Effective dose** for a body **PET** scan using **444-MBq (12 mCi)** ^{18}F-labeled FDG is **8 mSv.**
- In PET/CT, the **CT** component of a body imaging procedure is ~**12 mSv** when the CT scan is acquired for **diagnostic** purposes (i.e., $CTDI_{vol}$ (L) ~ 12 mGy).
  - A **low-dose CT** scan primarily for anatomy and **attenuation correction** (i.e., $CTDI_{vol}$ (L) ~ 2 mGy) results in an effective dose of **only 2 mSv.**
- Table 14.3 lists common organ and effective doses for imaging radionuclides.

B. Therapeutic Applications

- **Beta minus emitters** are **ideal** for **therapy applications** because the **beta particle energy** is primarily **deposited** in the **organ taking up** the **radionuclide.**
  - Beta particles in therapy typically have a range of 0.5 mm to a few millimeters.
- Large administered activities of sodium ^{131}I are commonly used for treatment of **hyperthyroidism** and **thyroid cancer,** resulting in high thyroid doses.
  - Thyroid dose to a patient receiving 370 MBq of ^{131}I with a 50% thyroid uptake is 200,000 mGy (200 Gy).
- ^{90}Y-labeled microspheres can be lodged in the small blood vessels of **liver neoplasms** to deliver therapeutic doses.
- ^{89}Sr is administered intravenously to treat painful **osseous metastases** from prostate cancer and breast cancer.
  - ^{89}Sr is a **pure beta emitter** and poses no hazard to medical staff or patient families, except for urinary excretions for a few days.

TABLE 14.2	Relative Dose to Target Organs When 1 MBq of Activity (e.g., ^{99m}Tc) is Taken up by Different-Sized "Organs" With No Biological Clearance		
Source Organ	**Source Organ Mass (kg)**	**Target Organ**	**Relative Target Organ Dose**
Whole body[a]	70	Whole body	1
Liver	2	Liver	20
Thyroid	0.02	Thyroid	2,000

[a]Uniform distribution.

TABLE 14.3	Organ and Effective Doses in Nuclear Medicine			
Procedure	Radiopharmaceutical	Administered Activity[a] (MBq)	Organ with Highest Dose (mGy)	Effective Dose (mSv)
Bone scan	^{99m}Tc MDP	925	Bone surfaces (57)	5
Liver/spleen scan	^{99m}Tc sulfur colloid	200	Spleen (15)	2.5
Biliary scan	^{99m}Tc mebrofenin	150	Gall bladder (16)	2.5
Cardiac MUGA scan	^{99m}Tc red blood cells	925	Heart (20)	6.5
Cardiac scan	^{99m}Tc sestamibi	1,100	Gall bladder (43)	10
Lung scan	^{99m}Tc MAA	150	Lungs (10)	1.5
Renal scan	^{99m}Tc MAG3	185	Bladder (20)	1.3
Thyroid scan	^{99m}Tc pertechnetate	185	Large intestine (11)	2.4

[a]Divide by 37 to obtain mCi. MAA, macroaggregated albumin; MAG3, mercaptoacetyltriglycine; MDP, methylene diphosphonate; MUGA, multigated acquisition.

- **^{223}Ra dichloride** is an alpha emitter that is used for osseous metastasis from prostate cancer.
- Table 14.4 lists key characteristics of radionuclides used for therapy in NM.

C. Patient Protection

- **Activity** in a **diagnostic unit dose** from a **radiopharmacy** can be **calculated** from the labeled activity and decay time.
  - **Radiopharmaceutical doses** prepared **in-house** must be **measured** in a **dose calibrator before injection.**
- **Doses from patients** after injection of most diagnostic radiopharmaceuticals **at 1 m** are about **10 μSv/h.**
  - For **^{18}F patients,** the dose rate is **100 μSv/h.**
- Dose rates from ^{131}I **therapy patients** are about **50 and 300 μSv/h** for **hyperthyroidism and cancer, respectively.**
- **Written directives** are **not required** for **diagnostic procedures** but are **mandatory** for all **therapy** procedures.
- NRC is **notified** for **medical events** where **unintended radiation** exposures exceed **50-mSv effective dose** or **500-mGy organ dose.**
- **Release** of ^{131}I NM patients (Nuclear Regulatory Commission [NRC] regulations) is **allowed** when their **activity** is **less than 1.2 GBq.**
  - **Patients** receiving ^{131}I may **activate** radioisotope **security alarms.**
- **Breastfeeding cessation** is used to ensure infant dose is less than 1 mSv.
  - Breastfeeding cessation for ^{99m}Tc **radiopharmaceuticals** is 24 hours and ^{18}F is 4 hours.

TABLE 14.4	Radionuclides Used for Therapy			
Radionuclide	Emissions	Half-Life ($T_{1/2}$; days)	Mean Particle Energy (MeV)	Gamma Ray Emissions (keV)
Radium 223	Alpha	11.4	5.8	10-1,000 (1%)
Strontium 89	Beta minus	51	0.58	<0.01%
Yttrium 90	Beta minus	2.7	0.93	None
Iodine 131	Beta minus	8.0	0.19	360 (82%)
Lutetium 177	Beta minus	6.6	0.13	208 (~11%)

- Breastfeeding cessation for ^{201}Tl, ^{111}In, and ^{67}Ga are 4, 6, and 28 days, respectively.
- ^{177}Lu and ^{223}Ra require discontinuation.
- Breastfeeding should be discontinued **6 to 8 wk before** ^{131}I **administration** to reduce dose to the maternal breast as well as the infant.

D. Operator Protection

- **Protective clothing** and handling precautions are **required** to minimize contamination.
- Personnel should **wear gloves** when handling radionuclides and dispose of them in radioactive waste receptors after use.
- Volatile radionuclides (^{131}I liquid and ^{133}Xe) should be stored in **fume hoods.**
- Handling of radionuclides requires **leaded syringes** to minimize extremity doses.
- **The dose rate** to the hands from **radiopharmaceutical syringes is 0.2 mGy/h/MBq.**
  - **Syringe shields** should be used, which **reduces extremity doses threefold.**
- **Extremity doses** need to be monitored using **ring dosimeters** worn on a finger.
- **NM operators** who risk intake of radionuclides (e.g., ^{131}I liquid) should undergo a mandatory **bioassay (e.g., thyroid monitoring** for **iodine uptakes).**
- The major source of **operator exposures** in NM is **patients** who generally have been administered **several hundred MBq** of ^{99m}Tc.
- **NM technologists normally do not wear lead aprons during their daily work.**
  - **Lead aprons** are **less effective** in **NM** than x-ray imaging because of the much higher gamma ray photon energies (e.g., 140 vs 40 keV).
- **The NM technologist's effective doses** range between **2 and 4 mSv** per year.

E. Miscellaneous Protection

- **The Radiation Safety Committee** must include authorized users of each type of radionuclide used, the **radiation safety officer (RSO),** nursing service member, and a manager who is neither an authorized user nor an RSO.
  - The RSO is the link between the committee and radionuclide users.
- All **packages** with radioactive labels must be **monitored** for **surface contamination** and at 1 meter upon receipt.
  - **Label** information includes the radiation trefoil symbol, the transportation index (TI) (dose rate at 1 m in mrem/h), radionuclide, activity, and the number "7" indicating the hazard is radiation.
  - A white "**Radioactive I**" label is used when surface readings are ≤0.5 mrem per hour and TI is 0.
  - A yellow "**Radioactive II**" label is used when surface readings are ≤50 mrem per hour and TI ≤ 1.
  - A yellow "**Radioactive III**" is above Radioactive II thresholds.
- **Wipe tests** or Geiger Counter surveys must be performed wherever radionuclides are prepared, administered, or stored at least weekly to test for contamination.
  - For wipe tests, small dampened filter papers are wiped over an area and checked in a well counter (threshold: 1,000 decays/min from a 100 cm^2 area).
- **Daily surveys** are required in areas where **written directive procedures** with unsealed materials are carried out and typically use a survey meter.
  - Battery voltage and accuracy testing using the Cs137 check source should be performed before each survey meter use.
- **Minor spills** require **containment, decontamination,** as well as **notification** of the **RSO.**
- **Major radiation spills** are based on activity released (e.g., **>4 GBq** of ^{99m}Tc or **>40 MBq** of ^{131}I).
  - Major spills require the **presence** of the **RSO.**
  - Only unit doses of **therapy agents or bulk amounts diagnostic agents** typically reach this level.
- Syringes used for injection are disposed of in special "hot sharps" receptacles.

- **Radioactive waste** of any radionuclide with a half-life <120 days can be **stored** for **10 half-lives** prior to being surveyed to confirm background activity and disposed of as regular waste.
- **Nuclear Regulatory Commission (NRC)** does **not regulate excreta** from people who have received radioactive materials for medical diagnosis or therapy.
  - **Disposal** of excreta in the **sewer system** in any amount is **legal.**

Chapter 14 (Nuclear Medicine II) Questions

14.1 What is a typical number of projections acquired in a dual-head SPECT system performing a cardiac SPECT study?
   A. 10
   B. 60
   C. 100
   D. 600

14.2 What is a typical matrix size for SPECT image?
   A. 32^2 or 64^2
   B. 64^2 or 128^2
   C. 128^2 or 256^2
   D. $\geq 256^2$

14.3 How does resolution change as iteration number increases during OSEM SPECT reconstruction?
   A. Increase
   B. No change
   C. Decrease

14.4 Use of low-pass filter to process SPECT images will likely _____ mottle and _____ resolution.
   A. reduce; improve
   B. reduce; degrade
   C. increase; improve
   D. increase; degrade

14.5 Bone SPECT (^{99m}Tc-labeled phosphonates) most likely uses _____ energy and a high-_____ collimator.
   A. low; resolution
   B. low; sensitivity
   C. medium; resolution
   D. medium; sensitivity

14.6 What radioisotope is used to perform extrinsic gamma camera flood (uniformity) testing?
   A. ^{57}Co
   B. ^{137}Cs
   C. ^{226}Ra
   D. ^{201}Tl

14.7 What section of the Jaszczak phantom is used for testing for artifacts such as ring artifact?
   A. Uniformity
   B. Spheres
   C. Rods
   D. Vials

14.8 Why do patients fast for 6 h before PET injection?
   A. FDG is competitive with glucose.
   B. Reduce radioisotope motility.
   C. Reduces brown fat activation.
   D. Reduces patient weight for dosing.

14.9 Patients are centered in the PET bore to optimize what image quality metric?
   A. Temporal resolution
   B. Noise
   C. Contrast
   D. Spatial resolution

14.10 What is a reasonable energy window in digital PET imaging?
   A. 300 to 500 keV
   B. 450 to 550 keV
   C. 200 to 800 keV
   D. 550 to 700 keV

14.11 Reducing coincidence window timing will improve what type of coincidence?
   A. True
   B. Scatter
   C. Random

14.12 What is time-of-flight PET technology?
   A. Models the point spread function and compensates
   B. Uses detector timings to localize emission along the line of response
   C. Utilizes >20 rings to rapidly image the entire body
   D. Segments the skin line to remove scatter outside the body

14.13 How does increasing the number of PET rings improve system sensitivity?
   A. More interring coincidences
   B. Fewer random coincidences
   C. Improved scatter rejection
   D. Reduces out-of-scanner coincidences

14.14 How does FDG localize in the body?
   A. Ligand binding
   B. Chemisorption
   C. Facilitated diffusion
   D. Embolization

14.15 Brown fat activation with FDG is most often seen in what demographic?
A. Geriatric men
B. Adolescent-to-young men
C. Geriatric women
D. Adolescent-to-young women

14.16 Attenuation correction artifacts near metal are commonly associated with what other artifact (sometimes too subtle to clearly see)?
A. Dead block
B. Truncation
C. Ring
D. Motion

14.17 What are typical effective doses for ^{99m}Tc-labeled radiopharmaceuticals?
A. 0.1 mSv
B. 4 mSv
C. 16 mSv
D. 55 mSv

14.18 What particle is responsible for dosing caregivers of I-131 NaI patients?
A. Beta minus (electrons)
B. Beta plus (positrons)
C. Gamma rays
D. Characteristic x-rays

14.19 The NRC would be notified if an NM patient received an unintended organ dose in excess of (mGy):
A. 5
B. 50
C. 500
D. 5,000

14.20 In NM, personnel *must* be provided with a dosimeter when their occupational dose may exceed _____% of a regulatory dose limit.
A. 1
B. 3
C. 10
D. 30

Answers and Explanations

14.1 B (60). A SPECT study would acquire about 60 projection images as a gamma camera rotates around the patient. This is a tradeoff between acquisition time and noise (number of counts).

14.2 B (64^2 or 128^2). Most SPECT images would use an image matrix of either 64^2 or 128^2. Lower count images tend to use smaller matrices to mitigate for high noise in the image.

14.3 A (Increase). OSEM is a common Iterative Reconstruction algorithm used to generate SPECT images from projection data (i.e., sinogram). As the number of iterations increases, the resolution improves, but the noise increases as well.

14.4 B (reduce; degrade). Use of low-pass filters reduces mottle and degrades resolution (i.e., blurrier).

14.5 A (low; resolution). SPECT and gamma camera images (99mTc) are generally obtained using low energy and a high-resolution collimators.

14.6 A (^{57}Co). Extrinsic gamma camera floods are obtained using large discs of ^{57}Co that have a 120 and 136 keV photon (close to 140 keV of 99mTc) and a half-life of 270 days, thus "lasting" a reasonable time before needing to be replaced.

14.7 A (Uniformity). The uniformity portion of the phantom is used to identify artifacts and to measure noise.

14.8 A (FDG is competitive with glucose.). Fasting reduces glucose, making it more likely cells uptake FDG instead of glucose from food sources.

14.9 D (Spatial resolution). Spatial resolution is generally best in the center of the bore and rapidly degrades as the patient is moved toward the bore wall.

14.10 B (450-550). Pulse height analysis window in digital PET imaging is roughly 20% and the peak is 511 keV.

14.11 C (Random). Requiring both detectors to trigger within a shorter time interval makes it less likely two random photons from two unrelated events will incorrectly trigger the system.

14.12 B (Uses detector timings...). TOF PET uses the exact photon interaction times to roughly localize the decaying radioisotope within the line of response.

14.13 A (More interring coincidences). With more rings, it is more likely that true coincidences will be detected between rings meaning that more detections will occur.

14.14 C (Facilitated diffusion). FDG localizes against the gradient using GLUTs to transport across the cell membrane.

14.15 D (Adolescent-to-young women). Brown fat is metabolically active and is more often seen in adolescent women. Cold temperature increases brown fat metabolic activity.

14.16 D (Motion). Attenuation correction factors are very high in the metal due to its density and high Z. Since there is no activity in the metal it typically does not matter. If the patient moves slightly between the CT scan and PET acquisition, the large correction factor multiplies the normal activity of metal-adjacent tissue, causing a false hot spot.

14.17 B (4 mSv). Average nuclear medicine patient effective doses are a couple of millisieverts for most 99mTc-labeled radiopharmaceuticals and are therefore deemed to be moderate (1-10 mSv).

14.18 C (Gamma rays). I-131 emits electrons and high energy gamma rays. The electrons kill off thyroid tissue and typically cannot escape the patient. Gamma rays are responsible for <10% of the dose to the thyroid and ~100% of the dose to people surrounding the patient.

14.19 C (500 mGy). NRC must be notified if an NM patient receives an unintended organ dose in excess of 500 mGy (or an effective dose in excess of 50 mSv).

14.20 C (10%). Personnel are provided with a dosimeter when their occupational dose is expected to exceed 10% of a regulatory dose limit.

Magnetic Resonance I

I. MAGNETISM AND RESONANCE

A. Magnetic Nuclei

- **Magnetic fields** exist as **dipoles** with the **north pole** the origin of the magnetic field and **south pole** the return (Fig. 15.1A).
- Some particles have property **(spin)** and behave like bar magnets.
  - Similar to how some particles have a property called charge.
- Nuclei with an **even number of protons** *and* an **even number of neutrons** have **no nuclear magnetization** because particles pair up and fields cancel.
  - Nuclei with an **odd number of protons**, or **odd number of neutrons**, have a **nuclear magnetization and can be imaged.**
  - **Magnetic particles or nuclei** may be called **dipoles, spins,** or **magnetic moments.**
- Abundance of **hydrogen** in the body (**~63% of atoms**) with its 1 proton makes it the basis of magnetic resonance imaging (MRI).
  - **Magnetic fields** associated with **electrons** are approximately **1,000 times stronger** than **protons** but are not used clinically used due to other implementation difficulties.
- In the **absence** of any **external magnetic field, protons** in tissues are **randomly oriented**, with **no net tissue magnetization.**
- In an external magnetic field, hydrogen **protons** will either **slightly align parallel** or **antiparallel** (Fig. 15.1B).
- The **parallel orientation** corresponds to a **slightly lower energy** level, and there are slightly **more protons** in this **parallel** orientation alignment.
  - The excess hydrogen protons that align parallel to the field give the tissue a **net magnetization (M_z)** (Fig. 15.1B).
- **Net tissue magnetization** is **proportional** to **magnetic field strength** (see Table 15.1).

B. Susceptibility

- **Magnetic susceptibility** is the extent to which **matter becomes magnetized** when placed in **an external magnetic field (B).**
- Local **(internal) magnetic fields** within tissues **change** because of the effect of atomic electrons, and are **quantified** by **tissue susceptibility.**
- **Diamagnetic materials** have **small negative values** of **susceptibility** and result in **small decreases** of the **local magnetic field.**
  - **Tissues** and plastic are **diamagnetic** with a very small negative **susceptibility.**
- At **interfaces**, *changes* in **susceptibility** result in **changes** in **local magnetic fields.**
  - Changes in **magnetic susceptibility** alter magnetic fields at interfaces that may result in **signal loss** due to spin dephasing.

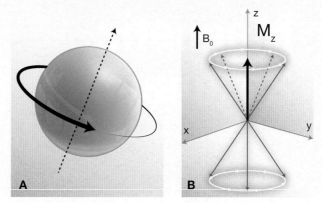

FIG 15.1 A: Each proton exhibits magnetic properties with the magnetization oriented along the dashed line. The arrow represents the North Pole and other side the South Pole of the field; **B:** In a magnetic field B_0 pointing along the z axis, protons align parallel ("up") and antiparallel ("down") to B_0 and precess at the Larmor frequency. Magnetization components in the x-y plane all cancel out so that only the longitudinal magnetization along the z axis contributes to the MR signal. The net magnetization (black vertical arrow) is the difference between the four that point "up" and the three that point "down."

- **Paramagnetic atoms** placed in external magnetic fields produce an **increase** in the **local (internal) magnetic field.**
  - **Paramagnetism** is caused by magnetism of **unpaired atomic electrons.**
- **Paramagnetic materials,** such as **gadolinium** and **deoxyhemoglobin,** have a small **positive** of **susceptibility.**
- **Ferromagnetic** substances **dramatically increase** the **local magnetic** field and have a very **large susceptibility.**
  - Examples include **steel** in some dental devices and **implanted medical devices.**
- **Ferromagnetic** materials can significantly **distort** acquired **signals.**

C. **Radiofrequency**
  - A **changing magnetic field can induce an electric field** in an antenna (coil) and be used to create a signal.
    - Net tissue magnetization is stationary and aligned with the external magnetic field, so there is no signal.
  - If the protons (net tissue magnetization) are pushed away from alignment, they will **precess similar to the wobbling of a spinning top** and create a changing magnetic field (Fig. 15.1B).
  - **Larmor (precession) frequency** for a magnetic nucleus is directly **proportional** to the **magnetic field** strength.
    - For **protons (i.e., hydrogen nuclei),** the Larmor frequency is **42 MHz at 1 T** (i.e., radiofrequency [RF]).

TABLE 15.1	Relative Number of Two Million Proton Spins (Parallel and Antiparallel) as a Function of Magnetic Field Strength (B)			
Magnetic Field (Tesla)	Parallel	Antiparallel	Net Longitudinal Magnetization (M_z)	Relative Longitudinal Magnetization
1.5	1,000,004	999,995	9	1
3	1,000,009	999,991	18	2
7	1,000,021	999,979	42	4.67

- A **radiofrequency pulse at the Larmor frequency resonates** with the hydrogen proton and pushes it away from alignment at a rate **proportional to the RF intensity and duration.**
  - **Doubling the RF pulse duration or intensity doubles** the flip angle.
- A **vector** at **angle θ°** can be **replaced** by two vectors that are directed **parallel** and **perpendicular** to the external **magnetic field** along the + z axis.
- The **vector parallel to the external magnetic field** is called **longitudinal magnetization (M_z)**, and the **perpendicular vector** is called **transverse magnetization (M_{xy}).**
  - **More M_z before RF pulse means more M_{xy} after the pulse, and more M_{xy} after the pulse means a stronger induced signal in the coil.**

D. Free Induction Decay

- After a **90° RF pulse**, the **net tissue magnetization** is all in the **transverse plane (M_{xy})**, and the **longitudinal magnetization (M_z)** is **zero.**
- The **transverse magnetization vector (M_{xy})** rotates at the **Larmor frequency.**
- This **rotating transverse magnetization** can be **detected** as an **induced voltage** in a **coil** wrapped around the tissue.
  - **RF coils (antennas)** produce stronger signals when placed closer to the source.
- **Voltages detected** in the coils **oscillate** at the **Larmor frequency** and are called the **free induction decay (FID) signal** (Fig. 15.2).
  - **Increasing the magnetic field** increases **FID signal frequency**, and vice versa.

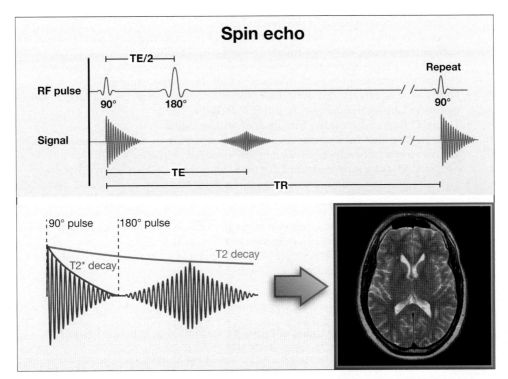

FIG 15.2 Top: Pulse sequence diagram showing acquisition of a Spin Echo signal. The initial 90° RF pulse creates the FID which rapidly decays away due to T2* dephasing. A 180° pulse at a user-selected time TE/2 causes the transverse magnetization to refocus and a spin echo to form at time TE. This then repeats at time TR to collect the next pulse. Bottom: FID signal demonstrating rapid T2* dephasing and signal loss. T2 losses alone are much slower and also represent the maximum signal that the echo can attain. A representative T2-weighted spin echo image is shown. FID, free induction decay; RF, radiofrequency; TE, echo time; TR, repetition time.

- **FID signals** are **weak** because of the small number of nuclei that contribute to the signal (Table 15.1).
  - The small number of nuclei contributing to magnetic resonance (MR) signals, and weakness of nuclear magnetism, results in **low signal-to-noise ratios (SNR)** in MR.
- The **FID is not typically used for image formation**; instead, **echoes** of the FID are created and collected after signal localization information is imprinted in the echoes.
- Transverse magnetization will always decay to zero as the system becomes disordered and relaxes.

▊ II. RELAXATION TIMES

A. **Spin-Lattice Relaxation (T1)**
  - **Protons** placed into **magnetic fields** produce a **net longitudinal magnetization** with a magnitude M_z parallel to the direction of the external magnetic field.
  - **Longitudinal magnetization** does not occur instantaneously but **grows exponentially** from zero to M_z characterized by a **time constant T1.**
    - At a time equal to T1, 63% of M_z will have formed, with essentially full **net longitudinal magnetization (i.e., M_z)** occurring **after 4 × T1.**
  - **T1** is the **longitudinal relaxation time** and is a result of **spin-lattice interactions.**
    - Only the presence of **atomic lattice motions** at the **Larmor frequency** can "encourage" spins to **give up their excess energy and realign with the external magnetic field.**
  - Table 15.2 shows T1 times for solids (long), tissues (intermediate), and fluids (long).
  - **T1 times are characteristic of the tissue type.**
  - **Large slow molecules** do *not* have motions that result in magnetic oscillations at the Larmor frequencies, so energy transfer is slow (i.e., **T1 long).**
  - **Tissues** have **faster molecular motions**, resulting in lattice motions at Larmor frequencies that do "encourage" nuclei to return to equilibrium (i.e., **shorter T1**).
  - **Fluids** have **extremely fast molecular motions**, with a corresponding **lack of lattice motion at Larmor frequencies**, resulting in **long T1.**
  - **Tissue T1 times are typically hundreds of milliseconds.**
  - **After** an **RF pulse** displaces the longitudinal magnetization, **net tissue magnetization always reverts (recovers)** to its equilibrium value (i.e., M_z) **after 4 × T1.**
    - In **liver, M_z fully recovers after 2,000 ms** (T1 is 500 ms) following any RF pulse.
  - Tissue **T1 increases** with **increasing magnetic field** strength.

B. **Spin-Spin Interaction (T2)**
  - In uniform magnetic fields, **transverse magnetization decays exponentially** with a **time constant T2**, resulting in a **reduction** in FID signal.
    - At time T2, the FID signal has decayed to 37% of its original value (M_{xy}), and **after 4 × T2**, the **transverse magnetization is essentially zero.**

TABLE 15.2	Representative Values of T1 and T2 for Protons in Different Types of Material			
Material	Molecular Size and Motion	Molecular Interactions	Longitudinal Relaxation Time T1 [ms]	Transverse Relaxation Time T2 [ms]
Solid (e.g., bone)	Large and slow	Bound	Long [>1,000]	Ultrashort [<0.01]
Soft tissue (e.g., Liver)	Intermediate	Intermediate	Moderate [500]	Short [50]
Fluid (e.g., CSF)	Small and fast	Free	Long [>1,000]	Long [>1,000]

- **Spin-spin interactions dephase transverse magnetization (M_{xy})** when they experience **each other's others magnetic field.**
  - **Spin** precession speed up in the higher fields and slows down in the lower fields caused by adjacent spins.
- **Increasing spin-spin interactions shortens T2**, and vice versa.
  - Once **spins** have **interacted (dephased)**, the **transverse magnetization is irretrievably lost.**
  - **Dephased** spins just means their fields **point in random directions and cancel** to leave no net transverse magnetization.
- Table 15.2 summarizes **T2** values, which are **characteristic of the tissue** and **roughly independent** of **magnetic field strength.**
- **Protons** in **large, slow,** and **bound molecules** in all **solids** (e.g., bone) have extremely **short T2** (<0.01 ms), and immediately dephase after a 90° RF pulse
  - It is very **difficult** to obtain a **signal** from **solids.**
- **Protons** in **molecules** with **intermediate size** and **speed** (e.g., tissues) have **short T2 (~50 ms).**
- **Protons** in **small, fast,** and **free molecules** (e.g., **water**) have **long T2 (>1,000 ms).**
- Figure 15.3 shows transverse magnetization **(M_{xy}) decaying** following a 90° RF pulse (i.e., **T2**) followed by longitudinal magnetization **(M_z) recovery** (i.e., **T1**).
  - For all **tissues T2 ≤ T1**, since transverse magnetization (M_{xy}) cannot be present when longitudinal magnetization (M_z) has fully recovered.

C. Magnetic Field Inhomogeneity (T2*)

- In MR, **transverse magnetization** in tissues is observed to **decay** much more **rapidly** than would be expected from **spin-spin interactions alone.**
- **FID signals** decrease exponentially with a **decay rate constant T2*** (Fig. 15.2).
- For a tissue with T2 50 ms, and T2* 5 ms, M_{xy} disappears after 20 ms (i.e., 4 × T2*).
  - In the absence of T2* effects, M_{xy} would disappear after 200 ms (i.e., 4 × T2).
- Any **magnetic field inhomogeneity increases spin dephasing** in the transverse plane (i.e., M_{xy}) **contributing to T2*.**
- **Variations** in **local magnetic fields** increase (or decrease) rotation rates of adjacent spins, so they point in different directions (i.e., spins are **dephased).**
  - This **dephasing results** in a **loss** of **transverse magnetization**, resulting in a rapid reduction in the FID signal (Fig. 15.2).
- **MR magnets** always have **magnetic field inhomogeneities** with slight differences (parts per million) in magnetic field at different locations.

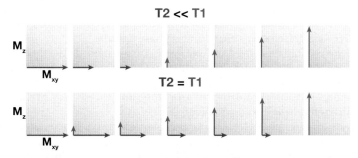

FIG 15.3 Following a 90° RF pulse, the net magnetization is all in the transverse plane (red arrows M_x) and decays exponentially with a time constant T2. When T2 << T1 (upper line), the transverse magnetization decays rapidly, and then longitudinal magnetization (blue arrows M_z) recovers exponentially with a time constant T1 and eventually returns to its full equilibrium value (see Fig. 15.1). When T1 and T2 are equal (lower line), we see exactly the same behavior because M_{xy} still decays exponentially with time constant T2, and M_z still recovers exponentially with time constant T1. RF, radiofrequency.

- **Inhomogeneities** are produced in the vicinity of **magnetic tissues** (e.g., **blood clots**).
- At **tissue boundaries, magnetic fields change** due to **differences** in **material suscep-tibility.**
- **T2* dephasing** is the **total** dephasing of **transverse magnetization (i.e., M$_{xy}$)** from all sources of **magnetic field inhomogeneity.**
  - **Magnet inhomogeneities, magnetic tissues,** and **interfaces** contribute to **T2*.**

E. **Spin Echoes**

- Following a **90° RF pulse**, net magnetization vector rotates into the transverse plane.
- In the transverse plane, net **magnetization (M$_{xy}$) rapidly dephases (T2* effects).**
- A **180° RF (refocusing) pulse** at a **time TE/2** generates a **spin echo (SE)** at time **TE, canceling** out **T2* dephasing effects.**
- Figure 15.4 shows an analogy based on soldiers who **start** of **in phase (lined up)** result-ing in an FID signal.
  - Soldier **marching speed** is analogous to the **Larmor frequency,** where a higher local field results in a higher Larmor frequency (spin rotation).
- Each soldier walks at a different speed, and they **rapidly dephase (out of step),** corre-sponding to reduction of the FID signal due to T2*.
  - Soldiers, like spins, always march at their own speed irrespective of direction.
- At time TE/2, a **refocusing 180° RF pulse** is applied, which rotates spins through 180°, analogous to soldiers performing a right about turn.
- At time TE, the **soldiers** are **perfectly lined up** to **generate** an **echo,** which **cancels** out **T2* dephasing.**
- **Some soldiers disappear (i.e., T2 effects),** and echo is **weaker** than the **FID signal.**
- **Echoes, not** the **FID,** are the signals generally **detected** in **MR** imaging.
  - As an **echo grows** and **decays,** it is **sampled (digitized),** providing one **row** of **data** in **k-space.**

III. IMAGING

A. **Time-Varying Gradients and Localization**

- In **uniform magnetic fields,** MR **signals** (e.g., echoes) originate from the **entire patient,** with **no spatial information** that permits generating images.
- **Signal localization requires magnetic field gradients** to modify the magnitude of the magnetic field at different locations.
  - A **gradient changes** the **Larmor frequency** along this **gradient direction by slightly altering the magnetic field strength a tiny bit.**
- **Identification** of the **Larmor frequency** enables the **location along** this the **gradient direction** (selected axis) to be **determined.**
- **Locating** the voxel producing a **signal** requires application of **three gradients,** known as the **slice-select, frequency encode,** and **phase encode.**
  - **Each echo** is obtained using a **unique set** of combinations of the **three gradients.**
- In MR, detected signals are generally echoes, which are **analogous** to **computed tomog-raphy (CT) projections** obtained at each x-ray tube angle.
  - **CT** acquires projections at **different x-ray tube angles,** whereas **MR** acquires echoes with **different phase encode gradient** values.
- To generate an **MR image (128^2) requires** acquisition of **128 echoes** and **sampling each echo 128 times.**
  - In this example, acquired data are a 128^2 matrix, with 128 × 128 numbers.

B. **Slice Select**

- **Slice** selection is achieved by **applying** a **gradient** in the desired direction (canonically z-direction) whenever an **RF pulse** is **applied.**
- Consider a magnetic field gradient along the (operator selected) z-direction so that the Larmor frequency increases with increasing z.

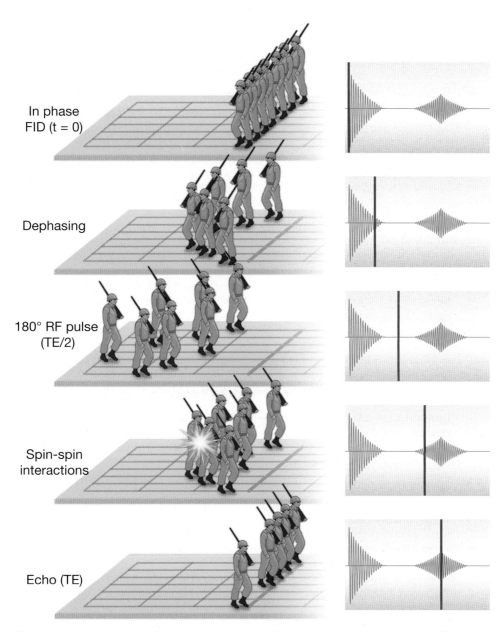

FIG 15.4 An analogy of echo formation based on marching soldiers who all start lined up (in phase) resulting in a signal (FID) from seven (in-phase) soldiers. Each soldier walks at a slightly different speed analogous to spins rotating at different speeds in slightly different magnetic fields, and the signal is rapidly lost (dephasing). At time TE/2, a refocusing 180° RF pulse is applied to rotate spins through 180°, analogous to soldiers performing a right about turn. Each soldier continues to walk at his own speed, with two soldiers lost to T2 effects (spin-spin interactions). At time TE, the remaining five soldiers are perfectly lined up to generate an echo (TE), which is weaker than the initial FID. FID, free induction decay; RF, radiofrequency; TE, echo time.

- When a **RF pulse** with a given frequency is applied, there is only **one location** along the **z-axis** where **longitudinal magnetization** will be **rotated** through 90° (Fig. 15.5A).
  - To the left of the selected slice (Fig. 15.5A), Larmor frequency is lower than the applied RF, and to the right of the selected slice the Larmor frequency is higher.

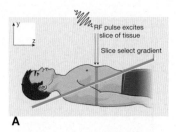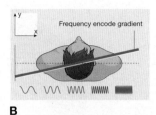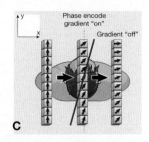

A   **B**   **C**

FIG 15.5 **A:** A slice select gradient is applied for each RF pulse to selectively excite protons in the slice located at a z value where the magnetic field corresponds to the Larmor frequency of the RF pulse; **B:** When echoes are formed, a frequency encode gradient is applied to encode spatial information along the x axis (i.e., low frequencies left and high frequencies right); **C:** Between RF pulses and echoes, a phase encode gradient is applied to encode spatial information along the y axis (i.e., large phase shifts at patient front and small phase shifts at patient rear). The encoded information is extracted mathematically using 2D Fourier transforms generating an MR image of each slice (see Fig. 15.6). MR, magnetic resonance; RF, radiofrequency.

- **Changing RF frequency adjusts** the **location** of the **selected slice** along this z-axis.
  - In Figure 15.5A, increasing the RF frequency would move the selected slice to the right (larger z-coordinate).
- **RF pulses** contain a **narrow range** of **frequencies (i.e., transmit bandwidth)** which **determines** the **slice thickness.**
  - For a given slice select gradient, **increasing** the **transmit bandwidth** (range of RF frequencies transmitted) results in **thicker MR slices,** and vice versa.
- At fixed RF bandwidth, **changing** the **slice select gradient strength** (i.e., mT/meter) **changes slice thickness.**
  - **Increasing** the strength of the **slice select gradient** results in **thinner slices,** and vice versa.
- Slice select gradient ensures **only protons in a single slice will be excited, thus localizing the signal in that direction.**

C. Frequency Encode

- A **frequency encode gradient** is **applied** during the time **echoes** are created.
  - The **frequency encode direction** (canonically x-axis) must be **perpendicular to** the **slice select** direction (Fig. 15.5B).
- Consider the pixels along the x direction when the echo is forming, and the frequency encode gradient is applied, as depicted in Figure 15.5B.
- The left pixels in Figure 15.5B have **lower magnetic fields,** with lower Larmor frequency, and therefore signals from this region have **lower frequencies.**
  - At the right end of Figure 15.5B, the **magnetic field is higher,** resulting in **higher frequencies** in the **detected signal.**
- **Frequencies** in the **echo** can be **extracted** using **Fourier techniques,** and the location of the signal along this direction can be determined.
- For a **128^2 MR image,** the **echo (signal)** is **sampled 128 times,** providing a row of data with 128 discrete values.
  - For a **256^2 MR** image, the **echo** is **sampled 256 times.**
- Application of the **frequency encode gradient** during echoes provides information where along the frequency encode gradient signals originate but **provide no y-axis information.**
  - Changing the number of data points (samples) in echoes does not affect image acquisition time.
- This is also called the **readout gradient,** since it is turned on when reading (sampling) the echo.

D. Phase Encode

- **Between** the **RF pulse** and **echo**, a **phase encode gradient** is **applied.**
  - **Phase encode direction** (canonically y-axis) must be **perpendicular to** both **slice select** and **frequency encode** directions.
- Consider a row of pixels along the y-axis in the absence of any gradient (Fig. 15.5C).
- Because **all spins** are in the same **uniform magnetic field**, they **all rotate** at the **same speed**, and **point** in **same direction.**
- Application of a gradient along the y-axis results in a **magnetic field** at the **bottom** that is **lower** than at the **top.**
  - **The spins** at the **bottom rotate** more **slowly** than the **spins** at the **top.**
- When the **phase encode gradient** along the y-axis is **switched off**, the **spins point** in **different directions** (i.e., they have **different phases**).
  - After the gradient is switched off (Fig. 15.5C), the **direction** in which a **magnetization** is **pointing** permits **y-axis location** of a signal to be **identified.**
- In Figure 15.5C, **spins** that point **upward** are at the **bottom**, and those that point to the **right** are at the **top.**
  - This is analogous to the frequency encode gradient (Fig. 15.5B) where low frequencies are at the left, and high frequencies are on the right.
- The exact phase to localize the signal cannot be determined from a single echo; instead, just the magnitude difference from the slight phase differences is recorded.
- By repeating this with slightly different phase encode gradient strength many times, the system gets many slightly different echoes for the same slice.
  - If there are 256 pixels desired in the phase encode direction, then 256 different echoes are collected to create a system of 256 equations that can be solved to give the signal strength at each position in the phase encode direction.

TABLE 15.3	Sequence of Events in a Generating a 128^2 Spin Echo Image			
Event	**Slice Select (SS) Gradient G_z**	**Phase Encode (PE) Gradient G_y**	**Frequency Encode (FE) Gradient G_x**	**Comment**
90° RF pulse	**On**	Off	Off	FID rapidly decays (T2*)
First PE gradient	Off	**On**	Off	First of 128 values
180° RF pulse (TE/2)	**On**	Off	Off	Refocusing pulse
Echo (TE)	Off	Off	**On**	Echo sampled 128 times
Wait (TR)	Off	Off	Off	Inactive period
90° RF Pulse	**On**	Off	Off	FID rapidly decays (T2*)
Second PE gradient	Off	**On**	Off	Second of 128 values
180° RF pulse (TE/2)	**On**	Off	Off	Refocusing pulse
Second Echo (TE)	Off	Off	**On**	Echo sampled 128 times
Wait (TR)	Off	Off	Off	Inactive period
90° RF pulse	**On**	Off	Off	FID rapidly decays (T2*)
....	....	....	....	....

FID, free induction decay; RF, radiofrequency; TE, echo time; TR, repetition time.
Sequence is repeated total of 128 times, resulting in 128 rows of data corresponding to 128 echoes generated using 128 different phase encode gradients. Each echo has 128 data points, and data acquisition takes 128 × TR seconds.

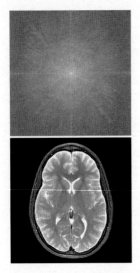 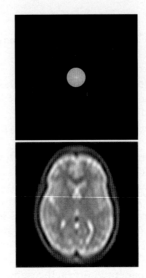 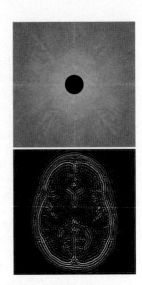

FIG 15.6 Images on the top line are k-space (acquired data), which show the spatial frequencies in an MR image. Each line corresponds to a digitized echo that has encoded spatial information, analogous to a CT projection in a sinogram (Fig. 11.3C). The lowest spatial frequencies (i.e., large objects) are in the center (origin), and the highest spatial frequencies (i.e., small objects and edges) are at the periphery. A 2D Fourier transform of k-space is used to generate the MR images shown on the bottom line. Using the central region of k-space (middle) results in an image showing large-scale contrast, whereas using the periphery of k-space (right) results in an image showing the corresponding "details." When the whole of k-space is used (left), the complete MR image is obtained. CT, computed tomography; MR, magnetic resonance; RF, radiofrequency.

E. k-Space

- An **echo** is **generated** and **sampled (digitized)**, resulting in a **row** of **discrete numbers.**
- **Slice select gradients (z-axis)** are applied whenever an **RF pulse** is generated, and a **frequency encode gradient (x-axis)** is applied during the **echo.**
- In between the initial RF pulse and echo, a phase encode gradient is applied (y-axis).
- Table 15.3 shows the sequence of events in obtaining a 128^2 MR spin echo image.
  - **Acquired data (128 rows each with 128 discrete numbers)** are **called k-space.**
- Figure 15.6 shows a schematic example of the acquired data (k-space), and how these are generated in spin echo imaging.
- **Each number** in **k-space** refers to a **spatial frequency.**
  - The **center (origin)** represents **low spatial frequencies,** and the **periphery** represents **high spatial frequencies.**
- **Low spatial frequencies** provide the **image contrast** data (large scale structures), and **high spatial frequencies** provide **small features** and **edges (detail)** (Fig. 15.6).
- **MR images** are **obtained** by performing a **two-dimensional Fourier transform (2D FT)** of **k-space.**
  - The **2D FT** extracts the **information encoded** into the **echoes,** analogous to **filtered back projection** algorithms extracting **data encoded** in **CT projections.**
- A 256^2 **MR** image would acquire **256 echoes, each echo** would be **sampled 256** times, and **k-space** would be a 256^2 **matrix.**

IV. INSTRUMENTATION

A. Static (Main) Magnet

- **Superconducting MR magnets** use a wire-wrapped cylinder (i.e., a solenoid) to generate a uniform magnetic field inside the bore.
  - **Superconducting magnets** are kept **cold using liquid helium.**

- A perpetually circulating electric current creates the **static (main) magnetic field (B_0)** that aligns protons in the body for imaging.
- The static **magnetic field** is **always** "on."
  - If the wire temperature rises, the system loses its superconducting properties and the stored magnetic energy is converted to heat resulting in a **magnet quench.**
- **Magnetic field** "strength" is the number of magnetic lines per unit area.
  - The **most common** clinical **MR magnet** is **1.5 T** (15,000 Gauss).
  - Earth's magnetic field is ~0.5 G and a refrigerator magnet's is ~10 to 100 G.
- **MR magnetic fields** must have a **homogeneity** of only a **few parts** per **million.**
- Large metallic objects (e.g., **elevators** and ferromagnetic structures) can **disrupt** the **uniformity** of the main magnetic field and degrade MR image quality.
  - **Magnetic shimming** is used to make small corrective changes to the main field to **improve** the **magnetic field uniformity.**
- Magnetic field inhomogeneities can result in **fat saturation artifacts**, where nonuniform areas result in bright signals because the fat saturation pulses were ineffective.
- Metallic objects in patients show artifacts due to **magnetic field distortions** and may result in bright areas (**pulse pile**) on **images.**
- **Ferromagnetic objects** (e.g., scissors, screwdrivers, oxygen cylinders) may be **pulled into** the powerful **magnet (missile effect).**

B. Gradient Coils

- MR systems have **three magnetic field gradient coil pairs** oriented in the x, y, and z directions.
- A combination of three orthogonal sets of gradient **coils allows gradients** to be **oriented** in **any arbitrary direction.**
  - This is different from CT where acquisition is always axial slices and other orientations are reconstructed using image processing later.
- Activated gradients superimpose a linear gradient along the selected direction.
- **Axial gradients (z)** are produced using **Helmholtz coils.**
  - **Gradients** that change the main field as a function of **x or y** distance are normally produced by **saddle coils.**
- On a 1.5 T scanner gradient strengths are **~30 mT** per **meter**, meaning the field increases 30 mT 1 meter from the center of the bore.
  - Gradients are always 0 in the center of the bore.
- **Gradients** may need to be **switched on** and off **rapidly (<500 μs).**
  - The **slew rate** is the time to achieve the required magnetic field amplitude.
- **Nonuniform gradients** result in image **distortions.**
- **Gradients** generate small, rapidly decaying **eddy currents** in other coils or **metal structures nearby.**
  - Induced **eddy currents** impair scanner performance and may **create image artifacts.**
- Actively **shielded gradient** coils **reduce problems** associated with **eddy currents.**

C. Radiofrequency Coils

- **Transmitter coils** are used to send in **RF pulses**, and **radio waves** from **patients** are **detected** by **receiver RF coils.**
  - **The range** of **emitted frequencies** is called the **transmit bandwidth,** and which determines the slice thickness.
- **Receiver coils** may be physically **separate** from the transmit RF coil or may be the **same coil** switched electronically **from transmit** to **receive mode.**
- **Receiver bandwidth** is the range of frequencies received in the echoes and is directly proportional to the applied gradient strength (mT/m).
  - Detected **noise** is **directly proportional** to receiver bandwidth, so using strong gradients generally reduces acquired SNRs.
  - Low bandwidth makes chemical shift artifact worse.

- **Volume coils** are designed to **transmit** and **receive** uniform RF signal throughout a volume, e.g., the **head coil** or **body coil built into the MR scanner.**
  - The large field of view (FOV) of the body coil means it receives lots of noise from random motion of protons in the body within the FOV.
  - The relatively large distance between the body coil and patient means the signal is relatively weak.
  - Head coil has a smaller FOV and is closer to the patient, meaning it will have less noise and higher signal.
- **Surface coils** have **increased sensitivity close** to the **coil,** but the signal drops off with increasing distance from the coil.
  - These have the largest SNR due to their small FOV and close proximity to the patient.
- **Linear volume coils** receive the signal from only one of the x- or y- axis of the rotating transverse magnetization.
  - **Quadrature volume coils** receive the signal in both the x- and y- axis, therefore increasing the overall SNR and reducing image artifacts.
- **Phased array coils** are a combination of many surface coils around the body part being examined and are used for parallel imaging.
- In **large patients** and at **higher frequencies**, there may be significant **attenuation** of the RF waves by the patient.
  - **Dielectric artifacts** are dark regions in the patient center where a **weaker RF** has **not achieved** the required M_z **rotation** (i.e., <90° following a 90° RF pulse).

D. RF and Magnetic Shielding

- MR imaging systems require **RF shielding** to prevent **RF signals** (radio broadcasts) **getting into** the coils and increasing the background noise.
  - **RF shielding** also prevents the powerful **RF pulses** from **escaping** and **interfering** with outside electronic equipment.
- The **RF shielding** is a **Faraday cage**, which consists of **conductive sheet/mesh** of **metal (e.g., copper)** lining the MR magnet room.
- **RF leakage** into the MR suite results in **zipper (RF contamination) artifacts**, intense **lines** along the **phase encode gradient direction from external signals (e.g., FM radio).**
  - Leaving the **MR room door open** or damaging the Faraday cage will result in **zipper artifacts.**
- The **magnetic flux lines** from the main magnetic field can extend out to a **large distance from** the **magnet.**
  - The **static gradient magnetic field (fringe field)** may affect magnetically sensitive devices.
- **Passive magnetic shielding** consists of **thick iron plates** or layers of special steel sheet metal embedded in the MR magnet room walls.
- An alternative to static shielding is the use of **active shielding.**
  - **Active shielding** makes use of magnetic fields created by additional **coils** (i.e., electromagnets) to **cancel** the **ambient field** within a volume.
- **Very old pacemakers** may be **deactivated** by magnetic **fields above 0.5 mT.**
  - **Access** is **restricted** in areas having **magnetic fields > 0.5** mT (i.e., **5 Gauss line**).
  - Since most old pacemakers are no longer in use this restriction will be updated to 0.9 mT (9 Gauss) in the near future.

E. Shim Coils and Cryogen

- **Shim coils** are active or passive magnets designed to improve B_0 homogeneity.
  - Inhomogeneities cause the Larmour frequency to vary by a few parts per million and are worse with higher field strengths.
- After the MR scanner is built, small defects in manufacturing cause inhomogeneities in the B_0 field.
  - **Tune-up shims** are typically passive and are designed to correct for defects and improve magnetic field homogeneity.

- When a patient enters the scanner bore, **they alter the magnetic field.**
  - **Static shims** are active and passive magnets that are adjusted based on measurements before scanning begins.
- Shimming is especially important in cardiac imaging, echo planar imaging, spectral fat suppression, and in areas of many susceptibility changes (e.g., hands).
  - Poor shimming causes **line broadening in spectroscopy.**
- Modern MRI systems use supercooled coils to generate B_0.
- **The cryogen** controls the temperature of the coils using liquid helium to keep coil wires superconducting.
- Slight increases above the **4 kelvin boiling point** of liquid helium will result in a massive expansion of helium into gas form, which may cause pressure explosions.
  - Even brief exposure to liquid or boiled gas helium may cause **frostbite.**

V. SPIN ECHO AND GRADIENT-RECALLED ECHO

A. Spin Echo

- **Spin echo (SE)** imaging commences with a **90° RF pulse** that **rotates longitudinal magnetization (i.e., M_z) into the transverse plane (i.e., M_{xy}).**
  - Slice select gradient is used to control which slices are excited.
  - **Magnetization (M_{xy}) rapidly dephases**, principally because of T2* effects.
- **Phase encode gradient localizes the signal in one dimension.**
- **Spin echoes** are obtained by applying a **refocusing 180° RF pulse** at a time **TE/2** to produce an **echo** at **time TE,** as depicted in Figure 15.2.
  - Frequency encode gradient is applied during echo readout to localize the signal in the final dimension.
- **Spin echoes** mitigate **T2* dephasing** as shown in Figure 15.4 but are **weaker** than the **FID** because of T2 losses (i.e., spin-spin interactions).
  - **Relative** to the **FID,** a tissue (**T2 = 50 ms**) would have an **echo intensity** of **60%** at a TE of **25 ms**, and **20%** at a TE of **80 ms.**
- **Each echo** is **digitized** and results in **one line** of **k-space** being stored in a computer.
  - **SE sequences** (i.e., 90° RF + refocusing 180° RF pulse) are **repeated** after a **repetition time (TR)** as shown in Figure 15.2.

B. TR, TE, and Contrast Weightings

- **T1** and **T2** are **tissue properties**, but it is *operator's choice* of **repetition time (TR)** and **echo time (TE) scan parameters** that introduces **T1, T2,** and **proton density tissue weighting.**
  - TR is the time between successive flip angle pulses (e.g., 90° to the next 90° pulse).
  - TE is the time from the flip angle pulse to the center of the received echo.
- **The choice** of **TR** affects the **contrast** between **tissues** that have **differences** in **T1** because tissues with **short T1** will **recover M_z** quickly, whereas those with **long T1 will not.**
  - **T1-weighted** images are obtained with a **short TE and short TR.**
- **Short T1 tissues** have close to the full longitudinal magnetization (M_z) on the second, third, and all subsequent acquisitions, and **echoes are strong.**
  - **Long T1 tissues** have little longitudinal magnetization (M_z) on the second, third, and all subsequent acquisitions, and **echoes are weak.**
- For **short TR times,** short T1 materials (e.g., **fat**) **appear bright,** and **long T1 materials (e.g., CSF) appear dark** as depicted in Figure 15.7.
- A **long TR** value permits the magnetization in all tissues to fully recover, and long TR times generate **no T1 weighting.**
  - A **short TR time is the average T1 time in the FOV** and a **long is about 3× the short.**
- **The choice** of **TE** affects the **contrast** between **tissues** that **differ** in their **T2** values.
  - **T2-weighted** images are obtained with a **long TE and long TR.**

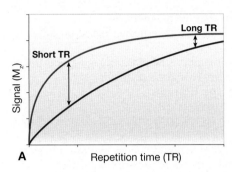

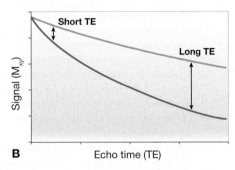

FIG 15.7 A: Following a 90° RF pulse, longitudinal magnetization (i.e., M_z) recovers rapidly when T1 is short (red curve) but much more slowly when T1 is long (purple curve). When short values of TR are selected, tissues with short T1 will result in much higher signals than those with long T1 resulting in high contrast (different signals) between these two tissues. Selection of a long TR will result in similar signals from both tissues irrespective of their T1 values, and thus exhibit little T1-weighted contrast. **B:** When echoes are created in T2 weighted spin echo imaging, selection of a long TE will result in a much greater signal (i.e., M_{xy}) from tissues with long T2 (yellow curve) than from tissues with much shorter T2 (blue curve). At short TE times, the signals from both types of tissue (yellow and blue) will be similar and thereby show little T2-weighted contrast. TE, echo time; TR, repetition time.

TABLE 15.4	Operator Choices of Echo Time (TE) and Repetition Time (TR), Flip Angle, and Their Effect on Tissue Contrast in Spin Echo and Gradient-Recalled Echo Imaging Performed at 1.5 T			
	Image Contrast	**TE (ms)**	**TR (ms)**	**Flip Angle (°)**
Spin echo	T1 contrast	25	600	90
	T2 contrast	90	1,800	90
	Proton density contrast	25	1,800	90
Gradient-recalled echo	T1 contrast	3	7	50
	T2* contrast	30	500	10
	Proton density contrast	3	300	10

- **Long TE** times **reduce transverse magnetization** for **tissues** with **short T2** more than for tissues with **long T2**, thereby providing **high contrast** (Fig. 15.7).
  - In **T2-weighted SE images**, **tissues** with **long T2 values appear bright**, and **tissues** with **short T2** values **appear dark**.
- **Short TE** values result in little T2 decay, with **minimal differences (contrast)** between **tissues**, thereby eliminating T2 weighting (Fig. 15.7).
- **Proton density–weighted images** have contrast dependent on the different densities of mobile hydrogen in the tissues.
  - **A long TR and short TE minimize T1 and T2 weightings.**
- Table 15.4 summarizes how **T1 and T2 weighting** is achieved by adjusting **TR and TE times** in spin echo imaging.

D. Acquisition Time and Fast Spin Echo

- A **spin echo sequence (128 × 128)** acquires **128 echoes** and **takes 128 × TR seconds.**
- In the **time interval** between **TE and TR**, MR hardware (coils and gradients) can be used to **acquire additional images** at **different slice locations.**
- With **TR of 550 ms,** and **TE of 100 ms, five 128^2 images** can be acquired in **70 seconds**, the **time** to **acquire one slice** (i.e., 128 × TR [0.55 s]).
- Initial echo (**100 ms**) pertains to **slice #1**, the next one at **200 ms** would pertain to **slice #2**, the one after at **300 ms** would pertain to **slice #3**, and so on.

- A **second echo** pertaining to **slice #1** would be obtained at **650 ms**, a **third echo** pertaining to **this slice** would be obtained at **1,200 ms**, and so on.
- With **square pixels, more pixels** are needed for the **longer AP** dimension (e.g., 192) in **head** images than for the **shorter lateral dimension** (e.g., 128).
  - The **longer dimension** is normally the **frequency encode direction**, with each echo sampled 192 times.
  - There is no time penalty for increasing frequency encode samples.
- Pulse sequences are repeated 128 times, generating 128 different echoes, with the **phase encode gradient** applied along the **shorter dimension.**
- In **head MR**, the **frequency encode gradient** is normally applied along the **(longer) AP** orientation and in **abdominal MR**, along the **lateral orientation.**
  - It is possible to make the longer dimension the phase encode gradient direction, but this would require longer imaging times (i.e., 192 × TR vs 128 × TR).
  - Typically, this is done only to avoid certain artifacts (e.g., motion) going through anatomy of interest.
- **Fast spin echo (FSE)** techniques **acquire multiple echoes** in **each TR interval.**
  - When **four echoes** are acquired in **each TR interval** (i.e., **echo train length [ETL] is four**), a **different phase encode gradient** is applied to **each echo.**
- Since each echo will generate a line of k-space, an **ETL** of **four reduces imaging time** by a **factor** of **four.**
  - **Intensities** of **later echoes** get **progressively weaker (T2 dephasing),** so the appearance of **FSE image edges may blur for large ETLs.**
  - **Larger ETLs** also increase effective TE resulting in **more T2 weighting.**

D. Gradient Recalled Echoes

- **Gradient recalled echo (GRE)** sequences are generally designed to be faster to acquire than spin echo and even fast spin echo.
- **GRE** is generally initiated with a **user-selected flip angle < 90°.**
- Table 15.5 shows the amount of magnetization in the longitudinal direction and transverse plane as a function of flip angle.
- **Longitudinal magnetization (M_z)** is still **present,** so it is **not necessary** to **wait for recovery** of **longitudinal magnetization.**
  - **Low flip angles** offer both **signal (M_{xy})** and **longitudinal magnetization (M_z)** (Table 15.5), permitting use of a short TR times.
- **GRE imaging** relies on **reversing** the **polarity** of an **applied magnetic field gradient** to dephase and then rephase the FID to **generate echoes** (see Fig. 16.2).
  - **Reversed gradients** are **applied** along the **frequency encode direction,** providing frequency encoding during echo creation and sampling (digitization).
- **GRE** does **not need 180° refocusing RF pulses** to generate echoes and usually has a **lower SAR** because of the absence of a 180° RF refocusing pulse and **flip angle < 90°.**

TABLE 15.5	Longitudinal and Transverse Magnetization Components as a Function of Flip Angle, and Where $[M_z^2 + M_{x-y}^2]^{0.5}$ Always Equals 100%	
Flip Angle (°)	Longitudinal Magnetization M_z (%)	Transverse Magnetization M_{x-y} (%)
0	100	0
30	87	50
45	71	71
60	50	87
90	0	100

Small Flip Angles Still May Result in Relatively Large Transverse Magnetization.

E. GRE Imaging

- **GRE pulse sequences** use **short TR** times, permitting **fast acquisition times.**
- GRE sequences (TR 5 ms and 256 acquisitions) can be acquired in 1.3 seconds.
- A major variable in determining **tissue contrast** in **GRE** is the choice of **flip angle.**
- Table 15.4 shows how selected flip angle, TE, and TR times, influences the type of contrast in GRE images (i.e., T1, T2, or T2*).
- **T1 weighting** uses **larger flip angles (e.g., 70°)**, and **T2* weighting** uses **smaller flip angles (e.g., 10°).**
  - **GRE images** have much **lower signals** than **SE sequences** and **appear noisy** due to the lower flip angles used.
- **T2* relaxation** is the main **determinant** of **image contrast** with some **GRE** sequences since gradients **do not mitigate inhomogeneity dephasing like in SE images.**
- Areas of **T2* dephasing (blood clots** and **hemosiderin)** appear **dark** on **GRE images.**
  - By contrast, in **SE imaging, T2* effects are mitigated** when echoes are generated and appear less dark.
- Figure 15.2 shows an SE and Figure 16.2 shows the corresponding GRE image.
- **T2*GRE** sequences are used to depict **hemorrhage, calcification,** and **iron deposition** in tissues.
- Changes in **magnetic susceptibility** distort magnetic fields and result in artifacts that **depict signal loss (i.e., T2* effects).**
- **Balanced steady-state free precession (bSSFP) is** widely used in **cardiac imaging** and demonstrates the unique **contrast weighting of T2/T1.**

Chapter 15 (Magnetic Resonance I) Questions

15.1 Which nucleus has a net magnetism?
A. Helium-4
B. Carbon-12
C. Oxygen-16
D. Phosphorus-31

15.2 What is the relationship between the Larmor frequency and magnetic field?
A. Linear
B. Exponential
C. Logarithmic
D. Inversely proportional

15.3 What is the susceptibility of paramagnetic materials (e.g., Gd)?
A. Negative
B. Zero
C. Positive

15.4 How would doubling the strength and duration of an applied RF field increase the net magnetization flip angle?
A. 180°
B. 270°
C. 360°
D. 720°

15.5 How does FID frequency change when the magnetic field increases?
A. Increased
B. Unchanged
C. Reduced

15.6 What is a typical TR for T1W SE abdominal imaging?
A. 5 ms
B. 50 ms
C. 500 ms
D. 5,000 ms

15.7 How does doubling the magnetic field strength from 1.5 to 3T impact T2 times?
A. Doubled
B. Unchanged
C. Halved
D. Quartered

15.8 What is a typical T2* time?
A. 5 ms
B. 50 ms
C. 500 ms
D. 5000 ms

15.9 How will doubling TR impact acquisition times in GRE abdominal imaging?
A. Quadruple
B. Double
C. Unchanged
D. Halved

15.10 What type of receiver coil generally has the best SNR?
A. Head
B. Body
C. Surface

15.11 What is not present in GRE imaging compared to SE imaging?
A. Susceptibility artifact
B. 180° pulse
C. Slice select gradient
D. Center of k-space

15.12 What coils are primarily used provide spatial information in MRI?
A. RF
B. Gradient
C. Shim
D. Magnet

15.13 In SE sequences, with an echo at time TE, a slice select gradient is most likely applied at what time?
A. TE/4
B. TE/2
C. TE
D. >TE

15.14 How does increasing the slice select gradient strength (mT/meter) impact slice thickness?
A. Increased
B. Unchanged
C. Reduced

15.15 What image property does the center of k-space control?
A. Contrast
B. Noise
C. Spatial resolution
D. Temporal resolution

15.16 To quickly generate a 128 × 192 SE MRI image most likely requires the acquisition of _____ echoes, and sampling each echo _____ times.
A. 128; 128
B. 128; 192
C. 192; 128
D. 192; 192

15.17 Magnetic field inhomogeneities are most likely to affect signal intensities in what sequence?
A. GRE
B. SE
C. FSE
D. IR

15.18 How does acquisition time change if ETL is doubled in fast spin echo imaging?
A. Quadruples
B. Doubles
C. Unchanged
D. Halves

15.19 What artifact may occur if the scanner door is left open during scanning?
A. RF Leakage
B. Wraparound
C. Dielectric
D. Chemical shift

15.20 What characterizes dephasing time due to interactions between spins?
A. TR
B. T2
C. TE
D. T2

Answers and Explanations

15.1 D (Phosphorus-31). Phosphorus-31, which has an odd number of protons (Z = 15) and therefore 16 neutrons (A = Z + N = 31), and is used clinically for MR spectroscopy.

15.2 A (Linear). Larmor frequency for protons is 42 MHz/Tesla and is directly proportional to the magnetic field (i.e., 63 MHz at 1.5 T).

15.3 C (Positive). Paramagnetic materials have a small positive susceptibility (e.g., +0.001), which increases the local magnetic field slightly (e.g., >0.1%) when they are placed in a magnetic field.

15.4 C (360°). If the RF strength doubles, the flip angle doubles, and if the RF pulse is on for twice as long, this also doubles the flip angle. Doing both will thus quadruple the flip angle from 90° to 360°.

15.5 A (Increased). The FID frequency is directly proportional to the applied magnetic field, so increasing the applied magnetic field increases the FID frequency.

15.6 C (500 ms). Short TR times are generally 500 ms similar to average T1 times, ten times longer than tissue T2 relaxation times, and a hundred times longer than T2* times.

15.7 B (Unchanged). Unlike T1, T2 times are generally unaffected by magnetic field strength.

15.8 A (5 ms). T2* times are generally 5 ms, and ten times shorter than tissue T2 relaxation times, and a hundred times shorter than T1 times.

15.9 B (Doubled). Acquisition times for SE and GRE are proportional to TR.

15.10 C (Surface). Surface coils have a limited field of view, so they receive less body noise, and they are very close to the body, which keeps signal strength high.

15.11 B (180° pulse). The 180° pulse in SE is replaced by a gradient that dephases and then flips to rephase spins rapidly.

15.12 B (Gradient coils). Spatial information in MR is obtained by using gradients. Because a point is defined by three coordinates (x, y, and z), and a gradient provides information along one direction, MRI requires three gradients to be applied, which are all perpendicular to each other.

15.13 B (TE/2). For an echo at time TE, a 180° refocusing pulse is applied at TE/2, and a slice select gradient is always applied when the RF pulse is switched on.

15.14 C (Reduced). Increasing the slice select gradient strength reduces the corresponding acquired image slice thickness, and vice versa.

15.15 A (Contrast). The center of k-space encodes image contrast, while the edges of k-space impact the edge sharpness (light-dark pixel transitions).

15.16 B (128 echoes, each sampled 192 times). To generate a 128 × 192 SE MRI image would most likely acquire 128 echoes, and sampling each echo 192 times, taking 128 × TR time. It is also possible to acquire 192 echoes, and sampling each echo 128 times, but this takes longer (i.e., 192 × TR time).

15.17 A (GRE). Magnetic inhomogeneities increase T2* effects, which are observed on GRE pulse sequences; by contrast, T2* effects disappear (cancel out) when echoes are created using 180° refocusing pulses (e.g., SE and IR sequences).

15.18 D (Halves). Doubling ETL also doubles the number of k-space lines acquired in each TR and so it will halve the acquisition time.

15.19 A (RF Leakage). When the door is left open electromagnetic from outside may be picked up by the coils and contaminate the image.

15.20 B (T2). T2 characterizes the time for dephasing to occur in a tissue due to spin-spin interactions.

Magnetic Resonance II

I. SIGNAL SUPPRESSION AND SWI

A. Inversion Recovery

- **Inversion recovery (IR)** uses an initial **inversion 180° RF pulse** (Fig. 16.1).
- **After** the **180° IR pulse**, the **longitudinal magnetization** is pointing in the **negative z direction (−z)** and **recovers** to the +z direction **after passing through zero.**
- In IR sequences, the initial **180° pulse** is **followed** by a **90° pulse** after **time TI (inversion time)** (Fig. 16.1).
- This rotates **(any) longitudinal magnetization (M_z)** into the **transverse plane (M_{xy}).**
  - Applying the **90° TI pulse** when a **tissue's magnetization** is transverse will rotate it into **longitudinal** the plane leaving **zero** transverse **magnetization** and **suppressing** he **tissue's** signal.
- Inversion recovery is the basis of **short time inversion recovery (STIR)** sequences for **fat suppression** (Fig. 16.1).
  - At 1.5 T **STIR** has a **TI** value of about **250 ms** to **nullify** the **signal** from **fat.**
- In **fluid-attenuated inversion recovery (FLAIR)** sequences, **signal** from **fluids** is **suppressed** (Fig. 16.1).
  - At 1.5 T, **FLAIR** has a **TI** value of about **1,700 ms** to **eliminate cerebrospinal fluid (CSF) signal.**
- TI is generally chosen to be $\sim0.7 \times T_1$ of tissue to null.
- IR sequences are **especially useful in the presence of implants** where other methods may encounter issues due to magnetic field inhomogeneities.
- IR is widely used in cardiac imaging to null **blood** (dual inversion recovery), **blood and epicardial fat** (triple inversion recovery), and **myocardium.**
- IR sequences have **low signal-to-noise ratio (SNR), increased acquisition time,** and **may unintentionally suppress other tissues with T1 times close to the tissue of interest.**

B. Chemical Fat Saturation

- Chemical fat saturation (fat sat) utilizes a radiofrequency (RF) pulse at the Larmor frequency of fat.
  - Fat has a **slightly lower Larmor frequency than water**: ~220 Hz at 1.5 T.
  - Fat protons are **saturated by RF and then a gradient dephases them.**
- Fat sat is the most widely used fat suppression method due to its ease of use and ability to be **prepended onto almost any acquisition sequence.**
- Fat sat is based on the Larmor frequency, which is proportional to the magnetic field.
  - Magnetic field **inhomogeneities cause a change in fat Larmor frequency** and can cause a failure in fat suppression.

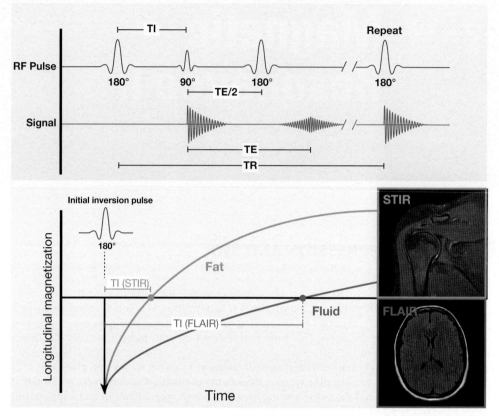

FIG 16.1 Inversion recovery (IR) sequences commence with an inversion radiofrequency (RF) pulse (180°), followed by a read-out 90° RF pulse at inversion time (TI) to "read out" (any) longitudinal magnetization (M_z) that has recovered and then "measured" in an echo formed following a 180° refocusing RF pulse. In IR sequences, the longitudinal magnetization is initially flipped 180°, so it points downward ($-M_z$) before recovering to the equilibrium value ($+M_z$) taking a time 4 × T1. As shown by the fat (orange) and fluid (blue) curves, M_z for each tissue has to pass through zero, so a judicious choice of TI (Fig. 16.2C) can suppress the signal from selected tissues. The choice of the shorter TI values can suppress the signal from fat (orange curve) in a STIR sequence (i.e., short tau IR), whereas the choice of a longer TI can suppress the signal from fluids (blue curve) in a FLAIR sequence (i.e., fluid-attenuated IR). FLAIR, fluid-attenuated inversion recovery; STIR, short time inversion recovery.

- **Implants** (e.g., biopsy clips) and **areas near the bore wall** (anatomy of large patients) often demonstrate fat suppression failure due to **inhomogeneities.**
- **Hybrid fat saturation methods** (e.g., STAIR [short repetition time adiabatic inversion recovery] and SPIR [spectral presaturation with inversion recovery]) combine fat sat with IR to **reduce sensitivity to magnetic field** inhomogeneities but retain the higher SNR, speed, and tissue selectivity.
- In many applications (e.g., musculoskeletal) fat signal is purposely attenuated instead of eliminated.
- Table 16.1 lists suppression methods and their dependencies on tissue properties and field homogeneity.

C. **Dixon Method and In-Out Phase**
- Water and fat have Larmor frequency differences of a few hundred Hertz.
- **Proper timing of TE** (echo time) can ensure that fat and water protons in the same pixel are pointing in the same direction, giving a **strong combined signal (in-phase).**

TABLE 16.1	Suppression Methods and Their Dependencies		
Suppression Method	**T1 Dependence**	**T2 Dependence**	**Main Field Inhomogeneity Dependence**
Chemical fat saturation	None	None	Strong
Dixon method	None	None	Weak
Inversion recovery	Strong	None	None
Hybrid (SPIR, SPAIR, etc.)	Strong	None	Moderate

- **Proper timing** (2.2 ms at 1.5 T and 1.1 ms at 3 T) **of TE** can also ensure that fat and water protons in the same pixel are pointing in opposite directions, causing **signal reduction (out-of-phase).**
- A **change in intensity** between in-phase and out-of-phase images can indicate the presence of **microscopic fat dispersed within other tissue.**
- Unintended out-of-phase imaging by poor TE choice can occur accidentally and is considered an artifact called **India ink (a type of chemical shift artifact).**
- **Dixon method** is a widely used fat suppression method based on in-phase and out-of-phase imaging.
- For each pixel, **two unknowns** (amount of fat signal and amount of water signal) in the pixel are solved using **two equations** and **two knowns** (in-phase and out-of phase pixel values).
  - Two new images are created: **fat image and water image (i.e., fat suppressed).**
  - Adding **extra "known" values** by acquiring more images at different TEs **improves the water-fat separation accuracy.**
- Dixon method is relatively insensitive to inhomogeneities compared to fat sat.

D. Saturation Bands

- Saturation bands are designed to **eliminate signal from a portion of the bore.**
- Extra RF pulses are spatially formed to only **excite a portion of the patient.**
  - **Gradients are then used to dephase protons and suppress signal** from that spatially selected region.
- Saturation bands are a **type of prepended pulse** and can be used before other acquisition sequences.
- Saturation bands are used in angiography to **remove signal from blood moving in a specific direction** (e.g., arterial or venous).
- They are also used to **remove motion artifact from areas** (e.g., spine) **of interest** by removing signal from nearby moving structures (e.g., swallowing throat).
- Suppression may fail if the RF saturation pulse does not fully penetrate the patient (B_1 inhomogeneity).

E. Susceptibility-Weighted Imaging

- Susceptibility-weighted imaging (SWI) is **based on T2*-weighted gradient-recalled echo (GRE)** imaging.
- Certain materials (e.g., hemosiderin or calcium) cause a **local inhomogeneity that dephases local signals and results in a signal void** (Fig. 16.2).
  - The larger the susceptibility difference of the material compared to surrounding tissue, the stronger the dephasing.
- Susceptibility-weighted imaging **modifies T2*-weighted GRE to accentuate the susceptibility-induced dephasing** and make it more sensitive to smaller amounts of material.

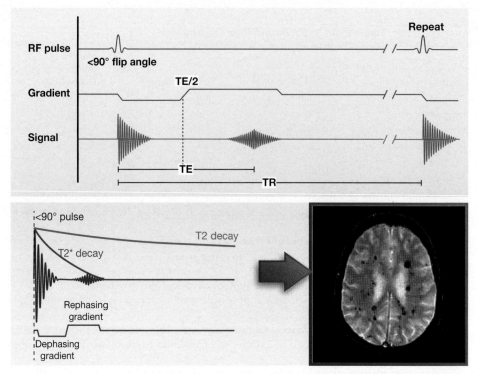

FIG 16.2 In gradient-recalled echo (GRE) sequences, an initial flip angle less than 90° and echoes formed by reversing an initial dephasing gradient, resulting in relatively weak echoes (compared to spin echo) and T2* instead of T2 dependencies. In GRE imaging, echoes fail to approach the maximum intensity determined by T2 loss because dephasing from field inhomogeneities is not reversed as in spin echo sequences. Failure to reverse dephasing due to field inhomogeneities can lead to T2* weighting where strong paramagnetic or diamagnetic materials cause signal loss from dephasing (as demonstrated by the microbleeds in the image). T2* weighting also forms the basis of susceptibility-weighted imaging.

- SWI also **incorporates the phase** of the signal (i.e., whether the Larmor frequency near the material increases or decreases).
  - **Paramagnetic material** (positive susceptibility) concentrates field lines causing **higher Larmor frequency.**
  - Diamagnetic material (negative susceptibility) disperses field lines causing **lower Larmor frequency.**
- SWI imaging is excellent at detecting **microbleeds.**

II. FLOW AND DIFFUSION

A. **Diffusion-Weighted Imaging**
- **Diffusion** depends on the **random motion** of **water molecules** in tissues.
- **Diffusion-weighted imaging (DWI)** typically uses **T2-weighted** echo-planar imaging (EPI) with **two additional gradients** applied in each dimension of interest to provide information regarding water diffusion through tissue.
  - **DWI gradients** are applied on **either side** of the 180° refocusing pulse.
  - Diffusion gradients are **characterized by a "b" parameter.**
- **At least two images** are **obtained, one** with **no diffusion gradients (i.e., b = 0),** and **the other** with **diffusion gradients** applied **(e.g., b = 1,000).**
  - **Higher b values** are more sensitive to diffusion but have lower SNR.

- **Without water diffusion,** water hydrogen protons are **dephased by the first gradient and then fully rephased by the second gradient,** so there is **no change in the image.**
  - When water hydrogen protons diffuse, **dephasing (signal loss) by the first gradient is NOT rephased fully by the second because the protons have moved and see different gradient strengths.**
- **Acquired images** are **used** to **compute** a value that quantifies the amount of water diffusion **(i.e., apparent diffusion coefficient [ADC])** at **each pixel.**
  - **Bright areas** on **DWI images and low ADC values** indicate **little diffusion.**
- However, a **bright** area on **DWI images (b = 1,000)** *and* **high ADC** values **show T2 shine-through,** reflecting **tissues** with very **long T2 values and not high diffusion.**
- Diffusion is **restricted by increased number and size of cells** as well as **reduced extracellular matrix.**
- Near areas of magnetic field **inhomogeneity,** a **fast spin echo (SE) version of DWI** is utilized to reduce the impact of susceptibility artifacts on the image.
- Advanced reconstructions using diffusion tensor imaging may highlight the degree of flow anisotropy **(fractional anisotropy)** on diffusion using a **0 (isotropic) to 1 (unidirectional) scale.**

B. **Contrast Media and Contrast-Enhanced Angiography**
- **Gadolinium** is a **paramagnetic contrast agent.**
  - **Gd** may be **extracellular fluid** (intravenous), **blood pool** (intravascular), or **organ specific.**
- **Gadolinium** acts as a **relaxation agent** of nearby protons, markedly **reducing T1.**
  - Relaxed water produces the enhancement on the image—Gd itself is not visible on the image.
- **Contrast agents** that **reduce T1** produce hyperintensity on T1-weighted images and are called **positive contrast agents.**
- Small **particles** of Fe_3O_4 consist of a **single domain** and are termed **superparamagnetic.**
- Materials such as **(super)paramagnetic** and **ferromagnetic contrast agents** disrupt the local magnetic field homogeneity and **shorten T2 and T2*.**
  - Excessive concentrations of Gd **may cause signal void** due to enhanced dephasing (shortened T2).
- **Contrast agents** that **reduce T2** produce hypointensity on T2-weighted images and are called **negative contrast agents.**
- **Contrast-enhanced magnetic resonance angiography (MRA)** is performed using **Gd contrast media.**
- **Contrast medium** is injected into a **vein** and **images obtained precontrast** and during a **first pass** through the arteries.
- **Subtraction** of the **two acquisitions** shows image of **only** the **blood vessels,** with the difference signal from the surrounding tissues being zero.
- Contrast agents that remain in the circulation up to an hour (i.e., **blood-pool agents)** **permit longer imaging times** and thereby **higher resolution.**
  - **Blood pool agents enhance** both **arteries** and **veins** at the same time.
- **MRA** images are produced by projecting the stack of sections onto a single two-dimensional image, called **maximum intensity projection (MIP).**

C. **Time-of-Flight Angiography**
- **Time-of-flight (TOF)** relies on **blood** being **tagged** in **one region** being **detected** in **another region.**
  - **TOF** is also known as **flow-related enhancement.**
- Tagging requires the **longitudinal magnetization** of the **flowing blood** to be **different** from the corresponding **longitudinal magnetization** of **stationary tissues.**
- Figure 16.3 A shows how **stationary tissues** become **saturated** when **short TR times** are used because **longitudinal magnetization (M_z)** does not have time to **recover.**

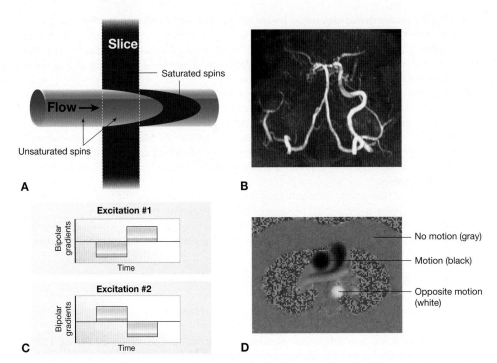

FIG 16.3 A: In time-of-flight (TOF) angiography, inflowing blood that is not saturated gives rise to a bright signal. **B:** TOF angiographic images are best viewed with a maximum intensity projection (MIP) format, which depicts blood vasculature. **C:** In phase-contrast angiography, an initial image is obtained with a set of bipolar gradients added along a selected direction. A second image is obtained but with the order of the bipolar gradients reversed. A comparison of each pixel in the two images provides information of the magnitude (and direction) of flow along the selected direction. **D:** In a phase-contrast image, gray values indicate no flow, with darker intensities depicting flow in one direction and brighter intensities depicting flow in the opposite direction. The mottled pattern in the lung where there is very little signal represents "noise."

- **Fresh blood** entering a slice (i.e., **not saturated**) results in **a higher signal** than the (saturated) stationary tissue (Fig. 16.3A).
- Because **blood** is continuously **refreshed** during image acquisition, it **never** experiences enough excitation pulses to become **saturated.**
- **TOF requires** the selection of **slices** that are **perpendicular** to the **blood vessel.**
  - **Venous** and **arterial flow** can be **selected** by using **saturation bands** either **above or below** the **slice** of interest.
- **TOF** is most commonly used in the **head** and **neck,** and gives detailed high-resolution images viewed using MIP displays.
- A limitation of **TOF** is **signal loss** because of **turbulent** and/or **slow flow.**
- TR is chosen **short enough to keep stationary tissue suppressed** but **long enough to allow fresh blood to flow into the slice.**

D. **Phase Contrast**
- **Phase-contrast MRA** encodes **blood velocities** by **applying bipolar gradient** between a standard excitation pulse and the readout.
  - A **bipolar gradient (e.g., negative gradient followed by positive gradient)** can be **applied along any axis,** or a combination of axes, as shown in Figure 16.3B.
- **Phase accrued** during the application of the gradient is **zero** for **stationary spins** but **nonzero** for **spins that move** (i.e., flowing blood).

- A **subsequent image** is **obtained** where the **sequence** of the **bipolar gradient** is **reversed** (e.g., positive gradient followed by negative gradient).
  - The **difference** of the **two images** is then **calculated**.
- **Static tissues** such as muscle or bone **subtract out**, but **moving blood** acquires a **different phase enabling flow velocities** to be **calculated**.
  - **Phase contrast** acquires **flow** in **one direction** at a time, so **three separate image acquisitions** are needed to provide a **complete image** of **flow**.
- Figure 16.3B shows an example of a phase-contrast image.
- **Black** represents the **maximum flow** in **one direction**, **white** corresponds to the **maximum flow** in the **opposite direction**, and **gray** indicates **stationary tissues**.
  - Phase-contrast images show **areas** giving **little signal** (e.g., **lung**) as **mottle (i.e., noise)**.
- A benefit of **phase-contrast** angiography is that **quantitative measurements** of blood flow can be obtained.
- An aliasing artifact causing very fast flows to appear to reverse direction can occur if the user-selected velocity encoding parameter is chosen too small.
  - It should be chosen to be a **larger velocity than the highest velocity expected to be measured**.
  - Setting the encoding velocity unnecessarily **high will cause excessive noise**.

E. **Perfusion**

- **Myocardial perfusion imaging** requires the rapid acquisition of a few slices through the heart for **multiple (e.g., 40) time points** after **gadolinium injection**.
  - Reconstructed slices are viewed in **cine mode** to view Gd uptake and washout.
- A special RF pulse is prepended to the acquisition to excite all spins in the volume of interest and then a gradient is used to **suppress the signals**.
  - **Gd-enhanced blood and tissue with a shortened T1** time will recover quickly and **demonstrate a signal during acquisition**.
- **Gradient echo or EPI** is used due to their short acquisition times to reduce motion artifact.
- Perfusion imaging requires **high temporal resolution** to freeze cardiac motion and **good spatial resolution** to localize and resolve small defects.
- If a **balanced steady-state free precession acquisition** sequence is used, **banding (off-resonance) artifacts** may occur, and care must be used not to interpret such artifact as myocardial defect.
- **Dark rim artifact** is a dark line in the myocardium present before contrast enhancement and thought to be related to truncation (Gibbs) artifact.

III. ADVANCED MAGNETIC RESONANCE

A. **Three-Dimensional Acquisition**

- **Three-dimensional Fourier transform (3D FT)** techniques permit imaging of stationary regions (i.e., volumes) such as the brain and knees.
- In three-dimensional imaging, a **nonselective RF pulse** simultaneously makes transverse magnetization for the entire sample volume.
- **Two sets of orthogonal phase encoding gradients** are used in addition to the frequency encoding gradient, which are applied along **z** and **y directions**.
  - Echoes are sampled with frequency encode gradient along the **x direction**.
- A **32 × 32 × 32 image** would require generating nearly **1,000 echoes (32 × 32),** each of which would be **sampled 32 times.**
- The acquired data are a **3D volume** set of **32 contiguous k-space slices**, with each slice having 32 pixels along each axis.
  - **Imaging time** would be **32 × 32 × TR**, where TR is the repetition time.
- **3D acquisitions** allow thinner slices to be reconstructed, so pixels may be isotropic and improved resolution is available for multiplanar reconstructions.

- **Gaps** generally occur when generating a series of **2D slices.**
- **Disadvantages** of **3D acquisition** techniques include **longer acquisition times** and more severe artifacts, since there are two phase encode directions.
- Three-dimensional acquisitions are typically used when all anatomy of interest can be encompassed in a single acquisition and is popular in angiography of the head.

B. Echo-Planar Imaging

- **EPI** starts with a **90° RF** pulse that rotates the longitudinal magnetization (i.e., M_x) into the transverse plane (i.e., M_{xy}).
- **Rapidly switched gradients** are applied to **produce** a **large number** of **echoes.**
  - **Each echo** generates **one line** of **k-space.**
- **Each echo** is **preceded** by a **different phase encode gradient**, and the image data are acquired line by line (k-space) within a single acquisition.
  - **Later echoes** have **progressively** more **T2* (and T2) weighting.**
- Special **high-performance gradients** are **required** for **EPI** with very **fast switching** and **settling times.**
- In a **single-shot echo-planar** sequence, **all phase encoding steps** are obtained in a **single TR interval.**
  - **Images** can be **acquired** in less than **100 ms**, allowing excellent temporal resolution required in cardiac imaging.
- In **multishot EPI**, the range of **phase steps** is **equally divided** into **several "shots"** or **TR periods.**
  - An image with 256 phase steps could be divided into 4 shots of 64 steps each.
- **EPI benefits** include **reduced imaging time** and **decreased motion artifact.**
  - **Susceptibility effects** from field inhomogeneity, geometric distortion, and blur generally **degrade EPI.**

C. Functional Magnetic Resonance Imaging

- **Functional magnetic resonance imaging (fMRI)** relies on **blood oxygenation, blood volume**, and/or **blood flow changes** in the brain associated with **neuronal activity.**
  - **Oxygenated hemoglobin (slightly diamagnetic) reduces T2*** effects because O_2 "shields" the hemoglobin iron atoms and reduces dephasing of adjacent protons.
  - **Deoxyhemoglobin is paramagnetic and causes dephasing by altering local field inhomogeneity.**
- **Brain activity increases local venous blood oxygenation**, which **increases** the **intensity** of the **detected T2*-weighted signal intensity** from these regions.
  - This is called **BOLD (blood oxygenation level–dependent)** imaging.
- **EPI** sequences with **T2* weighting** are commonly **used.**
- **Intensity changes** are **small (e.g., <5%)** but increase at higher magnetic fields.
  - **Data** are often **corrupted** by **noise,** requiring statistical procedures to extract the underlying signal.
- **Images** are **collected** during a **rest state** as well as the **activated state** then **compared** to generate functional maps.
  - **Mental activity** can include **visual, motor, auditory,** or other brain function.
- **Functional information** can be superimposed on high-resolution magnetic resonance images as **color overlays.**
- **Magnetic resonance functional imaging** has **better temporal** and **spatial resolution** than **positron emission tomography.**

D. Parallel Imaging

- **Coil channels** are the electronics needed to process a signal from a coil element.
  - More channels allow individual coil elements to act independently, increase SNR in conventional imaging, and are required for parallel imaging.
- In parallel imaging, a **multichannel and multicoil element coil is wrapped around the anatomy of interest.**

- There are several methods, but all generally **reduce the number of phase encode steps by undersampling k-space.**
  - **Wraparound artifact** occurs due to undersampling, but **measured sensitivity of each coil element and its position are used to correct the artifact.**
- An **acceleration factor** is chosen such that a **factor of 4 utilizes four independent channels, creates four groups of coil elements around the patient, acquires every fourth line of k-space and quarters acquisition time.**
  - Using coil and coil channels this way brings an **SNR reduction of the square root of acceleration factor,** and choosing a factor too large can lead to artifact when unwrapping fails.

E. **Magnetic Resonance Spectroscopy**

- **Magnetic resonance spectroscopy (MRS)** makes use of the slight **differences** in **resonance frequency** of **protons** or **other nuclei** found in **metabolites due to differing atomic arrangements in the molecule.**
- **Tetramethylsilane** acts as a baseline, and peaks at other frequencies are found due to their slightly different Larmor frequencies (**chemical shift**).
  - **Peak height** is related to the **number of chemical groups (e.g., methyl groups) present** and the static field strength—they do not necessarily represent concentration of the larger molecule.
- **MRS requires** more **uniform static magnetic** field than conventional hydrogen imaging to reduce line broadening.
  - **Water** and **fat** peaks are generally **suppressed** (e.g., STIR), so they do not overwhelm the weak metabolite signals.
  - **Short T2 metabolites will have broader lines than long T2 metabolites.**
- **The signal** of a **localized rectangular volume** can be **interrogated** by using a combination of gradients and RF pulses.
- Spectroscopy sequences include **STEAM (stimulated echo acquisition mode)** and **PRESS (point resolved spectroscopy).**
  - **Signals** are collected in the **absence** of any **gradients,** producing a **localized chemical shift spectrum.**
- ^{1}H and ^{31}P are the nuclei most often used for **in vivo localized spectroscopy.**
  - Typical voxel sizes used in MRS studies are ~1 cm^3 for ^{1}H and ~8 cm^3 for ^{31}P.
- **Proton spectroscopy** can be used to estimate concentrations of **N-acetyl aspartate, creatine and phosphocreatine, choline,** and **lactate** (Table 16.2).

IV. IMAGE QUALITY

A. **Resolution and Contrast**

- **Pixel/voxel sizes** generally determine the **spatial resolution.**
- In head magnetic resonance using a **25 cm field of view (FOV)** and **256^2 matrix,** the **pixel size** is about **1 mm,** double the pixel size in **head computed tomography (0.5 mm).**
- **Smaller FOVs and larger matrix sizes improve resolution but also increase noise.**
- Weak echoes typically fill the edges of k-space in fast SE and echo-planar imaging.
  - The edge of k-space encodes image edges (graylevel transitions), so weak signals will cause edge blurring.

TABLE 16.2	Metabolites in Magnetic Resonance Spectroscopy	
Metabolite	**Larmor Frequency Shift (ppm)**	**Biological Properties**
Phosphocholine (Cho)	3.2	Cell proliferation
Creatine (Cr)	3.0 and 3.9	Energy-rich phosphates
N-acetyl-L-aspartate (NAA)	2.0	Intact glioneural structures
Lactate	1.3	Anaerobic glycolysis

- **Tissue contrast** is determined by **tissue properties (T1, T2, and T2*).**
- In **SE** imaging, the **choice** of **TR** and **TE** values introduces **T1** and **T2 weighting,** as discussed in Chapter 15.
    - **Proton spin density (ρ)**–weighted images generally have the **worst contrast,** since there is little variation in the proton concentration across soft tissues.
- In addition to TR and TE, **contrast** in **GRE imaging** is **modified** by changing the **flip angle,** as discussed in Chapter 15.
- On T1-weighted SE images, **Gd uptake increases lesion contrast,** and on T2-weighted SE images, **Fe_2O_3 uptake increases lesion contrast.**
- **Contrast** is the percent difference between average graylevel values and **should not be confused with the SNR,** which compares signal strength to noise.

B.   **Signal-to-Noise Ratio**
- **The SNR** is often the **most important** determinant of image quality.
- **Magnetic resonance signal** is directly **proportional** to the **pixel volume** (i.e., number of spins).
    - **Halving** the **voxel size in each dimension reduces voxel volume (i.e., signal)** by a **factor of 8** (i.e., 2^3), and vice versa.
- **Increasing** the **FOV or decreasing matrix size increases the SNR.**
- **The signal** is roughly **proportional** the **magnetic field.**
    - Relative to a 1.5 T system, a 3 T system will generally have roughly double the SNR because of the increase in net tissue magnetization (see Table 15.1).
- Detected **noise** is increased when the **receiver bandwidth** is increased.
    - Quadrupling receiver bandwidth halves SNR.
- **RF coils** affect the amount of **image noise,** which is generally **highest** in (large) **body coils** and **lowest** in (small) **surface coils.**
    - **Coils with more channels will have better SNRs** but are more expensive.
- **Number of acquisitions (excitations)** is a user-selected parameter that acquires the same signal multiple times and averages it.
    - **Setting this to 4 will average four acquisitions** of the same anatomy and will quadruple the (deterministic) signal but will only double the (random) image noise **(doubles the SNR).**
- The **Ernst angle** in GRE imaging is the **flip angle that maximizes the SNR** for a selected tissue (but does not necessarily maximize the tissue contrast).

C.   **Patient-Based Artifacts**
- **Chemical shift artifacts** are caused by the slight difference in resonance frequency of protons in water and fat, resulting in misregistration of fat and water **along the frequency encode direction.**
    - **Increasing receiver bandwidth** reduces the severity.
    - **India ink artifact** is a type of chemical shift artifact caused by fat and water proton magnetization canceling at the specific choice of TE and is the basis of in-phase and out-of-phase imaging.
- **Motion artifact** occurs when the patient moves between successive signal acquisitions in the same scan.
    - Motion artifact creates less intense versions of the moving object to be repeated along the phase encode direction (ghosts).
    - In addition to restraints, suppressing the signal of the moving tissue, and faster imaging, a sequence called PROPELLER oversamples the center of k-space and allows for motion artifact mitigation.
- **Flowing blood** and **CSF** as well as **pulsing vessels** can result in **pulsation (motion) artifacts** as well.
- **Tendons and nerves** aligned at **55° (magic angle)** to the main field result in **artificially longer T2 times (e.g., 5 ms)** that can appear artificially **bright** on T1 and **proton density** SE images (i.e., short TEs).

TABLE 16.3	Selected Artifacts, Their Direction, and Mitigation	
Artifact	**Direction**	**Mitigation**
Motion/pulsation	Phase encode	Stop motion, image faster, and PROPELLER
RF contamination/zipper	Phase encode	Ensure RF shielding integrity and remove RF sources from scanner room
Chemical shift	Frequency encode	Increase receiver bandwidth
Truncation/Gibbs ringing	Phase encode (typically)	Increase resolution and smooth using postprocessing
Wraparound/aliasing	Phase encode (typically)	Increase FOV, suppress wrapped tissue, and "No Phase Wrap" option
Magic angle	None	Reposition patient and compare to long TE acquisitions
India ink	None	Modify TE
Susceptibility	None	SE sequences and reduce TE

FOV, field of view; RF, radiofrequency; SE, spin echo; TE, echo time.

- **Magic angle artifacts disappear** on **T2-weighted images** (i.e., TE 100 ms).
- **A susceptibility artifact** is the result of dephasing from paramagnetic and diamagnetic field inhomogeneities.
  - **SE sequences and reduced TE** can mitigate dephasing and thus susceptibility.

D. Equipment-Based Artifacts

- **Truncation artifact** exhibits a pattern of dark and bright bands adjacent to a sharp edge, which can be minimized by increasing the amount of data acquired (matrix size).
  - **Truncation artifacts** (e.g., may simulate a syrinx in spinal cord) are sometimes referred to as **Gibbs** or **ringing artifacts.**
- **Wraparound artifact** occurs when the FOV is smaller than the structure, and imaged objects outside the FOV are mapped to the opposite side of the image.
  - **Wraparound** is caused by **undersampling (aliasing)** and can be **reduced** by **increasing** the **FOV, nulling the overlapping tissue, or implementing "no phase wrap."**
- **K-space spike artifact (aka corduroy or herringbone)** occurs when an electrical issue causes a signal spike in k-space.
  - This causes an **alternating pattern of signal dropout** throughout the image (a consequence of the reconstruction process).
- **Dielectric artifact** occurs when the RF (B_1) field is not homogeneous, so not all spins are rotated the same amount into the transverse plane (M_{xy}).
  - **Saline or "dielectric" pads** around the patient may help as will transmitting RF from multiple directions (**multitransmit**).
- **Flare artifact** occurs for surface coils when tissue is very close to the coil and is common in breast magnetic resonance imaging (MRI).
  - The signal near the coil is so bright that contrast may be lost, so **padding between the patient and coil** is recommended to mitigate this.
- Table 16.3 lists select artifacts, their directional dependencies, and some methods for mitigation.

V. SAFETY

A. Zones, Personnel, and Labeling

- MRI departments are set up with consideration to safety zones where **danger increases as zone number increases** (Fig. 16.4).

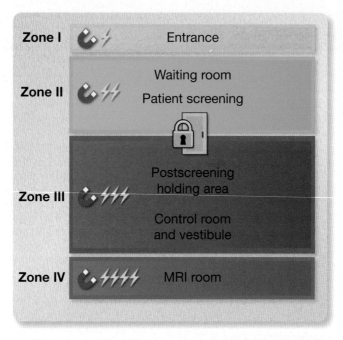

FIG 16.4 The magnetic resonance (MR) area is broken into four zones based on the risk from the main magnetic field. Zone I is outside the MR area and accessible to the public and includes things like hallways. Patients and staff do not expect to come into contact with magnetic fields. Zone II is accessible to the public but within the MR department, so patients and staff likely understand that they will be coming into contact with magnetic fields. Zone III is behind a locked door and cannot be accessed unless accompanied by safety-trained MR staff. This includes the MR control rooms. The 5G line must be contained within zone III. Zone IV is the MR scanner room and only patients undergoing MRI and select MR staff can enter the scanner room. This room has the highest levels of danger. MRI, magnetic resonance imaging.

- Zone I is public access, a **locked door separates zones II and III**, and zone IV is the magnet room.
- Workers must have **level 1 safety training** (not a danger to themselves) to be allowed access to **zones III and IV.**
  - Level II training is required so that the worker can oversee the safety of someone untrained in zones III and IV.
- The American Board of Magnetic Resonance Safety certifies a worker's safety knowledge.
  - The **MR medical director** is a safety trained physician overseeing MR safety.
  - The **MR safety officer** is typically a technologist and handles day-to-day safety under the authority of the MRMD.
  - The **MR safety expert** is typically a physicist who advises on policy, risk, and image quality issues for common and complex cases.
- Implants and other objects are labeled **MR safe, MR conditional, and MR unsafe** depending on the risk to the patient.
  - MR safe objects are safe in any MR environment and unsafe are unsafe or have not been tested.
  - MR conditional objects are **safe under specified field, gradient, RF, and other conditions.**

B. RF Effects

- The RF field is the **source of patient heating and the primary source of patient burns.**
- **Stronger magnets** have higher Larmor frequencies that utilize higher frequency (more energetic) fields that **increase heating (proportional to the square of B_0).**

TABLE 16.4	Magnetic Resonance Components and Their Primary Patient Safety Risks
Component	**Description**
Main field	Missile effect and implant torque
Time-varying gradient	Acoustic noise and peripheral nerve stimulation
Radiofrequency	Heating and thermal burns
Cryogen	Frostbite and asphyxiation

- **More and larger flip angles** require longer and **more intense RF (heating proportional to the square of flip angle).**
- Thermal burns are the most encountered safety issue after contrast reactions.
- Patient heating is commonly estimated by the vendor-specific specific absorption rate (SAR).
  - In normal mode imaging, whole-body heating is **limited to an SAR of 2 W/kg or 0.5°C.**
  - The SAR **does not account for implants,** so localized heating can be higher, and B_{1rms+} **(measured in μT) is a better risk indicator.**
- **Less RF (e.g., GRE instead of SE), lower field strengths, reduced scan range, and fewer sequences** can help a protocol meet MR conditional heating limit.
- **Limiting contact between metal (e.g., wires) and the body surface, not allowing the body to form loops (e.g., hand touching thigh or ankles touching)** will reduce chance of thermal burns.
- Table 16.4 lists major MR components and their primary safety risks.

C. Static Field

- The **missile effect** occurs when a ferromagnetic object is pulled into the scanner by the main magnetic field.
  - This has resulted in patient and worker death and serious injury.
- Magnetic field pull is **strongest at the entrance and exit of the scanner bore.**
  - **Larger and more ferromagnetic** objects feel **more pull.**
- The static field may cause rotation (torque), which can be dangerous for implants such as **aneurysm clips.**
  - Torque is typically **strongest along the centerline of the bore.**
  - **Geometry** can impact the torque and is typically strongest for **long thin rigid ferromagnetic structures.**
- **Patients should be placed into a gown and screened for implants prior to entering the scanning room.**
- Detrimental effects from static magnetic fields are not evident below 10 T.
  - **Hazards** exist for patients who have **ferromagnetic devices** implanted in their bodies.
- The static field can cause **malfunctions in machines (e.g., computes) and active implants (e.g., deep brain stimulators).**

D. Static Field Gradient and Time-Varying Gradient Effects

- **Time-varying gradients** refer to **gradients generated to localize the signal** during scanning.
  - Since these gradients turn on and off, the **slew rate** (field strength change per unit time dB/dt) is used to measure possible gradient effects.
  - A **larger slew rate means higher patient danger.**
- A changing magnetic field can **induce an electric field in the body** which can stimulate muscles and nerves.
  - Gradient strength is strongest at the bore periphery, so that is where **peripheral nerve stimulation** will be strongest.
  - Induced currents **can cause malfunctions in machines and active implants.**

- Time-varying gradients push and pull on the coils and other scanner pieces, **causing them to flex and produce loud sounds.**
  - Patient **ear protection is required** to **reduce sound intensity below 99 dB** to avoid hearing loss.
  - **Fetal hearing is not impacted** due to the sound attenuation produced by the mother's tissues.
- It is possible that induced currents in implants may cause **burns** in tissue, but this is a **minor cause compared to RF heating.**
- The **static gradient field (aka fringe field)** refers to the change in magnetic field strength as one moves away from the magnet bore.
- A patient moving toward or away from the bore can experience effects from **electric fields induced by the changing magnetic field.**
  - **Vertigo, magnetophosphenes, and a metallic taste** are all possible from time-varying or static gradient fields.

E. **Cryogen Quenching**

- The main magnetic field is sustained by a superconducting electromagnetic coil **kept cool by the cryogen and liquid helium.**
- In the event of a **person being pinned by the magnet or a large fire** approaching the scanner room, it might be necessary to **quench the magnet.**
- Quenching stops the cryogen sustaining the temperature, causing the helium to boil and the **magnetic field strength to drop.**
  - Quenching allows a person pinned to the magnet by a ferromagnetic object to be removed.
  - Quenching keeps the MRI scanner from becoming a **pressure bomb** in the presence of a large fire by **venting away the helium gas.**
- Helium boiling causes its **volume to expand over 1,000 times.**
- If the **helium gas** is not properly vented, it can return into the room causing **asphyxiation and frost bite.**
- Newer technology can produce scanners using **lower amounts of helium** to increase safety (especially at field strengths <1.5 T).

Chapter 16 (Magnetic Resonance II) Questions

16.1 What flip angle is typically used to initiate an inversion recovery sequence?
A. 10°
B. 30°
C. 90°
D. 180°

16.2 How does increasing matrix size impact image SNR?
A. Increases
B. No change
C. Decreases

16.3 What suppression method uses a system of equations to create fat- and water-only images?
A. Dixon method
B. Fat sat
C. STIR
D. SPIR

16.4 What sequence will mitigate suscepti-bility artifact?
A. Fast spin echo
B. bSSFP
C. GRE
D. Echo-planar

16.5 Increasing the acceleration factor in parallel imaging decreases acquisition time at what cost?
A. SNR
B. Contrast
C. Spatial resolution
D. Reduced chemical shift

16.6 How does doubling the main mag-netic field strength impact patient heating?
A. Quadruples
B. Doubles
C. Unchanged
D. Halves

16.7 What signal is suppressed in an IR sequence obtained at 1.5 T, applying a 90° "read out" pulse at TI time 250 ms?
A. Liver
B. Bone
C. Fat
D. CSF

16.8 In DWI imaging, restricted diffusion (e.g., stroke) would be expected when the DWI pixel values are _____ and the ADC values are _____.
A. low; low
B. low; high
C. high; low
D. high; high

16.9 How does Gd impact T2 times of surrounding tissues?
A. Increases
B. No change
C. Decreases

16.10 Who should be the head of the MR safety committee?
A. MR medical director
B. MR safety expert
C. MR safety officer
D. MR lead interpreting physician

16.11 What is a typical image acquisition time for a single-shot echo-planar sequence?
A. 1 ms
B. 10 ms
C. 100 ms
D. 1,000 ms

16.12 What is the consequence of choos-ing velocity encoding parameter arbitrarily high in phase-contrast imaging?
A. Increased chemical shift
B. Decreased resolution
C. Decreased image contrast
D. Increased noise

16.13 MR spectroscopy requires the use of exceptionally:
A. Uniform magnetic fields
B. Strong magnetic gradients
C. Intense RF coils
D. High RF frequencies

16.14 A locked door to keep out the public should be present between what two zones?
A. I and II
B. II and III
C. III and IV

16.15 Gd is generally a _____ contrast agent, whereas Fe_3O_4 is a _____ contrast agent.
A. positive; positive
B. positive; negative
C. negative; positive
D. negative; negative

16.16 What is the impact on SNR by doubling the number of excitations and doubling the receiver bandwidth?
A. Quadruples
B. Doubles
C. No change
D. Halves

16.17 How does SNR change when doubling each voxel dimension?
A. 2
B. 4
C. 8
D. 16

16.18 Magic angle artifacts are most likely to appear on images with a:
A. Short TE
B. Long TE
C. Short TR
D. Long TR

16.19 Chemical shift artifacts appear along what direction?
A. Slice select
B. Phase encode
C. Frequency encode
D. Any

16.20 What scanner-produced field is primarily responsible for patient burns?
A. Main
B. Radiofrequency
C. Gradient
D. Shim

Answers and Explanations

16.1 D (180°). Inversion recover inverts the net magnetization to start the sequence.

16.2 A (Decreases). Smaller pixels decrease image SNR.

16.3 A (Dixon method). Several images at different TE (in-phase and out-of-phase as well as others) are used to solve a system of equations allowing signal from fat to be separated from signal from water.

16.4 A (Fast spin echo). Spin echo and fast spin echo sequences mitigate susceptibility artifact by using a 180° refocusing RF pulse. bSSFP is a type of gradient echo sequence and does not have this. Echo-planar acquisitions may have a refocusing RF pulse but may not depending on if they are spin, gradient, or hybrid flavors of EPI.

16.5 A (SNR). SNR decreases with acceleration as detector channels are used to unwrap the image instead of adding to signal detection.

16.6 A (Quadruples). Patient heating is roughly proportional to the square of the magnetic field strength and is due to the increased frequency (and energy) of the applied RF at the increased Larmor frequency.

16.7 C (Fat). Choosing a TI time of 250 ms (i.e., STIR pulse sequence) will suppress fat.

16.8 C (high; low). In DWI imaging, restricted diffusion (e.g., stroke) has high (bright) DWI pixels and low values of apparent diffusion coefficient.

16.9 C (Reduces T2). Both T1 and T2 are reduced by Gd. With typical concentrations T1 reduction dominates causing increased signal, but at high concentrations T2 reduction dominates causing signal void (sometimes seen in arthroscopy).

16.10 A (MR medical director). The head of the MR safety committee should be a physician with MR safety knowledge and experience such as a certified MR medical director.

16.11 C (100 ms). Following the 90° RF pulse, gradients are rapidly switched to create multiple echoes which must be obtained before the echoes disappear because of T2 effects (i.e., within 100 ms; 1 and 10 ms are far too short a time interval to obtain EPI images).

16.12 D (Increased noise). Choosing the parameter smaller than the maximum flow velocity can result in aliasing artifact, but too high the parameter results in increased noise and decreased velocity estimate accuracy.

16.13 A (Uniform magnetic fields). MR spectroscopy requires the use of exceptionally uniform magnetic fields.

16.14 B (II and III). A locked door separates the relatively safe zones II and III from the more dangerous zones III and IV.

16.15 B (positive; negative). Gadolinium will result in bright pixels on T1-weighted SE sequences, and SPIO results in darker pixels on T2 weighted SE images.

16.16 C (No change). Quadrupling the number of excitations (acquisitions) doubles the SNR, while quadrupling the receiver bandwidth halves the SNR.

16.17 C (8). Doubling each voxel dimension most likely increases the MR SNR by a factor of 8 because the volume of tissue generating the signal is eight times bigger (i.e., 2^3).

16.18 A (Short TE). Magic angle artifacts arise because of reduced spin-spin interactions that increase T2 times. These longer T2 times, however, are still very short and will thus only appear when TE is short (e.g., T1-weighted images). Magic angle artifacts disappear on T2-weighted images.

16.19 C (Frequency encode). Chemical shift artifacts appear along the frequency encode gradient direction and are a result of differences in Larmor frequency for protons in fat and water (tissue).

16.20 B (Radiofrequency). Time-varying gradients can occasionally heat an implant/foreign object to the point of causing a burn, but most burns are due to the energy deposited by the radiofrequency field.

CHAPTER 17 Ultrasound I

I. SOUND

A. Sound Waves

- **Sound waves** are **pressure disturbances** that travel away from their source, as depicted in Figure 17.1.
- **Ultrasound waves** are transmitted through tissue as **waves of alternating compression (high pressure)** and **rarefaction (low pressure).**
- At a given point, the **pressure increases** and **decreases** in a **cyclical manner** as a function of time.
  - When a sound wave is frozen in time, the **pressure increases** and **decreases** as a function of **distance along** the **wave.**
- **Ultrasound waves propagate** at a **velocity** (meters per second), which is the **product** of the **wavelength and frequency.**
- **Frequency (cycles per second)** is the number of **oscillations** at a fixed point in **each second.**
  - **Wavelength (meters)** is the **distance** between **successive wave crests.**

B. Frequencies

- **Frequencies** are measured in **Hertz (Hz)**, where 1 Hz is **one oscillation per second.**

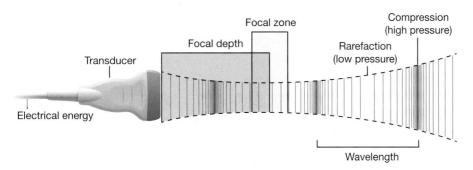

FIG 17.1 Sound waves are formed when electrical energy is converted into mechanical energy to form a pattern (i.e., wave) of varying pressure. The distance between two high pressure peaks is the wavelength, and the number of oscillations at a given point each second is the frequency. The wave travels at a speed equal to the product of the wavelength and frequency. A focused beam will narrow throughout the focal depth and has maximum lateral and elevational resolution in the focal zone. The beam then diverges.

- The **period** is the time between successive oscillations and is the **reciprocal** of the **frequency (i.e., 1/f).**
  - When the frequency is 10 Hz, the period is 0.1 second (i.e., 1/10).
- On a piano, **middle C** has a frequency of **256 Hz.**
- **Harmonic frequencies** are **integral multiples** of the **fundamental frequency.**
  - 512 Hz (2 × 256) and 768 Hz (3 × 256) are harmonics of middle C.
- **Audible sound** has frequencies ranging from **15 Hz to 20 kHz.**
  - 1,000 Hz equals 1 kHz and 1,000 kHz equals 1 MHz (1,000,000 Hz).
- In an orchestra, **small** instruments (e.g., **violins**) produce **high frequencies,** whereas **large** instruments (e.g., **double bass**) produce **low frequencies.**
- **Diagnostic ultrasound** generally uses transducers with frequencies ranging between **1 and 20 MHz.**
- Very high frequencies (**>20 MHz**) may be found in ophthalmologic transducers, and **intravascular transducers** inserted into **blood vessels** to image the vessel walls.
  - **Low frequencies** are associated with **good tissue penetration** for **deep imaging,** and **high frequencies** are associated with **good axial resolution** and **superficial imaging.**

C. Wavelengths

- Ultrasound wavelengths depend on the material compressibility.
- At **1.5 MHz,** the ultrasound **wavelength** in **soft tissue** is **1 mm.**
  - At this frequency, wavelength is **0.2 mm** in **air** and nearly **3 mm** in **bone.**
- Ultrasound **wavelength decreases** with **increasing frequency.**
  - In soft tissue, the ultrasound wavelength is 0.1 mm at 15 MHz, ten times lower than at 1.5 MHz.
- Ultrasound pulses are designed to be approximately two wavelengths long.
  - A **1.5 MHz** transducer generates **pulses** with a **2 mm spatial pulse length.**
- The **length** of the **ultrasound pulse** is the key determinant of **axial resolution.**
  - **Axial resolution** is generally the **wavelength** (i.e., half the spatial pulse length).

D. Sound Velocity

- For any given material, **sound velocity** is **independent** of **frequency.**
  - Different instruments in an orchestra produce different frequencies, but they all travel through air in a concert hall at *exactly* the same speed.
- **Sound velocity depends** on the type of **material** or tissue.
- **Materials** that are **not particularly compressible (e.g., bone)** have **high sound velocities.**
  - **Compressible materials (e.g., air)** have the **lowest sound velocities.**
- The **average velocity** of sound in **soft tissue** is **1,540 m/s.**
  - All ultrasound scanners always assume this value when estimating echo location using elapsed time.
- **Sound** travels more **slowly** in **air** and much **faster** in **bone,** as depicted by the data shown in Table 17.1.

TABLE 17.1	Relative Densities, Sound Velocities, and Acoustic Impedances Values of Materials of Interest in Ultrasound Imaging		
Material	**Physical Density**[a]	**Sound Velocity**[a]	**Acoustic Impedance**[a]
Air	<0.1	0.2	<0.01
Fat	0.9	0.95	0.9
Soft tissue (average)	1.0	1.0	1.0
Bone (skull)	1.9	2.6	5
Lead zirconate titanate (crystal)	7.5	2.6	20

[a]Relative to soft tissue.

- **Sound velocity** is about **5% lower** in **fat**, which results in imaging errors and artifacts when image creation assumes a fixed tissue velocity (i.e., 1,540 m/s).
- When velocity in a given tissue is fixed, frequency and wavelength are inversely related.
  - In **tissues**, **higher frequencies** have **shorter wavelengths**, and vice versa.

E. **Pressure, Power, and Intensities (dB)**

- **Intensity is the beam power per unit area and is proportional to the pressure squared.**
  - **Doubling the pressure quadruples the intensity.**
- **Relative intensities** in ultrasound are expressed using **decibels (dB).**
- **Decibels** are calculated using a **logarithmic scale.**
- **Negative decibel** values correspond to **signal attenuation**, and **positive** decibel values correspond to signal **amplification.**
- Intensity reduced to **10%** is **−10 dB**, that reduced to **1%** is **−20 dB**, that reduced to **0.1%** is **−30 dB**, and so on.
  - A **50% reduction** of sound intensity corresponds to **−3 dB.**
- Intensity increases of +10 dB correspond to a 10-fold increase, +20 dB to a 100-fold increase, +30 dB to a 1,000-fold increase, and so on.
  - **Doubling** of the sound **intensity** corresponds to **+3 dB.**
- Table 17.2 provides a summary of **relative intensities** expressed as **percentages** and **decibels.**

■ II. INTERACTIONS

A. **Acoustic Impedance**

- **Acoustic impedance (Z)** of a material is the product of the **density (ρ)** and the **speed of sound (v)** in the material, which is expressed in **rayls.**
- **Air** and **lung** have **low acoustic impedances**, because they both have low densities as well as low sound velocities (Table 17.1).
  - **Bone** and **piezoelectric crystals** have **high acoustic impedance** because they both have high densities as well as high sound velocity (Table 17.1).
- Table 17.1 lists relative values of acoustic impedance for materials and tissues of interest in ultrasound imaging.
- The **fraction** of **ultrasound reflected** at an interface **depends** on the **acoustic impedance** of the two tissues on either side of the interface.
- When there are **big differences** in **acoustic impedance** (i.e., acoustic impedance mismatch) at an interface, **most** of the ultrasound energy is **reflected.**
  - When the **acoustic impedances** are very **similar**, most of the ultrasound energy is transmitted, and **echoes** are **relatively weak.**

B. **Specular Reflections**

- **Specular reflections** are extremely strong reflections and occur from large **smooth surfaces** (Fig. 17.2A) similar to light reflected from a smooth mirror.

TABLE 17.2	Summary of Relative Intensities Expressed as Percentages and Decibels		
Relative Intensity	**Percentage (%)**	**Decibels (dB)**	
0.5	50	−3	
0.1	10	−10	
0.01	1	−20	
0.001	0.1	−30	
0.0001	0.01	−40	

- **Angle of incidence equals angle of reflection.** A **reflection** traveling back to a transducer is called an **echo** and is used to **create ultrasound images.**
  - **Transmitted** and **reflected ultrasound intensities** must **add** up to **unity** (conservation of energy).
- **Tissue/air interfaces reflect >99%** of incident ultrasound beam.
  - **Gel** is applied between the transducer and skin to displace air and **minimize large reflections** that prevent ultrasound transmission into patients.
- **Bone/tissue** interfaces also **reflect substantial fractions** of the incident intensity.
- In imaging the abdomen, the **strongest echoes** are likely to arise **from gas bubbles.**
  - **Imaging** through **air** or **bone greatly reduces image quality.**
- **Fat** and **tissue interfaces**, which both have similar acoustic impedances, result in **weak echoes.**
  - **Most** of the incident ultrasound is **transmitted** through a **fat/tissue** interface.
- Table 17.3 lists values of reflected intensities at interfaces encountered in ultrasound.

C. **Diffuse Reflection Scatter and Speckle**
- **Scattering** occurs when ultrasound encounters **objects** that are **smaller** than the ultrasound **wavelength** (Fig. 17.2C).
  - **Diffuse (nonspecular)** (Fig. 17.2B) reflections produce a similar effect since the scale of rough-surface microstructures are smaller than a wavelength.
  - The terms scatter and nonspecular reflections are **often used interchangeably.**
- At **1.5 MHz**, objects **smaller than 1 mm** result in **scattering.**
  - At **15 MHz**, objects smaller than **0.1 mm** are responsible for scattering.
- In scattering, most of the wave passes unperturbed, and a **scattered wave** is generated that **travels outward** in **all directions** from the scatter.
  - **Diffuse reflections are weak** because the reflected energy is spread over all directions.
  - Most reflections are diffuse reflections from organ parenchyma microstructures.

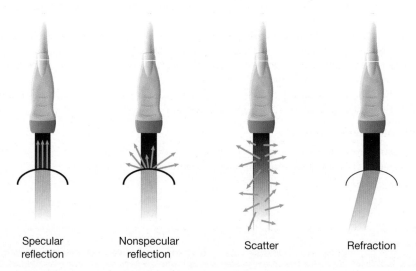

Specular   Nonspecular   Scatter   Refraction
reflection   reflection

FIG 17.2 Ultrasound interactions in ultrasound include specular reflection, nonspecular (diffuse) reflection, scatter, and refraction. Specular reflection, where the angle of incidence is equal to the angle of reflection, is responsible for generating organ boundaries. Scatter originates from structures that are smaller than the ultrasound wavelength and account for the speckle and low-intensity parenchymal reflections seen within organs. Nonspecular (diffuse) reflections are from a rough surface and are of low intensity due to the energy spread over multiple angles. Refraction, the bending of sound when passing from tissue to another, will give rise to location errors (i.e., artifacts).

TABLE 17.3	Reflection Intensities at an Interface Between Soft Tissue and the Specified Material	
Material Adjacent to Soft Tissue		**Reflected Intensity (%)**
Air		>99
Lung		50
Bone		40
Fat		0.8
Muscle		<0.1

- Organs such as the **kidney, pancreas, spleen,** and **liver** are composed of complex tissue structures that **contain many scattering sites.**
- **Speckle** is caused by **scattered** waves from small reflectors interfering with each other, creating a pattern characteristic of the **tissue structure (signature).**
  - Speckle **appears like noise but does not randomly change with time.**
- **The liver border (specular reflection) is stronger than the liver parenchyma (diffuse reflection).**
  - **Hyperechoic** means stronger echo strength (brighter image value) relative to the background signal.
- Organs that contain fluids such as the **bladder**, and **cysts** have no internal structure and almost **no echoes (i.e., show black).**
  - **Hypoechoic** means lower echo strength (darker image value) relative to the average background signal.

D. Refraction

- **Refraction** is the **change** in **direction** of an ultrasound beam when passing from one tissue to another (Fig. 17.2D).
  - **Refraction** is a result of **differences** in the **speed of sound** in the **two tissues.**
- When ultrasound passes from **one tissue** to **another** having a different speed of sound, the **frequency remains** the **same** but the **wavelength changes.**
  - Change of wavelength occurs to accommodate the different speed of sound in the second tissue and shortens when the speed is reduced.
- When the velocity of sound in tissue 2 is greater than that of tissue 1, the transmission angle is greater than the angle of incidence, and vice versa.
- **Ultrasound machines assume a straight line propagation**, and any **refraction effects** result in **image artifacts.**
- **Refraction** causes artifacts in the form of **spatial distortions.**
  - **Abdominal muscles can cause refraction that manifests as double structures (e.g., aortas).**
- **Refraction** can result in dark regions (i.e., **shadows**) in ultrasound images because the ultrasound **beam** is **"lost"** after it has been refracted.
  - Shadowing under the lateral edges of large vessel walls is due to refraction of the beam as it passes through the wall.

E. Attenuation

- **Attenuation** is a composite effect of **loss** of **ultrasound energy** in a given tissue because of scattering and absorption.
  - **Absorbed sound wave energy** is converted into **heat.**
- The **attenuation** of ultrasound in a homogeneous tissue is **exponential**, expressed in terms of **dB** (Table 17.2).
- **Attenuation** is generally taken to be directly **proportional** to the **frequency.**
  - **High-frequency transducers attenuate more** than low-frequency ones.
- **Attenuation** is also directly **proportional** to the **distance traveled in tissue**, so doubling the distance doubles the attenuation.

- Attenuation affects transmitted pulses into the patient and the echoes on their way out of the patient.
- **Fluids** have very **low** values of **attenuation** coefficient and will therefore transmit most of the incident ultrasound energy.
- An **attenuation coefficient** of **0.5 dB/cm/MHz** is commonly used to quantify the loss of power in ultrasound beams for clinical imaging.
  - Attenuation in soft tissue is 0.5 dB/cm at 1 MHz and 5 dB/cm at 10 MHz.
- **Lung** and **bone** have very **high attenuation** coefficients, and any ultrasound transmitted into these organs will be rapidly attenuated.
- Table 17.4 provides a summary of attenuation at different frequencies.

III. TRANSDUCER ELEMENTS

A. Transducer Operation

- A **transducer** is a device that **converts one form** of **energy** into **another** (Fig. 17.1).
- **Piezoelectric transducers** convert **electrical energy** into **ultrasonic energy**, and vice versa.
  - A common ultrasound transducer material is **lead zirconate titanate.**
- **High-frequency voltage oscillations** are produced by the scanner electronics and **sent** to the ultrasound **transducer.**
- **Transducer crystals** do **not conduct electricity,** but each side is coated with a thin layer of silver, which acts as an electrode.
  - **Nonconducting crystals change shape** in response to voltages at these electrodes.
- Crystal shape changes increases and decreases the pressure in front of the transducer, **producing ultrasound waves (transmitter).**
- When the crystal is subjected to **pressure changes** by the returning ultrasound **echoes,** the pressure changes are **converted back** into **electrical energy signals.**
  - **Voltage signals** from returning **echoes** are transferred from the receiver to a computer, which are used to **create ultrasound images.**
- A **notch or other indicator** on the ultrasound probe indicates what will **appear on the left side of the image display.**
  - Orienting the notch toward the patient's head will cause the anatomy in the field of view (FOV) toward the patient's head to be on the left side of the image.

B. Transducer Frequency

- Current transducers are multifrequency **broad bandwidth transducers** designed to generate more than one frequency.
  - Narrow-bandwidth transducers are used in Doppler where they improve flow measurement accuracy.
- For multifrequency transducers, **operators select** the **examination frequency** to match the **clinical requirements.**
- **Resonance** relates to the frequency at which the piezoelectric transducer is most efficient in converting electrical energy to acoustic energy.
  - **Resonance frequency** is determined by the **piezoelectric element thickness.**

TABLE 17.4	**Attenuation of Ultrasound in Soft Tissue Assuming the Attenuation Coefficient is 0.5 dB/cm per MHz and 100% Reflection**	
Round-Trip Distance[a] (cm)	**Attenuation (dB) at Transducer Frequency of:**	
	3 MHz	**10 MHz**
5	−7.5	−25
10	−15	−50
20	−30	−100

[a]Depth will be half of the round-trip distance.

- **Transducer crystals** are normally manufactured so that their **thickness (t)** is equal to **one-half** of the **wavelength** at resonance.
- **High-frequency transducers** are **thin** (e.g., 0.1 mm at 7.5 MHz).
  - **Low-frequency transducers** are **thick** (e.g. 0.5 mm at 1.5 MHz).
- Bandwidth refers to the number of frequencies present in a pulse.
  - A broad bandwidth (many frequencies) has improved axial resolution and is typically used in B-mode imaging.
  - A narrow bandwidth (few frequencies) has better sensitivity (ability to see weak reflectors) and improved flow measurement accuracy for Doppler imaging.
- **Q-factor** is the ratio of center frequency to bandwidth.
  - **A low-Q transducer has a lot of damping, short spatial pulse length, good axial resolution, a wide bandwidth, and reduced sensitivity.**

C. Backing and Matching Layers

- Virtually all medical ultrasound systems in **radiology** use **pulsed transducers.**
  - **Transducers** are designed to produce **short pulses.**
- **Blocks** of **damping material**, usually tungsten/rubber in an epoxy resin, are placed **behind transducers** to reduce vibration (ring down time) to **shorten pulses.**
- A **dampened transducer** generates a **broad range** of **frequencies**, whereas transducers without damping generate single (pure) frequencies.
  - **Pure frequencies** are always associated with **very long pulses**, and vice versa.
- A **matching layer** of material is placed on the front surface of the transducer to improve the **efficiency** of **energy transmission into** (and out of) the **patient.**
- **Matching layer material(s)** have an **impedance value** that is **intermediate** between that of the transducer and that of tissue.
  - **Matching layer thickness** is generally **one-fourth** the **wavelength** of sound in that material (**quarter wave matching**).
- **Multiple layers** allow better matching for wide bandwidth pulses but run into manufacturing difficulties above three layers.
- Figure 17.3 shows the essential components of a typical piezoelectric transducer.

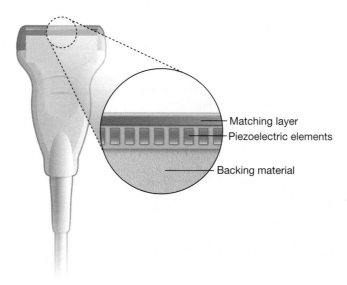

Matching layer
Piezoelectric elements
Backing material

FIG 17.3 Key components of ultrasound transducers include the piezoelectric crystal elements, transducer backing materials, and matching layer. Thickness of the crystal is one-half the wavelength, the backing material reduces the pulse length, and the matching layer improves the transmission of energy into the patient.

D. **Ultrasound Zones**
- The **near field** (Fresnel zone) of the ultrasound beam is **adjacent** to the transducer and is the primary region **used for ultrasound imaging.**
- The **length** of the **near field** is proportional to **frequency** and the **effective transducer size (r^2).**
  - For a transducer firing several elements at a time the effective diameter is roughly the diameter of the firing elements.
- **An unfocused beam** will converge to **approximately half its diameter at the end of the near field** before diverging.
- An ultrasound beam can be **focused** by using a **focusing cap**, element **timing delays,** or **shaping of the transducer face.**
  - A beam **can only be focused within the near field.**
- The **far field** (Fraunhofer zone) **starts** where the **near field ends.**
- In the **far field**, the ultrasound **beam diverges,** and the **intensity falls off very rapidly,** meaning echoes quickly become **too weak to detect** and lateral/elevational **resolutions are poor.**
- **Side lobes** are small beams of greatly reduced intensity that are emitted at **angles** to the **primary beam.**
  - Side lobes exist because **transducer elements expand in the lateral and elevational directions** as well as axial.
- **Grating lobes** are similar to side lobes but are caused by **interference patterns** from multielement transducers.
- The presence of **side and grating lobes** can bring objects outside of the FOV into the FOV, **increasing noise and creating "phantom" objects (usually visible only on anechoic backgrounds).**

E. **1.5D+ Arrays**
- **1.5D arrays** have a **large number** of **transducer elements** in the **scan plane** (e.g., 192) and a **small number** (e.g., 6) in the **slice thickness direction.**
- **Focusing** the small number (e.g., 6) **transducer elements** can be used to **reduce** the **slice thickness** and **improve elevational resolution.**
  - Generating **several lines**, each focused at a different depth, enables the **thinnest** part of each line be used for a composite image (**cherry picking**).
- **Lateral resolution** and **elevational resolution** in **1.5D arrays** are generally **comparable.**
- **Volume imaging** can be achieved using a **2D array** containing **thousands** of **transducer elements** (e.g., 50 × 50).
- With **2D arrays**, instead of the sound waves being sent straight down and reflected back, they are **sent** at **different angles.**
- Returning echoes are processed by a sophisticated computer program, resulting in a **reconstructed three-dimensional volume image.**
  - **3D imaging** electronic 2D arrays are now available for **superficial** and **breast applications.**
- **Mechanically scanned convex** or linear arrays can also be used to provide **3D** and **4D imaging** of **fetuses** in vivo.
  - **4D fetal ultrasound** allows a three-dimensional picture in real time and do **not exhibit** the **lag** associated with the **computer-constructed image.**

IV. TRANSDUCER ARRAYS

A. **Linear Arrays**
- **Arrays** consist of **multiple-element transducers** containing groups of transducer elements.
  - The **width** of **each element** is typically less than **half a wavelength** and the **vertical heights** are generally **several millimeters.**

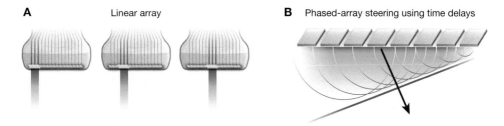

A   Linear array   **B**   Phased-array steering using time delays

FIG 17.4 A: Sequenced linear array generates each ultrasound pulse by firing several elements at a time to increase the near field depth. Pulses are sequentially fired along the linear array to cover the whole field of view. **B:** The ultrasound beam direction can be changed by varying the firing sequences of all the elements in a phased array. As the beam is swept out, pulses appear to originate from a single location with a very small footprint.

- **Linear arrays electronically scan** the ultrasound beam **without mechanical movement.**
  - A linear sequenced array explains both how the array is constructed (linear) as well as how it is operated (sequenced—firing in succession across the transducer).
- **Linear arrays activate** a group of **elements (~20)** to produce **one line** of **sight** and receive echoes along this single line of sight during a listening period (Fig. 17.4A).
  - A **group** of **elements**, rather than a single element, is used to **increase** the **near field distance.**
- The **next line** of **sight** is obtained by firing **another group** of **elements** that are **displaced** by **one or two elements.**
- The **complete frame** is obtained by **firing groups** of **elements** from **one end** of the linear array to the **other end.**
  - **Linear arrays** have roughly **128** to **256 elements** and generate rectangular looking fields of view (Fig. 17.5).
- **Linear arrays** tend to be of **higher frequency** and demonstrate good resolution of **small superficial structures.**
- One **limitation** of **linear arrays** is the **limited FOV** that is determined by the physical size of the linear array.
  - It is difficult to visualize a structure greater than ~10 cm due to the limited FOV.

B. Convex Arrays

- **Convex (curvilinear)** array operates in the **same manner** as the **linear array** with scan lines generated perpendicular to the transducer face.
- Up to 512 elements constitute a **convex sector array** in current scanners.
  - An aperture containing as many as 128 elements is selected to function at a given time.
- **Convex arrays** generate a **trapezoidal FOV** also called a **sector** image (Fig. 17.5).
  - **Wider fields of view** are obtained compared to a linear-array configuration.
- Convex arrays tend to be of **lower frequency** to allow for **deeper imaging** of larger structures due to their large FOV.
- **Convex sector systems** are capable of **lateral resolution** of less than **1 mm.**
- A drawback of the **curved array** (vs linear array) is **beam separation** at depth, which creates gaps and geometric distortion near the transducer face.
  - **At depth**, there will always be a **decrease in lateral resolution**, because structure could sit in the gap and be invisible.

C. Annular Arrays

- **Annular arrays** are created by taking a single crystal and cutting it into rings that get progressively smaller (cross section of an onion).
  - An **annular array transducer** is **focused** by applying an **electrical pulse** to **each element in turn.**

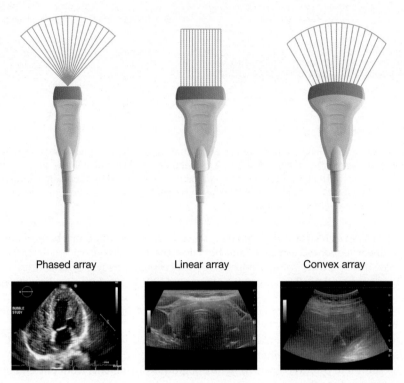

Phased array   Linear array   Convex array

FIG 17.5 Examples of clinical ultrasound transducers include phased arrays (left), linear arrays (middle), and curved arrays (right). Phased arrays have a small footprint and can be used in areas that are restricted in size (e.g., rib cage). Linear arrays are ideal for infants because of their limited fields of view, and the ability to depict superficial structures. Curved arrays offer a larger field of view than linear arrays, and are used to image adult abdomens.

- Individual pulses combine to create a composite pulse, focused to a point at a specific depth.
  - The **focal point depth** depends on the **time delay** between the **electrical pulses** applied to transducer elements.
- **Varying delays** between the pulses to each element permit the ultrasound beam to be **focused** to **different depths.**
- The resultant pulses can be focused to form well-defined beams for imaging.
- **Annular array transducers** allow ultrasound pulses to be **focused** in **two dimensions** rather than one.
- The ultrasound **beam** produced by **annular array** transducers is **symmetrical**, which means that it produces a **thinner scan slice** than other types of array.

D. Phased Arrays

- **Phased arrays** consist of many small ultrasonic transducers, each of which can be pulsed independently.
  - **Phased arrays** typically have **96 elements.**
- **Varying** the **timing (delays)** to **individual elements** results is a **beam** at a **set angle.**
- In effect, the **beam direction** can be **steered electronically** by adjusting the timing delays, as depicted in Figure 17.4B.
- As a result, the **ultrasound beam** is **swept through** the tissue or object being examined similar to a **searchlight.**
  - **Images** are generated by **detecting echoes** along **each line of sight.**

- **Data** from **multiple beams** are put together using sophisticated algorithms to **generate slices** through the object.
- Ultrasound images obtained with **phased arrays** always **originate** from a **single point** (Fig. 17.5C).
- **Phased-array** transducers are used for **cardiac imaging** because they have a **small footprint** (area of the beam origin) that can image **between** the **ribs.**
- **Phased arrays** are used when there is a **limited acoustic window** such as the ribs or encroaching lungs.
- Phased-array transducers also produce sector images with a very small superficial FOV.

E.   Focusing

- A **focused beam** can result from the interference of the multiple wavelets produced by each element.
- **Time delays determine** the **depth** of **focus** for the transmitted beam (Fig. 17.6).
  - The same delay factors are also applied to the elements during the receiving phase, resulting in a dynamic focusing effect on return.
- In this manner, a single scan line in the real-time image is formed.

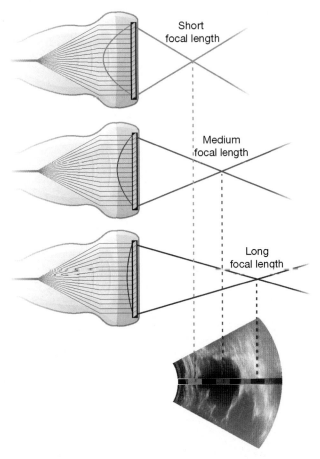

FIG 17.6 When focusing is achieved using a phased array, the focal depth can be varied for each pulse using different patterns of element activation (e.g., orange, red, and purple activation patterns). Improved imaging performance is achieved by generating several pulses with different focal depths, and then "cherry-picking" the best parts of each pulse to create a composite image. As the focal depth gets closer to the transducer, the beam diverges more quickly after the focus.

- To improve image quality, arrays can **electronically focus** the transmitted beam at **multiple depths** as depicted in Figure 17.6.
  - **Cherry-picking** the **focused regions** of multiple lines along a given direction will **increase** the **length** of the **focused region.**
- **Focusing** of **received echoes** is also **accomplished electronically.**
  - **Electronic focusing** can be used by **any array** of **elements**, including **linear** arrays, **curvilinear** arrays, and **phased** arrays.
- Virtually **all diagnostic ultrasound** beams **employ focusing** of the ultrasound beam.
- **Focusing** an ultrasound beam causes convergence and **narrowing** of the beam.
  - The major benefit of **focusing ultrasound beams** is to **improve lateral resolution.**
  - Focusing can only occur within the near field of the transducer.
- Using a **transducer face** that is **concave** can result in a **beam** that is **narrowed** at a predetermined distance from the transducer.
  - Placing a **concave acoustic lens** on the surface of the transducer can also **focus** the **beam** at a predetermined distance from the transducer.
- The point at which the **beam** is at its **narrowest** is the **focal point** and is the point of greatest intensity and best lateral resolution.
  - The **region** over which the **beam** is **relatively narrow** is referred to as the **focal zone.**
- In general, as the **focus is brought toward the transducer,** the beam will **diverge more quickly after the focal point.**

Chapter 17 (Ultrasound I) Questions

17.1 What is rarefaction?
A. Negative pressure of a sound wave
B. Bubbles formed from gas
C. A measure of tissue heating
D. Ratio of center frequency to band-width

17.2 What is the second harmonic frequency of a 2.5 MHz transducer?
A. 2 MHz
B. 4.5 MHz
C. 5 MHz
D. 7.5 MHz

17.3 Which of the following materials has the lowest velocity of sound?
A. Air
B. Fat
C. Tissue
D. Bone

17.4 Amplifying a signal hundredfold corresponds to a relative signal of (dB):
A. +20
B. +100
C. −20
D. −100

17.5 Materials with high acoustic impedances likely have a _____ density and a _____ sound velocity.
A. high; high
B. high; low
C. low; high
D. low; low

17.6 Big reflections occur at an interface when the acoustic impedances of the two materials are very:
A. Large
B. Small
C. Similar
D. Different

17.7 What is the intensity of the echo from a fat/tissue interface?
A. ≤1
B. 30
C. 70
D. ≥99

17.8 What beam property does NOT change when refraction occurs?
A. Sound velocity
B. Wavelength
C. Frequency
D. Travel direction

17.9 How does tissue attenuation change if transducer frequency doubles?
A. Doubles
B. Unchanged
C. Halves
D. Quarters

17.10 How does axial resolution change as the damping layer becomes thicker and more effective?
A. Decreases
B. No change
C. Increases

17.11 What thickness of an ultrasound transducer crystal generates sound with a wavelength λ?
A. $\lambda/10$
B. $\lambda/2$
C. 2λ
D. 10λ

17.12 What is the impedance of a matching layer given the impedance of a transducer ($Z_{transducer}$) and tissue (Z_{tissue})?
A. $>Z_{transducer}$
B. $>Z_{tissue}$ and $<Z_{transducer}$
C. $<Z_{tissue}$
D. Any value when $\lambda/4$ thick

17.13 How does near field length change when the effective transducer diameter doubles?
A. Not affected
B. Doubles
C. Triples
D. Quadruples

17.14 What does focusing improve?
A. Axial resolution
B. Lateral resolution
C. Dead zone volume
D. Speckle and noise

17.15 Which focusing method is likely to offer variable focal depths?
A. Acoustic lens
B. Shaped transducer
C. Phased array
D. Multitransmit array

17.16 Why are transducer elements fired in groups instead of individually?
A. To improve spatial resolution
B. To decrease side lobes
C. To increase temporal resolution
D. To improve damping

17.17 What is the term for firing groups of elements in rapid succession to sweep out an image?
A. Sector
B. Sequenced
C. Phased
D. Chirped

17.18 Linear arrays, rather than phased arrays or curvilinear arrays, would most likely be used to image:
A. Infants
B. Adults
C. Hearts
D. Brains

17.19 Transcranial imaging of the vasculature (via temples) would most likely use a(n) _____ array.
A. Linear
B. Curvilinear (convex)
C. Annular
D. Phased

17.20 What transducer is likely used for liver imaging?
A. Linear
B. Convex
C. Phased

Answers and Explanations

17.1 A (Negative pressure…). Sound waves have varying pressures along the wave, which oscillate in time. Compression is peak pressure and rarefaction is negative pressure (vacuum).

17.2 C (5 MHz). Five MHz is twice the transducer frequency (2.5 MHz) and would be the transducer second harmonic (the first harmonic is 2.5 MHz and is also called the fundamental).

17.3 A (Air). The velocity of sound in air (330 m/s) is lower than tissue (1,540 m/s), with bone having the highest velocity (>4,000 m/s).

17.4 A (+20 dB). A decibel value of +20 dB means a signal is a hundred times stronger, and −20 dB means the signal is a hundred times weaker (1%).

17.5 A (high; high). High acoustic impedance materials (e.g., bone) have both a high density and a high sound velocity.

17.6 D (Different). Big reflections occur at an interface when the acoustic impedances of the two materials are very different (i.e., acoustic impedance mismatch).

17.7 A (≤1 %). Fat/tissue interfaces reflect very little of the incident sound (<1%) because they have similar acoustic impedances which ensures most is transmitted (>99%).

17.8 C (Frequency). The frequency of a refracted sound wave is exactly the same as the frequency of the incident sound (all other factors change).

17.9 A (Doubles). Attenuation is proportional to sound frequency and is therefore a major problem for penetration when high frequency transducers are used.

17.10 C (Increases). As the damping layer becomes thicker and/or more effective it will stop ringing more which reduces spatial pulse length and increases axial resolution.

17.11 B ($\lambda/2$). Transducer thickness is generally half the wavelength, so the thickness of a 1.5 MHz transducer ($\lambda = 1.0$ mm) is 0.5 mm. Note that thin transducers generate high frequencies (i.e., short wavelengths), and vice versa.

17.12 B (>Z_{tissue} and < $Z_{transducer}$). Matching layer impedance will be the geometrical mean of tissue and transducer acoustic impedances (e.g., [$Z_{tissue} \times Z_{transducer}$]0.5) and will likely have a thickness of $\lambda/4$.

17.13 D (Quadruples). Doubling the effective transducer element diameter will quadruple the transducer near field distance, so using very small elements limits the imaging depth.

17.14 B (Lateral resolution). Use of focusing in ultrasound most results in narrower beams that will always improve lateral resolution.

17.15 C (Phased array). Multielemental transducers (e.g., phased arrays) can adjust the focal depth by varying the time delays of electrical pulses to individual elements, whereas the focal depth of acoustic lens and shaped transducers is generally fixed.

17.16 A (To improve spatial resolution). Individual elements in multielemental arrays mostly have a very small size meaning they have a very short near field and diverge quickly limiting spatial resolution even close to the transducer.

17.17 B (Sequenced). Liner or convex sequenced transducers fire groups of elements in rapid succession from one side of the transducer to the other to sweep out the image. This is different from phased arrays.

17.18 A (Infants). Linear arrays are most likely used to image infants because a large field of view is not required and superficial regions will be more visible.

17.19 D (Phased array). Transcranial imaging of the vasculature would use a phased array, which has a small "foot print" and can be applied via an acoustic window (e.g., eye lens or temple).

17.20 B (Convex). A convex transducer produces a sector image that has a large field of view at depth, allowing for imaging of a larger portion of the liver in a single view.

CHAPTER

18 Ultrasound II

I. CLINICAL IMAGING

A. **Lines of Sight**

- **Each ultrasound pulse** provides information for a **single line of sight**, resulting in a **single line** of an **ultrasound image.**
  - **Images** are built up by generating a **large number of lines of sight** that are **sequentially directed** to cover the region of interest in a patient (Fig. 18.1).
- **Pulse repetition frequency (PRF)** refers to the number of **separate pulses** (i.e., lines of sight) sent out **every second.**
  - **Common PRF** value is ~**4 kHz** (i.e., 4,000 pulses per second).
- Image **frame rates** are generally about **30 frames per second**, which permits ultrasound imaging where motion can be followed in real time.
  - The **product** of **frame rate** and **lines per image (N)** is equal to the **PRF.**
- The **line density (LD)** is the number of **lines per image divided** by the corresponding **field of view (FOV),** as depicted in Figure 18.1A.
- **Increasing** the **line density** generally **improves lateral resolution.**
- One way of **increasing** the **line density** is to **reduce** the **FOV,** as depicted in Figure 18.1B.
- Another way to **increase LD** is **reducing** the **frame rate,** as depicted in Figure 18.1B.
  - Reducing frame rates also **reduces temporal resolution.**
- **LD** can also be **increased** by **increasing** the **PRF,** as depicted in Figure 18.1B.
  - When **PRF increases**, the **listening time** is **reduced**, and **imaging depth decreases.**

B. **Depth Information**

- **Each pulse** has an extremely short duration (~1 μs).
- During the long **interval between pulses,** called the **listening interval,** transducers act as a receiver.
- For a **4 kHz PRF,** the **listening interval** between pulses is 1/4 kHz = **250 μs.**
  - **Increasing** the **PRF** always means a **reduced listening interval** for echo detection, and vice versa.
  - Sending out a pulse before the listening period ends would result in echoes with ambiguous location and depth.
- The **time interval** between an **emitted pulse** and the **returning echo** enables the **depth** of the **interface** producing the echo to be **determined.**
- For soft tissue (v = 1540 m/s), a **return time** of **13 μs** corresponds to a **depth** of **1 cm.**
  - A imaging depth of 1 cm corresponds to a round-trip distance of 2 cm.
  - When determining attenuation, the round-trip distance is used since both transmitted pulse and echo are attenuated.

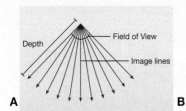
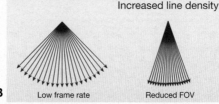

FIG 18.1 **A:** The pulse repetition frequency (PRF) is the total number of lines that are created in any second and is the product of the line density and frame rate. PRF also determines the waiting interval (depth), with increased PRF resulting in a shorter listening interval and reduced depth. **B:** The number of lines in an image divided by angular field of view defines the line density (i.e., lines per °). Increased line density can be achieved by reducing the frame rate (left), reducing the field of view (middle), or by increasing the PRF (right), which also results in a reduced imaging depth.

- Echoes 13 µs after the pulse was sent out thus correspond to an echo depth of 1 cm, echoes at 26 µs to an echo depth of 2 cm, and so on.
  - At a **PRF** of **4 kHz,** the **listening period** is **250 µs,** which corresponds to an **echo depth** of nearly **20 cm.**
- Table 18.1 shows the relationship between the PRF, echo listening time, and imaging depth.

C. **Depth Gain Compensation**
- An **echo** from a perfect reflector (e.g., air bubble) at the **surface travels no distance** and **undergoes no attenuation.**
- An echo from the same reflector at a **depth of 1 cm** will be **weaker** because the ultrasound echo has **traveled 2 cm** round trip and has been **attenuated.**
  - **Echoes** from this reflector at a **depth** of **10 cm** will be **extremely weak** because of attenuation in **traveling** a round-trip **distance of 20 cm.**
- **Uncorrected echo data** would thus show **distant echoes** as being **much weaker** than superficial echoes (Table 18.2).
- **Ultrasound scanners compensate** for **increased attenuation** with image depth.
  - This is accomplished by **increasing** the **signal gain** as the **echo return time increases.**
- Correcting for echo attenuation is known as **depth gain compensation (DGC).**
  - DGC is also known as **time gain compensation, time varied gain,** and **swept gain.**
- **DGC** makes **equal reflectors** have the **same brightness** in the ultrasound images, as illustrated by the data in Table 18.2.
  - **DGC controls** can be **adjusted** by the **operator** during the imaging procedures.
- Amplifying the echo also **amplifies noise** in the image, which becomes more noticeable as the echo intensity decreases (i.e., deeper echoes).

D. **Image Display Modes**
- The **strength (intensity)** of **returning echoes** along a **line** provides information about **differences** in **acoustic impedances** between tissues.

TABLE 18.1	Relationship Between the Pulse Repetition Frequency, Echo Listening Interval, and Penetration Depth	
Pulse Repetition Frequency (kHz)	**Echo Listening Time (µs)**	**Penetration Depth (cm)**
4	250	20
6	167	13
8	125	10

TABLE 18.2	Echo Attenuation and Time Gain Compensation Factors, for a 2 MHz Transducer and an Interface That Reflects 1% (–20 dB) of the Incident Sound		
Interface Depth (cm)	5	10	20
Distance traveled by echo (cm)	10	20	40
Echo attenuation (dB)	–10	–20	–40
Detected echo intensity (dB)	–30	–40	–60
Time gain compensation correction factor (dB)	+10	+20	+40
Displayed echo intensity (dB)	–20	–20	–20

- **A-mode (amplitude)** displays **depth** on the **horizontal axis** and **echo intensity** (pulse amplitude) on the **vertical axis.**
  - **Ophthalmology** is the only diagnostic application of **A-mode imaging.**
- **T-M mode (time-motion)** displays **time** on the **horizontal axis** and **depth** on the **vertical axis** (aka **M-mode [motion]**).
  - **T-M mode** displays time-dependent motion, which is valuable for studying rapid movement (e.g., **cardiac valve motion**).
- In **B-mode**, **echo intensity** is displayed as a **brightness value (B)** along **each line of sight.**
  - **B-mode** is used for **M-mode** and **gray scale** imaging.
- **Acquired data** from transducers are **sent** to a **scan converter** for processing.
  - Scan conversion is required because the format of image acquisition and display are different.
- **Scan converters compute two-dimensional images** from echo data from distinct beam directions, which are **subsequently displayed** on a monitor.
- Image creation based on echo information is shown schematically in Figure 18.2.
- B-Mode data are stored and displayed in a **512^2 matrix (1 byte [8 bit] per pixel).**
  - Each **ultrasound frame** (image) generally contains **0.25 MB** of information, and the frames are often shown in rapid succession for video loops.

E. Other Ultrasound Settings

- Many machine settings are automatically set by an **"optimize image" button** and then manually adjusted by the user as needed.

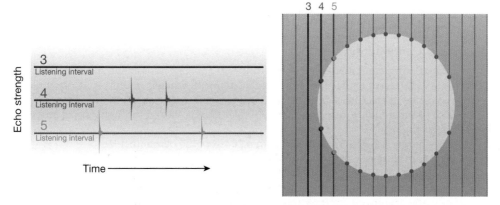

FIG 18.2 Ultrasound image creation occurs one line at a time after a very short duration pulse is emitted by the transducer, and echoes are recorded in a much longer time interval (pulse repetition period). In this figure, echoes received during three consecutive listening intervals (i.e., 3, 4, and 5) are depicted on the left, which appear as the corresponding three image lines depicted on the right. Note that scatter echoes are not shown.

- **Center frequency** is chosen either by transducer choice and/or setting the center frequency in multiselect transducers.
  - **Convex arrays** typically operate at low-to-moderate frequencies (2-6 MHz).
  - **Linear arrays** typically operate at moderate-to-high frequencies (6-14 MHz).
- **Depth** should be set a **little below the object of interest,** so it **fills the FOV** and there is **room for "diagnostic" artifacts** (e.g., shadowing) to be visualized.
- **Gain** is an amplification that increases the overall signal strength, causing the image to be brighter.
  - It should be set so that **background parenchyma is middle gray** and not too high where **amplified noise** may make anechoic structures to have signal.
- **Focus** (in electronic focus transducers) should be set at or slightly below the object of interest to optimize spatial resolution.
- **Read zoom** (magnify), like zoom on a workstation, makes a portion of the image larger but does not improve image quality.
- **Write zoom** acquires new data only in the new smaller region of interest while making it fill the screen.
  - Smaller region of interest laterally allows increased line density and **lateral resolution.**
  - Smaller region of interest axially allows **higher frame rates** due to shallower depth.

II. ADVANCED TECHNIQUES

A. Elastography
- Elastography was originally developed to image palpable masses that appeared **invisible on B-mode imaging.**
- Two types of elastography are used clinically: **strain and shear wave.**
- **Strain** elastography requires the **periodic compression** of the area of interest using the ultrasound transducer.
- Transducer compression forces cause **softer tissues to deform but harder tissues to only displace.**
  - A semiquantitative color overlay of tissue hardness is displayed on top of B-mode imaging.
- **Shear wave elastography** uses a transducer **ultrasound pulse to compress tissue.**
- The same transducer then images the **tissue re-expanding and the resultant shear wave** then moves through the patient perpendicular to the ultrasound beam.
- The **velocity of the shear wave** can be estimated and is an indication of tissue hardness.
  - Shear wave velocities are typically a **few meters per second and are lower in softer tissues.**

B. Spatial Compounding
- **Spatial compound imaging** (aka **multibeam** imaging) combines **multiple lines** of **sight at different angles** to form a **single composite image.**
  - In conventional ultrasound, tissue is imaged from a single direction.
- Each beamlet from a group of transducer elements is steered through a set of predetermined angles.
  - The **range** of **angles** is generally within **20°** from the perpendicular.
- **Echoes** from these **different directions** are **averaged** together (compounded) into a single composite image, which **reduces noise.**
- **Spatial compound imaging reduces angle-dependent artifacts, speckle,** and **clutter,** providing **improved contrast** and **margin definition.**
  - **Compound imaging** reduces frame rate due to the multiple angle acquisitions.
- All angles are present within the central triangular region of overlap to generate images using full compounding.
  - **Corners** of the image receive only a **subset** of all the **views,** which **reduces** the resultant **image quality.**

C. Extended FOV

- **Extended FOV (panorama)** uses **static B**-mode techniques to permit a **large subject area** to be viewed on a **single static image.**
- **Extended FOV** images are acquired by **sliding** the **probe** over the **area** of **interest.**
  - As the **images** are acquired, they are **"stitched"** together electronically.
- This results in a **single slice image** covering the area of interest, such as a **full-length view** of the **Achilles tendon.**
- **Extended FOV** imaging is beneficial where large patient areas need to be visualized on a single image and there is limited motion (e.g. musculoskeletal [**MSK**]).
  - **MSK abnormalities** (fluid collections, muscle injuries, and tumors) can be **visualized** relative to more **distant landmarks** such as **joints** or **tendons.**

D. Harmonic Imaging

- Harmonic imaging **transmits at the center (fundamental) frequency** but receives signals at the **second and sometimes third harmonic.**
  - **Harmonic imaging** requires very **broadband transducers.**
- Harmonic frequencies arise in the transmitted pulse from **nonlinear deformation of the pulse as it moves through the tissue.**
- **Harmonic imaging reduces side and grating lobe artifacts,** since they lack the power to generate strong harmonic signals.
- **Clutter and superficial reverberation artifacts are minimized** because harmonics do not form until deeper in the patient.
- **Lateral resolution is improved** because harmonics form in the central part of the fundamental beam.
- **Temporal and axial resolution may be diminished** due to the use of multiple and possibly longer pulses.

E. Contrast Agents

- **Contrast agents** for **vascular** and **perfusion imaging** are **encapsulated microbubbles** (e.g., 3 μm) containing air, nitrogen, or insoluble gases (perfluorocarbons).
  - They are **purely intravascular** due to large size compared to magnetic resonance imaging and computed tomography contrast agents, which move into the extracellular space.
- Ultrasound **signals (reflections)** are generated by nonlinear resonance and the large **difference** in **acoustic impedance** between the **gas** and surrounding **fluids/tissues.**
  - **Contrast agents** (microbubbles) also **produce harmonic frequencies.**
- Flow dynamics and perfusion are observed by watching **uptake and washout** of the contrast agent.
- **Low mechanical index protocols** must be used to avoid unintentional bubble destruction.
  - **Flashing** is when a high mechanical index beam is **purposely used to destroy the bubbles** so wash-in and wash-out can again be observed.
- **Bubbles popping do not cause tissue damage.**

III. DOPPLER

A. Doppler Physics

- The **Doppler effect** refers to **changes** in **frequency** resulting from a **moving sound source,** as depicted in Figure 18.3.
  - Objects **moving toward** the **detector** reflect sound at **higher frequencies,** and those **moving away** from the detector reflect sound at **lower frequencies.**
- The **shift** in **frequency** is proportional to **cos(θ)**, where θ is the angle between the ultrasound beam and the moving object (**Doppler angle**), as shown in Figure 18.3.
  - **Maximum frequency shift** occurs when the reflector is moving directly toward the transducer (i.e., **θ is equal to 0°**) or directly away (i.e., θ is equal to 180°).

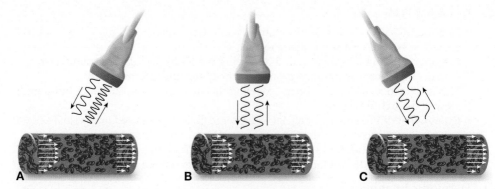

FIG 18.3 Illustration of the Doppler angle between the ultrasound beam, and the direction of flow which is critical for the resultant Doppler frequency shift. **A:** When blood flows towards the transducer the flow is typically colored red. **B:** When the Doppler angle is 90°, there is no Doppler frequency shift (i.e., zero) and an artifactual flow void may be seen. **C:** When the blood flows away from the transducer the flow is typically colored blue on the image. When the Doppler angle is 0°, the Doppler frequency shift is a maximum. Flow direction and measured value depend on the doppler angle.

- At a **90° Doppler angle**, there is **no Doppler shift** no matter how fast reflectors move.
  - **Doppler** only **measures** the **shift** in **frequency,** *not* the **reflector velocity.**
- At a **given Doppler angle**, the **Doppler frequency shift** is directly **proportional** to the **reflector velocity.**
  - Doubling the reflector velocity generally doubles Doppler frequency shifts.
- **Ultrasound Doppler shift frequencies** are in the **audio range,** as shown in Table 18.3.
  - Doppler frequency shift is proportional to the ultrasound frequency (f).
- The **simplified Bernoulli principle** says the **change in pressure** (mmHg) across an opening is equal to four times the square of the **velocity after the opening** (m/s).
  - This is useful for measuring pressure across a valve or stenosis, but **accuracy is limited due to turbulent flow, adding uncertainty to the velocity reading.**

B. **Blood Flow and Doppler**
- **Laminar flow** normally exists in vessels with faster flow in the center and lower flow near the vessel walls (frictional forces).
  - **Plug (blunt) flow** is a form of laminar flow found in **large vessels** and is characterized by **most blood moving at the same velocity and diminishing only at the vessel wall.**
  - **Parabolic flow** is a form of laminar flow found in **smaller vessels** and is characterized by blood **velocity gradually diminishing from the center of the vessel to the wall.**
- As the **vessel narrows,** flow **velocities increase,** and vice versa (**Bernoulli principle**).
  - **Turbulent flow** may occur when the vessel is narrowed by **stenoses.**
  - **Pressure is low at the stenosis where velocity is high and pressure is high before and after the stenosis where velocity is low.**
- **Doppler ultrasound** is used to identify and **evaluate blood flow** in vessels based on the **backscatter** from **blood cells.**

TABLE 18.3	Maximum Doppler Frequency Shifts (Hz) for Moving Blood (i.e., 0° Doppler Angle)	
Blood Velocity (cm/s)	**Transducer Frequency (MHz)**	
	2	**5**
10	260	650
30	780	2,000
100	2,600	6,500

- **Pulsed Doppler** provides **depth information** in addition to the Doppler frequency shift.
  - **PRF values** are generally **higher** in **Doppler** than in B-mode imaging (e.g., 8 kHz).
- Signals are processed so that **only echoes** from a **region of interest** contribute to the **Doppler signal.**
  - **Pulses** are **repeatedly directed** along the same scan line to **obtain multiple signals** for each pixel.
- **Duplex scanning** combines **real-time B-mode imaging** with **Doppler** detection.
  - **B-mode images** allow **selection** of a **region of interest** as well as an estimate of the Doppler angle.
- **B-mode images** provide information on **stationary reflectors**, and **Doppler shifts** provide information on **flow present** in a selected region of interest.

C. Spectral Analysis

- **Spectral analysis** selects a small region of interest in a B-mode image to be investigated for flow using **pulsed Doppler.**
- **Spectral analysis** shows **frequency shift** as a **function of time** that can provide information regarding blood flow (Fig. 18.4).
  - The **horizontal axis** is **time** and the **vertical axis** is **Doppler frequency shift (typically transformed to show estimated velocity).**
- **Echo intensity** at a given **frequency shift**, and at a given moment in time, is displayed as a **brightness value.**
  - Velocities (i.e., frequency shifts) in one direction are placed above the horizontal axis, and in the reverse direction below the horizontal axis.
- The effects of **Doppler angle** can be corrected by **estimating the flow angle to get a better velocity measurement.**
  - **Doppler angle should be kept below 60°** because velocity measurement uncertainty increases rapidly with angle (even after angle correction).
- **Blood flow** is **pulsatile**, and the spectral characteristics vary with time (Fig. 18.4).
- **Plug flow exhibits a thin waveform, parabolic flow has a thicker waveform, and turbulent flow exhibits an extremely broad waveform** due to the many velocities in the flow.

D. Color Doppler

- **Color Doppler** provides a **2D visual display** of **moving blood**, with measured Doppler **frequency shifts encoded** as **colors.**
- **Flow information** is provided by taking the **average Doppler shift** a number of **samples** obtained from **each pixel (location).**
  - **Color Doppler** provides information on the **direction** and **magnitude** of the **flow** over a selected region of interest.

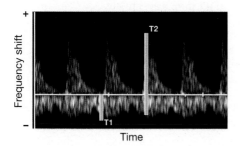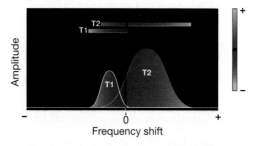

FIG 18.4 Spectral display showing detected frequency shifts on the vertical axis as a function of time (left). The right figure shows that the pattern of frequency shifts detected at T1 contains mainly negative values (blue), whereas the pattern of frequency shifts detected at time T2 contains mainly positive values (red).

- **Red** typically signifies **motion toward** the **transducer,** whereas **blue** signifies **motion away from** the **transducer.**
  - **Turbulent flow** may be displayed as **green or yellow.**
- **Color Doppler information** is displayed on **top** of the **B-mode image.**
  - Color Doppler can detect flow in vessels too small to see by imaging alone and allows complex blood flow to be visualized.
- Color Doppler displays are **not typically corrected for Doppler angle,** so **absolute velocities may underestimate true flow.**

E. **Power Doppler**

- **Power Doppler** uses the **same acquired** data as in **color Doppler.**
  - Ultrasound intensities (power) are identical in power and color Doppler.
- **The differences** between **power** and **color Doppler** relate to **how information** is **processed** and **displayed.**
- Consider **100 pulses** sent out at approximately **90°** to a blood vessel.
  - Assume that **45 show small negative frequency shifts, 45 small positive frequency shifts,** and 10 exactly zero.
- **Color Doppler** would interpret these 100 values as a **mean frequency shift** of **zero** and show this as a dark region indicating no flow.
  - **Power Doppler,** however, interprets the **same input data** as **90 frequency shifts.**
- Power Doppler exhibits this as an **orange color** that has **90%** of the **maximum intensity** observed in the blood vessel.
  - The **Doppler angle** has **very little effect** on the displayed color intensity, with the intensity at 90° only being slightly less than that at 0°.
- **Power Doppler signal** does **not vary** with the **direction of flow,** with the same color intensity for flow toward the transducer as away from the transducer.
  - **Power Doppler** does **not exhibit aliasing artifacts.**
- **Power Doppler** is **more sensitive** than standard color flow imaging and used to **detect slow flows.**

IV. IMAGE QUALITY AND SAFETY

A. **Axial Resolution**

- **Axial resolution** is the ability to **separate two objects** lying along the **axis** of the **beam,** as depicted in Figure 18.5.
  - **Axial resolution** is towards and away from transducer (depth in the image).
- **Axial resolution** is solely determined by the **spatial pulse length** and is independent of depth.
  - **Axial resolution** is approximately equal to one half of the pulse length, which is the **ultrasound wavelength** in tissue (assuming 2 waves making 1 pulse).
- **Increasing transducer frequency reduces pulse length** and **improves axial resolution.**
  - At 1.5 and 15 MHz, axial resolution is ~1 and 0.1 mm, respectively.
- Although **increasing transducer frequency improves axial resolution,** attenuation also increases resulting in **poor penetration.**
- **Ultrasound** imaging **trades off between spatial resolution** and **imaging depth.**
  - **High resolution** implies **poor penetration,** and vice versa.
- Breasts are relatively thin, with good penetration, and high resolution is achieved in breast ultrasound using high-frequency transducers (>10 MHz).
  - **High-frequency intracavitary ultrasound** probes permit **intravascular imaging** with **excellent resolution** in visualizing adjacent blood vessels.

B. **Lateral and Elevational Resolution**

- **Lateral resolution** performance is the ability to **resolve (separate) two adjacent objects,** as depicted in Figure 18.5.
  - **Lateral resolution** is typically the horizontal resolution on the image.

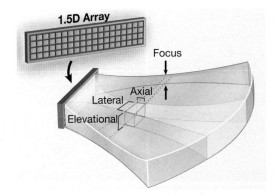

FIG 18.5 A 1.5D array and transmitted beam. The axial resolution is the ability to resolve two close objects with one deeper in the patient than the other. This is the vertical resolution on the image. The lateral resolution is the ability to resolve two close objects next to each other along the long face of the transducer. This is the horizontal resolution on the image. The elevational resolution is the slice thickness and impacts whether any partial volume artifact appears (an objects only partially in the thickness of the beam).

- **Ultrasound beam width** is the most important **determinant** of **lateral resolution** performance.
  - **Increasing** the number of **lines** per frame also **improves lateral resolution.**
- **Focused transducers** produce **narrow beams** and **improve lateral resolution.**
- **Multiple focal zones** may be used to **improve lateral resolution.**
  - Use of multiple focal zones is generally at the expense of a **reduced frame rate.**
- Lateral resolution usually becomes worse at a large distance from the transducer.
  - **Lateral resolution** is about **four times worse than axial resolution.**
- **Elevational resolution** is the resolution in the **plane perpendicular** to the **image plane,** as depicted in Figure 18.5.
  - **Slice thickness** is another term for elevational resolution.
- **Height** of **transducer elements** is directly related to **elevational resolution.**
- Elevational resolution generally depends on the distance (depth) from the transducer surface (Fig. 18.5).
  - **Elevational resolution** can be **improved by focusing.**

C. Ultrasound B-Mode Artifacts

- Ultrasound artifacts occur because **assumptions** made in creating images are **violated** (e.g., echoes are only created by the main beam, and there is only one reflection).
  - Additional **assumptions** include echo **velocity is 1,540 m/s,** sound travels in **straight lines,** and **attenuation** is **uniform.**
- **Mirror artifact** occurs when sound is reflected off a large specular reflector such as the surface of the liver causing parts of the image to be duplicated on the other side of the interface.
  - **Changing angle** will eliminate the mirror image.
- **Speed displacement** (speed of sound) artifacts are caused by the variability of the speed of sound in different tissues and typically appear as a sudden change in depth of a continuous structure.
- **Reverberation echoes** (Fig. 18.6) are the result of **multiple reflections** occurring between two adjacent interfaces.
  - The reverberation between transducer and skin is eliminated with gel and good contact.
- **Comet tail artifacts** (Fig. 18.6), a type of reverberation, occurs when the gap between reverberation echoes becomes very small (e.g., opposing walls of a simple cyst), and the reflections from one comet tail–like structure.
  - **Harmonic imaging** can mitigate this artifact.
- **Ring down artifacts** (Fig. 18.6) show a streaklike appearance from mixtures of **gas (air)** and **fluids.**
  - **Gas bubbles resonate a**nd create strong signals similar to contrast agents.

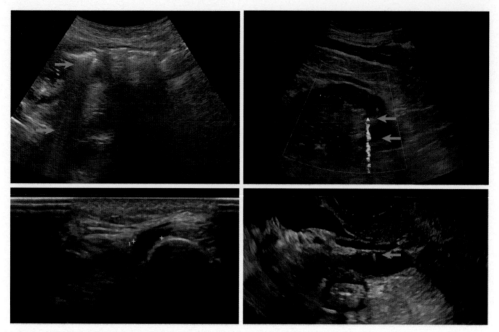

FIG 18.6 Select Ultrasound artifacts. Top-Left: Arrows indicate ring down artifact from pneumobilia post surgery. Top-Right: Color Doppler demonstrating twinkle artifact from a calcification (stone). Bottom-Left: Anisotropy causing a reduced tendon signal (between plus signs) due to specular reflections missing the transducer. Note also reverberation artifact between the transducer and skin visualized as horizontal lines at the skin line and clear in the image edges. Bottom-Right: Comet tail artifact due to reverberations between top and bottom surfaces of the anechoic structure.

- **Acoustic shadowing** is the **reduced echo intensity** distal to a highly attenuating or reflecting object such as a stone creating a "shadow."
- **Acoustic enhancement** is the **increased echo intensity** distal to a minimally attenuating object such as a cyst or blood vessel.
- **Anisotropy** (Fig. 18.6) occurs where the beam is incident on striated tissue that causes specular reflections (e.g., tendons).
  - If the beam is perpendicular to the tissue interface the reflection is strong, but at an angle the **echo will not hit the transducer and thus the tendon will appear artificially hypoechoic** (only scatter reaches the transducer).
  - **Changing angle and compound** imaging help.

D. **Doppler Artifacts**
- **Aliasing artifacts** occur with **high velocities** in the center of a vessel appearing to have reverse flow.
- **Aliasing artifacts** are overcome by increasing the **PRF,** which must be at least *twice* the highest **Doppler frequency shift (Nyquist limit).**
  - To **avoid aliasing**, a **1 kHz Doppler shift** requires a minimum **PRF** of **2 kHz.**
  - Changing the baseline, reducing frequency, and increasing Doppler angle can also help.
- **Twinkle artifacts** (Fig. 18.6) occur **behind** a **strong attenuator** (e.g., calcifications) and exhibit a pattern of rapidly fluctuating reds and blues where there is no flow (i.e., only tissues).
  - This artifact is **maximized** by placing **focus** below the calcification, **decreasing PRF,** and **changing color priority** (threshold where machine displays color values instead of gray level values).

- **Flash artifacts** fill the image with a **sudden burst of color**, which is a result of **sudden movement** of the transducer or the patient (e.g., kicking fetus).
- **Tissue vibration** artifact occurs when tissue motion from strong pulsatile or turbulent flow causes **surrounding tissue motion that is mistaken as flow** by the scanner.
  - **Reducing the color gain** and **changing color priority** can **mitigate** this.

E. **Bioeffects and Safety**

- The **spatial peak (SP) intensity** is the highest intensity in the beam cross section (typically in the **center** of the **beam) and spatial average (SA) is over the transducer face.**
- **Temporal average (TA) intensity** is the **time average** intensity (i.e., averaged over pulse and listening time).
  - **Pulse average (PA)** intensity is the time average only for the pulse.
- Representative intensities (SPTA) in **B-mode** ultrasound are about **20 mW/cm².**
  - **M-mode** and **Doppler** have intensities **4** and **50 times higher,** respectively.
- **Cavitation** is the creation of bubbles during rarefaction that can cause damage when popped.
- **Mechanical index (MI)** is a parameter that estimates the **chance** of **inducing cavitation** effects and is displayed during acquisition.
  - **High power and low frequencies** increase MI.
- The **thermal index (TI)** predicts the **rise** in **tissue temperature** in degrees **Celsius.**
  - A **TI of 1** is estimated to increase **tissue temperatures by 1°C.**
- **TI** can be specified for **soft tissue (TIS), bone (TIB),** or **cranial bone (TIC) (i.e., bone near the skin surface).**
  - **Bone and cranial bone heat more quickly.**
  - **Heating** from **B-mode < color Doppler < M-mode < spectral Doppler**
- Despite an excellent safety profile for adult, pediatric, and obstetric imaging, it is still recommended that **unnecessary exposures be eliminated (ALARA principle).**
- Table 18.4 **lists safety quantities and their advisory or regulatory limits.**

TABLE 18.4	List of Some Safety Quantities and Their Limits		
Quantity	**Limit**	**Advisory or Regulation**	**Comments**
Derated intensity SPTA[a]	720 mW/cm²	Regulation	Lower for ophthalmologic; exceptions can be granted
Mechanical index	1.9	Regulation	Lower for ophthalmologic; exceptions can be granted
Adult thermal index 15 min maximum	3	Advisory	AIUM; decrease 33% for pulsed Doppler near bone
Adult thermal index 4 min maximum	4	Advisory	AIUM; decrease 33% for pulsed Doppler near bone
Obstetric thermal index 15 min maximum	2	Advisory	AIUM; decrease 33% for pulsed Doppler near bone
Obstetric thermal index 4 min maximum	2.5	Advisory	AIUM; decrease 33% for pulsed Doppler near bone

[a]Derated indicating a 0.3 db/cm/MHz worst-case attenuation assumption.
AIUM, American Institution of Ultrasound in Medicine; SPTA, spatial peak temporal average.

Chapter 18 (Ultrasound II) Questions

18.1 Increasing gain increases echo amplitude but has what disadvantage?
A. Reduced contrast
B. Increased shadowing
C. Decreased axial resolution
D. Amplified noise

18.2 What is the listening period for a PRF of 4 kHz?
A. 2.5 μs
B. 25 μs
C. 250 μs
D. 2,500 μs

18.3 An increase in line density improves which resolution?
A. Axial
B. Lateral
C. Elevational
D. Temporal

18.4 Increasing the PRF implies a _____ listening period and a _____ ultrasound imaging depth.
A. longer; increased
B. longer; reduced
C. shorter; increased
D. shorter; reduced

18.5 What is the term for amplifying later echoes more than earlier echoes?
A. Color priority
B. Harmonic frequency
C. Multiple focal zones
D. Depth gain compensation

18.6 What frequency transducer is typically used for breast imaging?
A. Low (2 MHz)
B. Moderate (5 MHz)
C. High (10 MHz)
D. Very high (20 MHz)

18.7 What does spatial compounding improve?
A. Axial resolution
B. Temporal resolution
C. Power deposition (i.e., less)
D. Lesion contrast

18.8 What ultrasound mode is ideal for investigating the opening and closing of valves?
A. A-mode
B. Color Doppler
C. M-mode
D. Shear wave elastography

18.9 What parameter should be kept low during contrast-enhanced imaging?
A. Mechanical index
B. Effective wavelength
C. Pulse repetition frequency
D. Greyscale gain

18.10 What color is typically shown for color Doppler imaging with a Doppler angle of 90°?
A. Blue
B. Red
C. Black
D. Green

18.11 What flow in a large blood vessel is characterized by a thin spectral waveform?
A. Parabolic
B. Blunt
C. Turbulent
D. Uniform

18.12 Brightness in the spectral waveform is proportional to what quantity?
A. Blood cell quantity
B. Frequency shifts
C. Blood velocity
D. Mechanical index

18.13 What artifact can be used to characterize lesion calcification?
A. Ring down
B. Aliasing
C. Refraction
D. Twinkle

18.14 What is the maximum Doppler frequency shift that a color Doppler acquisition can faithfully measure (i.e., without aliasing) using a PRF of 4 kHz?
A. 1 kHz
B. 2 kHz
C. 8 kHz
D. 16 kHz

18.15 Temporal resolution is most likely independent of what acquisition parameter?
A. Pulse repetition frequency
B. Image line density
C. Imaging depth
D. Pulse length

18.16 For images obtained using a convex array, slice thickness is most closely related to which type of resolution?
 A. Axial
 B. Lateral
 C. Elevational
 D. Temporal

18.17 What artifact is the result of specular reflection?
 A. Aliasing
 B. Mirror
 C. Enhancement
 D. Flash

18.18 Ultrasound intensities (e.g., 20 mW/cm^2) most likely refer to a spatial _____ and a temporal _____.
 A. peak; peak
 B. peak; average
 C. average; peak
 D. average; peak

18.19 A thermal index of 3 is an estimate of what Celsius temperature increase?
 A. 1.5°
 B. 3°
 C. 4.5°
 D. 9°

18.20 What safety guidance should *always* be followed when generating US images?
 A. MI < 1
 B. TI < 1
 C. I_{spta} < 50 W/cm^2
 D. ALARA

Answers and Explanations

18.1 D (Amplified noise). Increasing gain can make weak echoes visible but also amplify noise.

18.2 C (250 μs). For a PRF of 4 kHz, the ultrasound listening period is 250 μs (i.e., 1/4,000 seconds).

18.3 B (Lateral resolution). Line density *always* affects lateral resolution but *may* also impact of temporal resolution (i.e., more lines per frame may result in fewer frames per second).

18.4 D (shorter; reduced). Increasing the PRF implies a shorter listening period, and a reduced ultrasound imaging depth. Increasing the PRF from 4 to 8 kHz reduces the listening interval (250-125 μs) and reduces imaging depth (20-10 cm).

18.5 D (Depth gain compensation). Time gain compensation (TGC), depth gain compensation (DGC), and time varied gain (TVG) all refer to the practice of electronically amplifying later echoes more than earlier echoes.

18.6 C (High, about 10 MHz). Breast imaging most likely uses high transducer frequencies (e.g., 10 MHz) that offer good axial resolution and can penetrate a typical compressed breast thickness (6 cm).

18.7 D (Lesion contrast). Spatial compounding reduces angle-dependent artifacts and noise/speckle, providing improved contrast and margin definition.

18.8 C (M-mode). M-mode is designed to assess motion in a single location and displays a single image line over time.

18.9 A (Mechanical index). A large mechanical index is likely to burst the ultrasound bubbles.

18.10 C (Black). At a Doppler angle of 90°, there is no frequency shift (i.e., cos [90°] is zero), so the measured signal would always appear black (no flow) in any color Doppler display.

18.11 B (Blunt). Flow in normal blood vessel exhibits a "flat" velocity profile but is reduced at vessel walls (i.e., blunt or plug flow).

18.12 A (Blood cell quantity). The brightness represents the intensity of the echo, which will be proportional to the number of blood cells traveling at a given velocity at a given moment in time.

18.13 D (Twinkle). Twinkle artifact will appear on and below calcified lesions during color Doppler imaging.

18.14 B (2 kHz). The maximum frequency shift (kHz) Color Doppler can faithfully measure without aliasing is 2 kHz with a PRF of 4 kHz (i.e., half the PRF).

18.15 D (Pulse length). Temporal resolution is most likely independent of the pulse length but can be affected by changes in PRF, line density, and imaging depth.

18.16 C (Elevational). Slice thickness is another name for elevational resolution on an image obtained using a convex array.

18.17 B (Mirror). Specular reflection from a surface such as the liver can cause a duplicate structure to be seen on the other side of the reflector. Scatter and diffuse reflections would be too weak to generate a mirror image.

18.18 B (peak; average). Ultrasound intensities refer to a measured spatial peak and a temporal average, as these best relate to maximum tissue heating.

18.19 C (3°). A TI of 3 means that the vendor's mathematical models believe a heat increase of 3 °C is possible. Actual temperature increase may be lower due to actual versus modeled thermal conditions.

18.20 D (ALARA). ALARA means elimination of unnecessary imaging and using only MI and TI necessary to produce a diagnostic image (i.e., benefit greater than risks).

Examination Guide

"I did then what I knew how to do. Now that I know better, I do better."

-Maya Angelou

These two practice examinations, each consisting of 100 questions and answers, cover the material summarized in this book. The examinations, which should be taken under examination conditions without access to a textbook, will help students to:

Practice for the real examination. Taking practice examinations helps you develop a strategy for dealing with difficult questions. Guessing *after* eliminating all "wrong" answers is one option, and temporarily skipping difficult questions to return at a later time is another option.

Highlight weaknesses and strengths. Taking these examinations should help identify your weaknesses as well as strengths. Weaknesses need to be corrected by consulting the appropriate chapter in this review book or, if greater depth is required, by consulting a textbook.

Build confidence. Successful completion of the examinations demonstrates that the subject material has been understood, which will ease preexamination nervousness.

The following guidelines should assist readers to perform successfully in any examination.
1. *Read and follow all examination instructions*.
2. Read each question *carefully*.
3. *Never* assume information.
4. Focus on keywords.
5. Eliminate obviously incorrect answers.
6. Reread the questions and verify your answers.
7. Answer *all* questions, even if you have to guess.
8. Do not spend more than <u>2 minutes</u> on any one question.
9. Assume the question is NOT trying to trick you.
    9.1. Physics is hard enough and typically does not require trickery.

PRACTICE EXAMINATION A:
Questions

A.1 How does doubling exposure time impact image noise?
A. Increase 100%
B. Increase 40%
C. No change
D. Decrease 30%

A.2 What percentage of a 120 kV spectrum is from characteristic x-rays?
A. ≤10%
B. 30%
C. 70%
D. ≥90%

A.3 In what direction do photons scatter after Compton interactions?
A. Primarily at 45°
B. Primarily at 90
C. Primarily backscatter
D. Essentially isotropic

A.4 What is a typical fetal dose from an AP abdominal radiograph?
A. 0.1 mGy
B. 1 mGy
C. 10 mGy
D. 100 mGy

A.5 How does increasing x-ray tube voltage impact quality and quantity?
A. Quality increases; quantity increases
B. Quality increases; quantity decreases
C. Quality decreases; quantity increases
D. Quality decreases; quantity decreases

A.6 Increasing what parameter will minimize scattered radiation impacting image quality?
A. Tube voltage
B. Beam area
C. Grid ratio
D. Focal spot

A.7 Roughly how much scatter is transmitted through a grid in radiography?
A. 10%
B. 30%
C. 60%
D. 80%

A.8 How does blood appear on 2D t1W spin echo imaging?
A. Black/Dark gray
B. Neutral/Middle gray
C. Bright/Light gray

A.9 What is the dynamic range of digital detectors used in radiography?
A. 10:1
B. 100:1
C. 1,000: 1
D. >1,000:1

A.10 What single image is likely to require the most storage space?
A. Chest x-ray
B. Mammogram
C. Abdominal CT
D. Prostate MR

A.11 What is the primary reason for the high attenuation of bone in fluoroscopy?
A. High density
B. High atomic number
C. Low atomic mass
D. Low specular reflection

A.12 Reducing x-ray tube filtration in abdominal x-ray imaging (+AEC), will most likely _____ contrast and _____ patient dose.
A. increase; increase
B. increase; decrease
C. decrease; increase
D. decrease; decrease

A.13 How does quadrupling the number of detected photons change noise?
A. Quadruple
B. Double
C. Halve
D. Quarter

A.14 A patient has a head CT and an abdominal x-ray. Which dose metric from these scans can be added to give an combined dose?
A. Effective dose
B. Equivalent dose
C. Skin dose
D. Absorbed dose

A.15 What measure is used to quantify changes in lesion visibility when adjusting radiography acquisition parameters?
A. Lesion contrast
B. Image noise
C. Noise/Contrast
D. Contrast/Noise

A.16 What are the units of Kerma-area product?
A. Gy/cm
B. Gy/cm^2
C. $Gy*cm$
D. $Gy*cm^2$

A.17 How does patient skin dose compare to entrance K_{air}?
A. Skin dose lower than K_{air}
B. Skin dose equal to K_{air}
C. Skin dose higher than K_{air}

A.18 What particle has a radiation weighting factor (W_R) different from 1.0?
A. X-rays
B. Gamma rays
C. Beta particles
D. Protons

A.19 What is the effective dose of a dual-energy x-ray absorptiometry?
A. Very low (<0.1 mSv)
B. Low (0.1-1 mSv)
C. Moderate (1-10 mSv)
D. High (>10 mSv).

A.20 The average annual effective dose from natural background in the United States is most likely:
A. 1 mSv
B. 2 mSv
C. 3 mSv
D. 5 mSv

A.21 What is the primary source of DNA damage for indirect action?
A. Hydroxyl radicals
B. Photoelectrons
C. Compton electrons
D. Scattered photons

A.22 What biological effect of radiation is modeled as having no threshold?
A. Cataractogenesis
B. Epilation
C. Erythema
D. Carcinogenesis

A.23 Cerebrovascular syndrome occurs for acute whole-body doses above what amount?
A. 0.5 Gy
B. 5 Gy
C. 50 Gy
D. 500 Gy

A.24 What acute absorbed dose results in permanent sterility for premenopausal women?
A. 0.15 Gy
B. 2 Gy
C. 15 Gy
D. 50 Gy

A.25 What organization uses radiation risks estimates to set regulatory dose limits for radiation workers?
A. NRC
B. ICRP
C. FDA
D. IAEA

A.26 What population has demonstrated radiation-induced genetic effects?
A. Atomic bomb survivors
B. Radiotherapy patients
C. Uranium miners
D. Mouse and drosophila studies

A.27 How does the atomic number of the gas used in an ionization chamber impact its sensitivity?
A. Higher Z is better.
B. Z does not impact sensitivity.
C. Lower Z is better.

A.28 What detector is typically used to measure dose from an x-ray tube?
A. Ionization chamber
B. Geiger counter
C. OSLD badge
D. Proportional counter

A.29 NCRP recommends lifetime dose stays below worker age X ____.
A. 1 mSv
B. 2 mSv
C. 5 mSv
D. 10 mSv

A.30 What is the current US regulatory dose limit for the extremities?
A. 5 mSv/y
B. 50 mSv/y
C. 150 mSv/y
D. 500 mSv/y

A.31 What radiation protection tool is NOT typically utilized for patients?
A. Optimization
B. Justification
C. ALARA
D. Dose limits

A.32 What parameter is increased most by automatic exposure rate control systems in "low-dose" mode when imaging a large patient?
A. Tube current
B. Tube voltage
C. Filtration
D. Pulse rate

A.33 What artifact is found only in image intensifier fluoroscopy systems?
A. Vignetting
B. Dead pixels
C. Lag
D. Motion blur

A.34 What is the disadvantage of small focal spots?
A. Decreased image uniformity
B. Increased heating
C. Increased patient dose
D. Decreased photoelectric interactions

A.35 What radiographic examination is likely to use a grid?
A. Skull (infant)
B. Chest (ICU)
C. Abdomen (adult)
D. Extremity (adult)

A.36 What kV is typically used for a fixed-room chest radiography?
A. 50 kV
B. 80 kV
C. 130 kV
D. 190 kV

A.37 What is worse in continuous-mode fluoroscopy vs 30 pps pulsed-mode acquisitions?
A. Temporal resolution
B. Image noise
C. Patient dose
D. Pin-cushion artifact

A.38 What percentage of US women are likely to get breast cancer in their lifetime?
A. 3%
B. 6%
C. 13%
D. 20%

A.39 What parameter is typically fixed for all screening mammography scans?
A. Filtration
B. Tube voltage
C. Tube current
D. Collimation

A.40 What is the disadvantage when the half-value layer of a mammography beam is too low?
A. Too many low-energy photons
B. Decreased spatial resolution
C. More severe halo artifact
D. Decreased image contrast

A.41 What happens to mammogram image quality if the AEC cell selected for sensing is at the nipple?
A. Decreased focal blur
B. Extended exposure time
C. Increased image noise
D. Induced halo artifact

A.42 In digital breast tomosynthesis, increasing what parameter will improve through-plane resolution?
A. Beam filtration
B. Focal spot size
C. Tube current
D. Arc extent

A.43 A copper filter in an interventional fluoroscopy system is applied primarily to reduce what dose?
A. Effective dose
B. Skin dose
C. Operator dose
D. Fetal dose

A.44 What is the typical effective dose delivered for a spine embolization?
A. 0.5 mSv
B. 20 mSv
C. 90 mSv
D. 250 mSv

A.45 What dose may produce skin erythema in the most radiosensitive individuals?
A. 0.5 Gy
B. 2 Gy
C. 13 Gy
D. 50 Gy

A.46 How does increasing collimation (smaller FOV) during fluoroscopy improve imaging?
A. Improved resolution
B. Fewer artifacts
C. Less mottle
D. Reduced doses

A.47 How does resolution for image intensifier–based fluoroscopy in standard mode likely compare to resolution at the highest Mag mode?
A. Standard mode has four times the resolution of Mag mode.
B. Standard mode has two times the resolution of Mag mode.
C. Mag mode has the same resolution as Standard mode.
D. Mag mode has two times the resolution of Standard mode.

A.48 An image Intensifier system attempts to keep what quantity constant?
A. Receptor dose
B. Image contrast
C. Patient dose
D. Image brightness

A.49 What quantity best correlates with peak skin dose?
A. Reference point air Kerma
B. Kerma-area product
C. Fluoroscopy beam-on time
D. Number of acquisition images

A.50 IRP K_{air} (Gy) currently displayed by vendors is most likely to:
A. Be measured free in air
B. Include backscatter
C. Correct for tissue/air differences
D. Be actual patient peak skin doses

A.51 What is the minimum skin dose that could possibly produce necrosis?
A. 5 Gy
B. 15 Gy
C. 50 Gy
D. 150 Gy

A.52 How much does a 0.5 mm lead apron (0.5 mm) reduce operator exposure?
A. <30%
B. 50%
C. 80%
D. >90%

A.53 How does the focal spot size in CT compare to radiography?
A. Larger than radiography
B. Comparable to radiography
C. Smaller than radiography

A.54 How many axial x-ray tube rotations of a 64-slice scanner (0.5 mm detector width) would be needed to completely cover a chest (320 mm long)?
A. 5
B. 10
C. 15
D. 20

A.55 How will image mottle change when increasing CT pitch while keeping the effective mAs constant?
A. Increase
B. Maintain
C. Reduce

A.56 The CT reconstruction kernel is always a trade-off between what two properties?
A. Contrast and resolution
B. Contrast and noise
C. Noise and resolution

A.57 Which tissue most likely has the highest HU value?
A. CSF
B. White matter
C. Kidney
D. Blood clot

A.58 How will CTDIvol change if x-ray tube voltage is doubled?
A. <2×
B. 2×
C. 4×
D. >4×

A.59 What is a reasonable CTDIvol for a routine head CT scan?
A. 15 mGy
B. 25 mGy
C. 40 mGy
D. 60 mGy

A.60 Dual-source scanners allow what parameter to be higher than single source?
A. Tube voltage
B. Pitch
C. Focal spot
D. Rotation time

A.61 What is a typical fetal dose for a single-phase abdomen/pelvis CT exam?
A. 0.2 mGy
B. 2 mGy
C. 20 mGy
D. 200 mGy

A.62 How does dose for a dental cone-beam CT compare to a routine head CT?
A. Higher than
B. Comparable to
C. Lower than

A.63 How will noise change if pitch is doubled while tube current modulation is utilized?
A. Increase
B. Keep constant
C. Reduce

A.64 Increasing what parameter will mitigate motion artifact?
A. Focal spot
B. Rotation speed
C. Detector area
D. Image magnification

A.65 What quality control failure results in too much Mo 99 being present in a Tc-99m study at the time of injection?
A. Radionuclide
B. Chemical
C. Physical
D. Radiochemical

A.66 What is the average range of an electron from I 131?
A. 0.01 mm
B. 0.5 mm
C. 10 mm
D. 50 mm

A.67 Which radionuclide is not a fission product?
A. ^{18}F
B. ^{131}I
C. ^{133}Xe
D. ^{90}Sr

A.68 What is the most activity that a 1 GBq ^{99}Mo/^{99m}Tc generator will produce after 66 hours?
A. 1,000 MBq
B. 500 MBq
C. 250 MBq
D. 125 MBq

A.69 What radionuclide is used for bone scintigraphy scans?
A. Fluorodeoxyglucose
B. Florbetaben
C. Monoclonal antibodies
D. Methylene diphosphonate

A.70 The pulse height analysis window for a ^{99m}Tc study would most likely accept gamma rays with energies between _____ and _____ keV.
A. 112; 140
B. 126; 154
C. 140; 168

A.71 What is an advantage of increasing the time per projection during SPECT scanning?
A. Decreased image mottle
B. Increased temporal resolution
C. Increased spatial resolution
D. Decreased motion artifact

A.72 What is the highest gamma camera flood uniformity acceptable for clinical use?
A. ±1%
B. ±5%
C. ±95%
D. ±99%

A.73 What property of PET detectors should be as low as possible?
A. Atomic number (Z)
B. Physical density (ρ)
C. Detector length (mm)
D. Light decay time (τ)

A.74 What is the disadvantage of post-processing PET images with a Butterworth filter?
A. Decreased maximum SUV for small lesions
B. Increased noise for large lesions
C. Extended acquisition times
D. Increased misregistration artifact

A.75 How do photon energies in SPECT compare to those in CT?
A. Lower than CT
B. Comparable to CT
C. Higher than CT

A.76 What is the critical organ dose for FDG?
A. 0.06 mGy
B. 0.2 mGy
C. 4 mGy
D. 60 mGy

A.77 How much stronger is an electron's magnetic field than a proton's magnetic field?
A. 10×
B. 100×
C. 1,000×
D. 10,000×

A.78 What is the susceptibility of most human tissues?
A. Negative
B. Zero
C. Positive

A.79 What is a typical spin-spin relaxation time for soft tissues?
A. 5 ms
B. 50 ms
C. 500 ms
D. 5,000 ms

A.80 What causes spin refocusing in spin echo imaging?
A. Radiofrequency pulse
B. Phase encode gradient
C. Frequency encode gradient
D. Shim fields

A.81 How will patient heating change as B_0 increases?
A. Decrease
B. No change
C. Increase

A.82 What artifact is caused by nonuniform gradients?
A. Geometric distortion
B. Fat sat failure
C. Increased eddy currents
D. Zipper artifacts

A.83 Why is nerve stimulation found primarily in the periphery instead of the center of the MR bore?
A. Gradients are strongest at the periphery
B. B_0 is weakest at the periphery
C. RF is weakest in the center
D. Shim magnets are strongest in the center

A.84 To eliminate both T1 and T2 weighting, the operator must choose TR to be _____ and TE to be _____.
A. long; long
B. long; short
C. short; long
D. short; short

A.85 Why is SAR lower for GRE MR sequences compared to SE sequences?
A. Increased RF frequency for SE
B. Reduced acquisition time for GRE
C. Increased gradient strength for SE
D. Reduced RF use in GRE

A.86 In DWI imaging, T2 shine though occurs when DWI pixel values are _____ and the corresponding ADC values are _____.
A. low; low
B. low; high
C. high; low
D. high; high

A.87 Functional MRI typically uses what acquisition sequence?
A. Echo-planar
B. Spin echo
C. Fast spin echo
D. Inversion recovery

A.88 How does quadrupling the receiver bandwidth impact image SNR?
   A. Quarter
   B. Halve
   C. Double
   D. Quadruple

A.89 What kind of reflection will a 15 MHz ultrasound beam undergo when interacting with a smooth 10 mm surface?
   A. Rayleigh
   B. Specular
   C. Diffuse
   D. Compton

A.90 What tissue has the lowest acoustic impedance?
   A. Lung
   B. Fat
   C. Tissue
   D. Bone

A.91 What is the ultrasound artifact created by interference pattern among transducer elements?
   A. Reverberation
   B. Enhancement
   C. Grating lobes
   D. Ring-down

A.92 What has the lowest ultrasound attenuation?
   A. Bladder contents
   B. Adipose tissues
   C. Soft tissues
   D. Cortical bone

A.93 What is the consequence of placing the ultrasound beam focus too shallow during imaging?
   A. Reverberation artifact
   B. Increased TIS
   C. Reduced speckle
   D. Poor lateral resolution

A.94 What happens to the beam intensity of the system if power is reduced 3 dB?
   A. Quarters
   B. Halves
   C. No change
   D. Doubles

A.95 What artifact is more likely as pulse repetition frequency decreases?
   A. Aliasing
   B. Shadowing
   C. Mirror
   D. Refraction

A.96 An echo arriving 40 µs after an earlier echo implies the distance between the two interfaces is most likely (cm):
   A. <1
   B. 1
   C. 2
   D. >2

A.97 What resolution is improved by using at least a 1.5 D ultrasound arrays?
   A. Axial
   B. Lateral
   C. Elevational
   D. Temporal

A.98 What parameter should be kept low for ultrasound contrast imaging?
   A. Pulse repetition frequency
   B. Mechanical index
   C. Thermal index
   D. System gain

A.99 Ultrasound intensities in color Doppler are likely _____ higher than in conventional B-mode imaging.
   A. 1.2x
   B. 3x
   C. 10x
   D. 50x

A.100 What is the effect of using a large Doppler angle during Doppler imaging?
   A. Increased velocity uncertainty
   B. Decreased lateral resolution
   C. Increased aliasing artifact
   D. Reduced flash artifact

PRACTICE EXAMINATION A:
Answers and Explanations

A.1 D (Decrease 30%). Mottle (noise) goes at 1/square root of detector dose. Doubling the exposure time while making no other changes will double the detector dose.

A.2 A (≤10%). For tungsten targets, characteristic x-rays never contribute more than a few percent to any clinical x-ray spectrum.

A.3 D (Essentially isotropic). When x-ray photons undergo Compton scatter in tissue, all scatter angles are approximately equally likely (i.e., isotropic).

A.4 B (1 mGy). Fetal dose from radiography is ~100× too low for deterministic effects.

A.5 A (Quality increases; quantity increases). Changes in x-ray tube voltage always affect the x-ray beam quantity and quality. As a result, whenever kV is adjusted, the mAs also needs adjusting to ensure the appropriate K_{air} at the image receptor.

A.6 C (Grid ratio). Using higher grid ratios reduces scatter, whereas increasing tube voltage and beam area increases scatter (focal spot does not affect scatter).

A.7 A (10%). On average, 70% primary transmission and 10% scatter are transmitted through a 10:1 grid in body radiography.

A.8 A (Black/Dark gray). In 2D SE imaging blood is hit by the initial 90° pulse but moves out of the slice before 180° pulse. As a result, it never refocuses to produce a signal. GRE produces bright blood.

A.9 D (>1,000:1). Digital x-ray detectors are likely to have dynamic ranges (i.e., maximum to minimum detectable signal) of at least 10,000:1.

A.10 B (Mammogram). Images in mammography are generally the largest of all medical images (e.g., 25 Mbyte), which is two to three times more than a chest x-ray (10 Mbyte).

A.11 B (High atomic number). The high atomic number greatly increases the number of photoelectric interactions, leading to large attenuation.

A.12 A (increase; increase). Reduced filtration means lower average energies and reduced patient penetration that increases both contrast and patient doses for x-rays that use automatic exposure control.

A.13 C (Halve). Quadrupling the number of x-ray photons used to create an image will likely halve the amount of random noise (mottle).

A.14 A (Effective dose). Effective dose is an equivalent whole body dose and so can always be added. Equivalent and absorbed doses must expose the same piece of tissue otherwise they cannot be added. Skin dose is absorbed dose to the skin.

A.15 D (Contrast/Noise). Contrast divided by noise (contrast-to-noise ratio) is an indicator of the relative lesion visibility because it accounts for both changes in lesion contrast and image noise (i.e., contrast-to-noise ratio or CNR).

A.16 D ($Gy*cm^2$). Kerma (Gy) multiplied by the x-ray beam cross-sectional area (cm^2) gives the Kerma-area product in $Gy*cm^2$. This is also written $Gy-cm^2$.

A.17 C (Skin dose higher than K_{air}). K_{air} is measured in air without any patient present, whereas patient skin doses are higher because tissues absorbs more than air (+10%) and includes backscatter from the patient (+30%).

A.18 D (Protons). Protons have a radiation weighting (W_R) factor of 2.

A.19 A (Very low (<0.1 mSv)). Dual-energy x-ray absorptiometry has a very low effective dose of ~0.001 mSv.

A.20 C (3 mSv/y). The current average exposure to all sources of natural background in the United States, including ubiquitous background and radon, is 3 mSv/y.

A.21 A (Hydroxyl radicals). Indirect action is when energetic electrons interact with water to produce hydroxyl radicals that are chemically reactive and may damage DNA.

A.22 D (Carcinogenesis). Genetic effects and carcinogenesis are stochastic effects with no threshold, whereas cataracts, epilation, and erythema are all deterministic (tissue) effects with a threshold dose.

A.23 C (50 Gy). Cerebrovascular syndrome occurs for acute whole-body doses of about 50 Gy.

A.24 B (2 Gy). Permanent sterility is induced at 6 Gy in men (single dose) and at 2 Gy in premenopausal women.

A.25 A (NRC). Only the NRC is a regulatory body in the United States. The other organizations listed are advisory bodies and have no legal authority in the United States.

A.26 D (Mouse and drosophila studies). There are no epidemiological studies that have demonstrated genetic effects in humans exposed to radiation.

A.27 A (Higher Z is better.). To absorb as many x-rays as possible, you need a high atomic number gas (e.g., xenon) at high pressure (increase density).

A.28 A (Ionization chamber). X-ray tube outputs are measured by medical physicists using an ionization chamber that is accurate but requires "billions and billions" of x-ray photons.

A.29 D (10). For a 60-year-old radiation worker, the NCRP recommends that their lifetime occupational dose is less than 600 mSv. In practice, an IR operator who receives 5 mSv/y for 20 years has a lifetime exposure of 100 mSv.

A.30 D (500 mSv/y). The current US regulatory dose limit for the extremities is 500 mSv/y (equivalent dose), and which is designed to prevent the induction of deterministic effects.

A.31 D (Dose limits). In general, there are no regulatory dose limits for performing diagnostic examinations. The only regulatory limits pertain to fluoroscopy K_{air} rates and mammography phantom doses (not to patients).

A.32 B (Tube voltage). Increasing voltage increases patient penetration and decreases noise but also lower contrast.

A.33 A (Vignetting). Vignetting is unique to image intensifiers due to their curved input and flat output surfaces.

A.34 B (Increased heating). The small area makes it less efficient at dissipating heat meaning either lower technique must be used or a larger focal spot must be used for large patients.

A.35 C (Abdomen (adult)). All adult abdomen scans use a grid to reduce scatter.

A.36 C (130 kV). Fixed-room chest radiography is taken against the wall Bucky with a long SID and high kV. The tube voltage is generally between 115 and 135 kV.

A.37 A (Temporal resolution). Continuous mode acquires a single frame in ~33 ms, but pulsed mode decreases the exposure time per pulse to 10 ms or less improving temporal resolution and better freezing motion. The pulse must have a higher mA to compensate for the lower exposure time, but the overall dose stays the same.

A.38 C (13%). It is estimated that 1 in 8 US women get breast cancer in their lifetime.

A.39 C (Tube current). Tube current is typically fixed to 100 mA in screening mammography, but will change for magnification mammography. All other parameters listed change based on breast size.

A.40 A (Too many low-energy photons). A low HVL means the beam is less penetrating. This occurs if there are too many low energy photons which are easily blocked. This implies that the beam will have a higher than normal patient dose (as the low energy photons interact) with no image quality improvement (low energy photons never reach the receiver to make an image).

A.41 C (Increased image noise). At the nipple very little tissue overlaps the AEC cell so most radiation hits it directly. This will cause the system to shut off early and deliver a fraction of the dose needed for good image noise.

A.42 D (Arc extent). As the arc increases (e.g., 50° instead of 15°), it samples more of angle space and improves through-plane resolution.

A.43 B (Skin dose). Use of copper filtration cuts low-dose photons to reduce skin dose, but such systems require a strong generator to compensate for the overall loss of photons.

A.44 C (90 mSv). Most IR procedures are in the tens of mSv with IVC filter around 15 mSv and spine embolization up at 90 mSv.

A.45 B (2 Gy). At a peak skin dose of 2 Gy there is a small chance of erythema in the most radiosensitive individuals, but the vast majority of patients will show no skin reaction.

A.46 D (Reduced doses). A collimated x-ray beam area means that fewer x-rays are incident on the patient (i.e., KAP is lower) and the patient carcinogenic risk will be lower.

A.47 D (Mag mode has two times the resolution of Standard mode). Though it will vary between make and model, in general the spatial resolution will roughly double between the standard mode and highest Mag mode.

A.48 D (Image brightness). An image intensifier system has automatic brightness control that attempts to keep the brightness in the image consistent.

A.49 A (Reference point air Kerma). K_{air} at the at the reference point best correlates with peak skin dose, but for an accurate skin dose estimate corrections must still be made.

A.50 A (Be measured free in air). IRP cumulative doses (Gy) that are currently displayed by vendors are measured free in air, so exclude backscatter and do not account for tissue/air differences. Most cumulative doses overestimate peak skin doses, but may occasionally be underestimates as well.

A.51 B (15 Gy). Necrosis could possibly form in the most radiosensitive individuals at 15 Gy of absorbed skin dose (15 Sv of skin equivalent dose).

A.52 D (>90%). Most medical physicists assume that dose reduction by wearing lead aprons is at least 90%.

A.53 B (Comparable to radiography). Focal spots in CT and radiography are both 0.6 mm (small) and 1.2 mm (large).

A.54 B (10 rotations). A 64-slice CT scanner has a beam width of 64 × 0.5 mm (i.e., 32 mm), which covers a 320 mm chest in 10 rotations.

A.55 B (Maintain). The amount of mottle in helical CT is dependent on the effective mAs, and so is unchanged. Since the effective mAs is the mAs divided by pitch, to maintain the effective mAs at higher pitch values requires the mAs to be increased.

A.56 C (Noise and resolution). When using filtered back projection, the choice of reconstruction kernel allows a radiologist to obtain better resolution and higher noise, or lower noise and worse resolution.

A.57 D (Blood clot). A blood clot will have an elevated HU value of about 80 (blood is 40), which means x-ray attenuation is increased by 4% (i.e., 40 HU).

A.58 D (>4). CT x-ray tube output is roughly proportional to $kV^{2.6}$, which means that when tube voltage doubles, CT radiation output (air Kerma) increases sixfold (X 6).

A.59 D (60 mGy). Adult head exams will typically be between 50 and 65 mGy.

A.60 B (Pitch). Dual-source CT scanners allow the use of exceptionally high values of CT pitch (e.g., >2), which reduces image acquisition time as required in cardiac imaging.

A.61 C (20 mGy). In modern scanners, the typical fetal dose is about 20 mGy, but this can change based on many factors.

A.62 C (Lower than). Dental cone-beam CT has very low (<0.1 mSv) or low dose (0.1-1 mSv), whereas patient dose in routine head CT are generally moderate (1-10 mSv).

A.63 B (Keep constant). As pitch increases, the photons per slice would decrease, but TCM automatically increases mA to compensate.

A.64 B (Rotation speed). Increased rotation speed will complete the scan faster, reducing the probability of motion. Further, motion that does occur will be small for any given image reducing motion artifact severity.

A.65 A (Radionuclide). Radionuclide purity tests determine the activity of unwanted radionuclides (like Mo 99). Too much Mo 99 present during injection will dose the patient unnecessarily.

A.66 B (0.5 cm). I 131 emits beta in a spectrum. At the average energy, an electron will travel ~0.5 mm.

A.67 A (^{18}F). The nuclide ^{18}F is positron emitter made using a cyclotron, whereas fission products are all β^- emitters.

A.68 B (500 MBq). The half-life of ^{99}Mo is 66 hours, so 66 hours will decay the parent to half of the initial activity (500 MBq), and this is the approximate amount of ^{99m}Tc that will be present when equilibrium has been established.

A.69 D (Methylene diphosphonate). FDG labeled with ^{18}F is used to assess metabolism. Florbetaben is a receptor-binding agent. Monoclonal antibodies are used to investigate antibody antigen reactions, and methylene diphosphonate measures physicochemical adsorption by bone.

A.70 B (126 and 154 keV). The window width for ^{99m}Tc is typically 20% (i.e., 28 keV) with the window centered on 140 keV, so gamma ray events with energies more than 126 keV, but less than 154 keV, would be accepted.

A.71 A (Decreased image mottle). A longer time per projection will collect more photons and reduce noise; however, it cannot be extended much for short-lived isotopes and it increases the likelihood of motion artifact.

A.72 B (±5%). A uniformity greater than 5% results in unacceptable clinical images, and gamma cameras generally have uniformities of 2% to 3%.

A.73 D (Light decay time). The ideal PET detector material would a very short light decay time (τ), but high atomic number (Z) and physical density (ρ), and a long detector length (mm).

A.74 A (Decreased SUV for small lesions). Postprocessing filters used in PET are blurring filters that decrease spatial resolution and noise. The blur on small lesions will decrease the maximum SUV value measured.

A.75 C (Higher than CT). CT images are obtained at an average energy of 60 to 70 keV, whereas the photons used in SPECT (^{99m}Tc and ^{123}I) are 140 and 160 keV, respectively.

A.76 D (60 mGy). Critical organ doses in nuclear medicine are tens of mGy.

A.77 C (1,000×). Magnetism associated with electrons is about 1,000 times stronger than that of protons. The weak proton field is one reason why the detected signals in MR are extremely weak.

A.78 A (Negative). Tissues are diamagnetic and have a very small negative susceptibility (e.g., −0.0001), and the local magnetic field will be slightly lower than the applied magnetic field (i.e., 0.01% lower).

A.79 B (50 ms). T2 times are generally 50 ms, ten times shorter than tissue T1 relaxation times and ten times longer than T2* times.

A.80 A (Radiofrequency pulse). Following an initial 90° RF pulse, a refocusing 180° RF pulse applied after 10 ms results in an echo at 20 ms.

A.81 C (Increase). As B_0 increases, so does Larmor frequency. This means RF frequency must increase and thus its energy also increases.

A.82 A (Geometric distortion). Gradients localize the signal location. Nonuniform gradients place signals in the wrong place causing geometric distortion in the image (e.g., too wide in one dimension).

A.83 A (Gradients are…). Gradients are strongest at the periphery and zero at the bore center. As they flip on and off, they induce electric fields in the nerves.

A.84 B (long; short). T1 weighting is eliminated when TR is long, and T2 weighting is eliminated when TE is short.

A.85 D (Reduced RF use in GRE). GRE sequences have lower specific absorption rates (SARs) because these do not employ 180° refocusing RF pulses and use an initial flip angle smaller than 90°.

A.86 D (high; high). In DWI imaging, T2 shine though results in high (bright) DWI pixels as well as high (bright) values of apparent diffusion coefficient.

A.87 A (Echo-planar). Functional MRI most likely uses echo-planar imaging sequences with T2* weighting.

A.88 B (Halve). SNR goes as 1/square root of receiver bandwidth. As the receiver bandwidth increase more frequencies are collected from the body which increases the received noise as well.

A.89 B (Specular). A 1.5 MHz transducer has a 1 mm wavelength, so the wavelength of a 15 MHz transducer ten times lower (i.e., 0.1 mm). This is much smaller than the surface and so likely specular reflection will occur.

A.90 A (Lung). It is lung that has the lowest acoustic impedance (density x sound velocity) because it has the lowest density and also the lowest sound velocity.

A.91 C (Grating lobes). The interference pattern creates weak beams (lobes) around the main beam but at a different angle.

A.92 A (Bladder contents). Fluids such as the bladder contents and simple cysts have very little attenuation, whereas attenuation in bone and lung is very high.

A.93 D (Poor lateral resolution). Objects away from the focus will be hit with a larger beam diameter resulting in reduced lateral resolution. Echo intensity deep in the patient will also decrease since the beam diverges quickly.

A.94 B (Halves). 3 dB down means an intensity reduction of 50%.

A.95 A (Aliasing). As repetition frequency goes down the sampling rate for motion is decreased making it more likely fast flows will exhibit aliasing.

A.96 D (>2). A waiting time of 13 µs for an echo corresponds to a depth of 1 cm, waiting 26 µs corresponds to a depth of 2 cm, so waiting 40 µs longer implies a separation distance of >2 cm.

A.97 C (Elevational). 1.5 D ultrasound arrays offer improved elevational resolution, which is likely to be at the expense of reduced temporal resolution.

A.98 B (Mechanical index). A low mechanical index ensures bubbles are not popped during imaging.

A.99 D (50). Ultrasound intensities in color Doppler are generally 50 times higher than in conventional B-mode imaging.

A.100 A (Increased velocity uncertainty). At large Doppler angles, a small error in specifying the angle of flow will produce a large (>25%) error in velocity measurements.

PRACTICE EXAMINATION B:
Questions

B.1 X-rays are produced when energetic electrons are decelerated in the electric field of tungsten ____.
A. Atomic nuclei
B. Outer electrons
C. Inner electrons
D. Inner or outer electrons

B.2 For an abdominal x-ray, about what percentage of x-ray photon energy incident on a patient is scattered out of the patient?
A. ≤10%
B. 30%
C. 70%
D. ≥90%

B.3 What energy allows for the highest transmission through a silver filter (K-edge energy 25 keV)?
A. 5 keV
B. 24 keV
C. 26 keV
D. 30 keV

B.4 What metric is allowed for comparison of stochastic radiation risk across examination types?
A. Equivalent dose
B. Shallow dose
C. Effective dose
D. Committed

B.5 If 3 mm Al attenuates an x-ray beam by 50%, approximately how much additional Al would attenuate the beam an additional 50%?
A. 0.1 mm
B. 3 mm
C. 10 mm
D. 30 mm

B.6 How many gene mutations are needed to deactivate tumor suppressor genes?
A. 1
B. 2
C. 3
D. 4

B.7 What is the meaning of the threshold dose in tissue (deterministic) effects?
A. >99% chance of effect for average people
B. >0% chance of effect for average people
C. >0% chance of effect for the most radiosensitive people
D. >99% chance of effect for the most radiosensitive people

B.8 In radiography, a chest x-ray acquired at 130 kV will have what image quality benefit?
A. Improved contrast
B. Decreased magnification
C. More transparent ribs
D. Fewer dead pixels

B.9 What bit depth is necessary to encode an image that uses 1,024 shades of gray?
A. 8 bits
B. 9 bits
C. 10 bits
D. 15 bits

B.10 What image processing technique reduces noise at the cost of reduced spatial resolution?
A. Low-pass filtering
B. Unsupervised deep learning
C. Low-pass filtering
D. Unsharp masking

B.11 Why is AEC not typically used when performing radiography of the finger?
A. Decreases image contrast
B. Increases magnification
C. Creates unnecessary dose
D. Body part too small

B.12 Mottle is most likely to limit detection of lesions that are:
A. Very small
B. Very large
C. Low contrast
D. High contrast

B.13 A bar phantom is used to measure what image property?
A. Quantum mottle
B. Image contrast
C. Temporal resolution
D. Spatial resolution

B.14 How does dose change for fluoroscopy systems when increasing image intensifier–system Mag mode and digital system zoom (i.e, reduced FOV)?
A. Image intensifier systems and digital systems increase.
B. Image intensifier systems increase, but digital systems stay constant.
C. Image intensifier systems stay constant, but digital systems decrease.
D. Image intensifier systems and digital systems decrease.

B.15 When testing two systems using ROC analysis, how is area under the curve interpreted?
   A. Larger area under the curve is better.
   B. The area under the curve is not used to compare systems.
   C. Smaller area under the curve is better.

B.16 Why is a 34 keV beam ideal for interventional fluoroscopy imaging?
   A. Minimizes glare artifact
   B. Minimizes patient dose
   C. Maximizes iodine contrast
   D. Maximizes spatial resolution

B.17 Conversations regarding therapeutic abortion are not recommended below what conceptus dose?
   A. 10 mGy
   B. 50 mGy
   C. 100 mGy
   D. 500 mGy

B.18 What organ has the highest tissue weighting factor (w_T)?
   A. Colon
   B. Thyroid
   C. Bladder
   D. Liver

B.19 The effective dose of chest CT examination would most likely be classified as:
   A. Very low (<0.1 mSv)
   B. Low (0.1-1 mSv)
   C. Moderate (1-10 mSv)
   D. High (>10 mSv).

B.20 What category of imaging has the highest effective dose?
   A. Ventilation-perfusion nuclear medicine scans
   B. CT head perfusion imaging
   C. Dual-energy x-ray absorptiometry
   D. Fluoroscopic interventional procedures

B.21 What is the Oxygen Enhancement Ratio if aerated cells in 2 Gy, but hypoxic cells neet 8 Gy to achieve the same level of cell kill?
   A. 2 Gy
   B. 4 Gy
   C. 6 Gy
   D. 8 Gy

B.22 What is the threshold for GI acute radiation syndrome?
   A. 0.1 Gy
   B. 1 Gy
   C. 10 Gy
   D. 100 Gy

B.23 What is the threshold for moist desquamation?
   A. 2 Gy
   B. 5 Gy
   C. 15 Gy
   D. 50 Gy

B.24 What cancer was increased in the radium dial painters?
   A. Breast cancer
   B. Thyroid cancer
   C. Leukemia
   D. Bone cancer

B.25 The cancer sensitivity of a young child is most likely _____ times higher than that of a 25-year-old.
   A. 1.5
   B. 3
   C. 8
   D. 12

B.26 What is the standard for storing, transferring, and displaying radiology image data?
   A. Integrating the Healthcare Enterprise (IHE)
   B. Health Level 7 (HL7)
   C. Digital Imaging and Communications in Medicine (DICOM)
   D. International Organization for Standardization (ISO)

B.27 Why isn't a 20 kV beam used to maximize contrast in a barium meal?
   A. Can melt the anode
   B. Photons penetrate through the detector
   C. Excessive scatter
   D. Too much attenuation

B.28 Dosimeters worn above the lead apron _____ operator effective doses, whereas those worn under a lead apron _____ operator effective doses.
   A. overestimate; overestimate
   B. overestimate; underestimate
   C. underestimate; overestimate
   D. underestimate; underestimate

B.29 What is the annual occupational dose limit for the eye lens?
   A. 5 mSv
   B. 20 mSv
   C. 50 mSv
   D. 150 mSv

B.30 What is the total radiation the fetus of a radiation worker can receive without exceeding a dose limit?
A. 0.5 mSv
B. 5 mSv
C. 50 mSv
D. 500 mSv

B.31 When are patient shields recommended during CT imaging?
A. Pregnant patients
B. Never recommended
C. Women chest scans (breasts)
D. Men pelvic scans (gonads)

B.32 What interaction transfers no dose to the patient?
A. Compton scatter
B. Rayleigh scatter
C. Photoelectric interaction
D. Pair production

B.33 What percentage of electrical energy is converted into x-rays in a radiographic x-ray tube?
A. 99%
B. 90%
C. 10%
D. 1%

B.34 Increasing what parameter will increase Heel effect severity?
A. SID
B. FOV
C. Anode angle
D. Tube current

B.35 What is a reasonable exposure index (EI) for an adult chest radiograph?
A. 0.25
B. 2.5
C. 25
D. 250

B.36 What occurs if the television frame rate is below 30 during fluoroscopy?
A. Reduced contrast
B. Flicker artifact
C. Reduced patient dose
D. Smooth patient motion

B.37 Why is the output port window in mammography made of beryllium instead of glass?
A. Less attenuation
B. Better focusing
C. More characteristic x-rays
D. Better image contrast

B.38 What change must be made when magnification mammography is utilized to improve spatial resolution??
A. Increase filtration
B. Utilize grid with high grid ratio
C. Decrease focal spot size
D. Increase compression

B.39 What artifact is responsible for artificial skin thickening in tomosynthesis imaging?
A. Halo
B. Dead pixels
C. Accordion
D. Stair step

B.40 How is beam energy changed when imaging thicker and denser breasts?
A. Increase tube current
B. Decrease tube voltage
C. Decrease SID
D. Increase filter K-edge

B.41 How does mAs in magnification mammography compare to contact screening mammography?
A. Increased
B. Kept constant
C. Reduced

B.42 What is the primary concern for very high-dose radiation delivered to the conceptus in the fourth week of gestation?
A. Spontaneous abortion
B. Organ malformation
C. Reduced IQ
D. Microcephaly

B.43 What is the goal of an image intensifier?
A. Decrease image lag
B. Increase spatial resolution
C. Decrease pincushion distortion
D. Increase light brightness

B.44 Which imaging chain most likely has the x-ray tube *above* the patient and table?
A. R/F
B. Urological
C. C-arm
D. IR

B.45 Switching from Normal to Mag 1 mode using an image intensifier fluoroscopy system roughly increases skin doses by _____% and Kerma-area products by _____%.
A. 0; 0
B. 0; 100
C. 100; 0
D. 100; 100

B.46 What is the maximum regulatory entrance K_{air} rate incident on a patient undergoing high-level control (HLC) fluoroscopy?
A. ~10 mGy/min
B. ~50 mGy/min
C. ~100 mGy/min
D. ~200 mGy/min

B.47 What is a reasonable peak skin dose in a barium enema examination?
A. 5 mGy
B. 50 mGy
C. 500 mGy
D. 5,000 mGy

B.48 Patient doses using FPDs with small fields of view are most likely _____ to those resulting from corresponding images obtained using image intensifier mag modes.
A. higher than
B. comparable to
C. lower than

B.49 According to the NRC, how long should breastfeeding cease after Tc-99m injection?
A. <5 hours
B. 1 day
C. 5 weeks
D. Permanently

B.50 Which of the doses below can be added together?
A. Effective dose of bone scintigraphy and mammography
B. Skin dose of a head CT and ankle radiograph
C. Equivalent dose of right breast and left breast in screening mammography
D. Absorbed dose of DXA and sinus CT

B.51 Last image hold is a dose reduction technique utilized in what modality?
A. Fluoroscopy
B. Ultrasound
C. DXA
D. CT

B.52 How much eye lens dose reduction is typical when wearing leaded glasses?
A. <10%
B. 35%
C. 65%
D. >90%

B.53 What is the purpose of the bow tie filter in CT?
A. Improve radiation uniformity
B. Decrease image noise
C. Increase temporal resolution
D. Mitigate truncation artifact

B.54 What image metric is much worse in cone-beam CT utilized in dental and interventional radiology compared to conventional CT?
A. In-plane resolution
B. Through-plane resolution
C. Soft tissue contrast
D. Quantum mottle

B.55 Statistical iterative reconstruction in CT greatly reduces what artifact or quality metric?
A. Image noise
B. Spatial resolution
C. Ring artifact
D. Motion artifact

B.56 Hounsfield units compare a tissue's linear attenuation with that of:
A. Air
B. Soft tissue
C. Aluminum
D. Water

B.57 Increasing the x-ray tube voltage does what to the HU value of water?
A. Increases
B. Does not affect
C. Reduces

B.58 What type of scan requires a negative pressure room?
A. FDG PET
B. VQ scan
C. Thyroid scintigraphy
D. MUGA

B.59 Retrospectively gated CT coronary angiography most likely makes use of a very low:
A. Tube rotation
B. Output (mAs)
C. CT pitch
D. Beam filtration

B.60 Compared to adults, CT scans of infants most likely use _____ mAs and _____ kV.
A. increased; increased
B. increased; decreased
C. decreased; increased
D. decreased; decreased

B.61 How does dose rate from DSA compare to dose from high-level controlled (HLC) fluoroscopy?
A. DSA dose is larger.
B. DSA and HLC fluoroscopy are comparable.
C. HLC dose is larger.

B.62 Where should the operator stand during cross-table (lateral) fluoroscopy?
A. Next to the detector
B. Next to x-ray tube
C. Either next to detector or x-ray tube

B.63 What is the purpose of a validation set when training an artificial intelligence algorithm?
  A. Train new features
  B. Reduce overfitting of the model
  C. Produce final sensitivity and specificity metrics
  D. Decrease training time

B.64 What is a reasonable estimate of eye lens dose in a routine head CT examination?
  A. 1 mGy
  B. 4 mGy
  C. 25 mGy
  D. 60 mGy

B.65 In the expression ^{99m}Tc, what does the letter m stand for?
  A. Metastable
  B. Magnetic
  C. Meson
  D. Moderated

B.66 How much activity remains after 10 half-lives?
  A. 0.1%
  B. 5%
  C. 10%
  D. 50%

B.67 Radionuclide equilibrium most likely occurs after four _____ half-lives for secular equilibrium and four _____ half-lives for transient equilibrium.
  A. parent; parent
  B. parent; daughter
  C. daughter; parent
  D. daughter; daughter

B.68 What agent localizes through phagocytosis?
  A. Labeled sulfur colloids.
  B. GI bleed studies
  C. Bone uptake of pyrophosphates
  D. Labeled leukocytes.

B.69 What is the energy resolution of ^{123}I (160 keV) using a typical gamma camera?
  A. 1%
  B. 10%
  C. 25%
  D. 50%

B.70 Parallel-hole collimator sensitivity is _____ with increased distance from the radiation source, whereas the corresponding spatial resolution performance is _____.
  A. constant; constant
  B. constant; degraded
  C. degraded; constant
  D. degraded; degraded

B.71 How long are radionuclides typically stored in hot storage before disposal in normal trash or drains?
  A. 1 half-life
  B. 10 half-lives
  C. 100 half-lives
  D. 1,000 half-lives

B.72 What is the FWHM spatial resolution in nondigital SPECT?
  A. 2
  B. 4
  C. 8
  D. 16

B.73 How does the dose from dual-energy acquisitions compare to the dose from single-energy acquisitions for a single-phase abdomen CT?
  A. Dual energy is much higher.
  B. They are about the same.
  C. Single energy is much higher.

B.74 What suppression method is most sensitive to inhomogeneities caused by implants during MR imaging?
  A. Inversion recovery
  B. Dixon method
  C. Saturation bands
  D. Chemical fat saturation

B.75 In phase-contrast MRI how should the velocity encoding parameter be set?
  A. Just below the receiver bandwidth
  B. Just above the fastest expected flow
  C. Just above the readout gradient strength
  D. Just below the SAR level

B.76 Which facility likely requires the most amount of lead shielding?
  A. CT
  B. SPECT
  C. PET
  D. ^{131}I room

B.77 At a magnetic field of 1 T, the number of protons contributing to the net magnetization is most likely _____ per million.
  A. 3
  B. 30
  C. 300
  D. >300

B.78 Hemosiderin and ferritin will cause signal loss due to what type of decay?
  A. T1
  B. T2
  C. T2*

B.79 Bone has a _____ T1 and a _____ T2.
A. long; long
B. long; short
C. short; long
D. short; short

B.80 What happens to slice thickness if the transmit RF bandwidth is increased?
A. Increased
B. Unchanged
C. Reduced

B.81 What happens to the MR image if periphery of k-space is removed before reconstruction?
A. Blurrier
B. Less contrast
C. Noisier
D. More artifacts

B.82 What artifact is likely to occur if the MR suite door is left open during scanning?
A. Gibbs ringing
B. Zipper
C. Magic angle
D. Susceptibility

B.83 To obtain T1 weighting, the operator must choose TR to be _____ and TE to be _____.
A. long; long
B. long; short
C. short; long
D. short; short

B.84 How does the SNR in gradient-recalled echo images compare to spin echo imaging?
A. Higher than
B. Comparable to
C. Lower than

B.85 In head inversion recovery sequences obtained at 1.5 T, applying a 90° "read out" pulse at 1,700 ms would most likely suppress the signal from:
A. Brain
B. Schwannoma
C. Fat
D. CSF

B.86 Parallel acquisition in MRI with an acceleration factor of 4 will reduce imaging time by a factor of _____ and SNR by a factor of _____.
A. 4; 4
B. 2; 4
C. 4; 2
D. 2; 2

B.87 A fast/turbo spin echo sequence with a large echo train length will likely have what type of contrast weighting?
A. T1
B. T1/T2
C. Proton density
D. T2

B.88 How can SAR be reduced in MR imaging?
A. Larger flip angles
B. Higher static field strengths
C. Using more gradient directions
D. Using GRE instead of FSE

B.89 How can anisotropy artifact be mitigated in ultrasound imaging of a tendon?
A. Increase power
B. Utilize compound imaging
C. Increase write zoom
D. Turn on speckle reduction

B.90 How much power does a tissue-air interface transmit?
A. <1%
B. 20%
C. 80%
D. >99%

B.91 What is the difference between speckle and noise?
A. Noise is caused by clock jitter.
B. Speckle impacts spatial resolution.
C. Speckle is not random.
D. Noise.

B.92 What increases when a damping block is added to an ultrasound transducer?
A. Pulse length
B. Mechanical index
C. Axial resolution
D. Sound velocity

B.93 How does near-field distance depend on transducer footprint?
A. Small footprint gives a short near-field distance.
B. Footprint and near-field distance are not related.
C. Small footprint gives a long near-field distance.

B.94 Changing color priority has what impact on the ultrasound image?
A. Increases speckle
B. Alters where color Doppler is displayed
C. Increases brightness of spectral Doppler waves
D. Decreases side lobe artifacts

B.95 What is the product of the lines per image and the image frame rate?
   A. Pulse repetition frequency
   B. Transducer operating frequency
   C. Nyquist frequency
   D. Angular sweep frequency

B.96 If the maximum velocity across the valve is measured by Doppler as 2 m/s, what is the pressure difference across the valve?
   A. 2 mmHg
   B. 4 mmHg
   C. 8 mmHg
   D. 16 mmHg

B.97 What is a major benefit of harmonic imaging?
   A. Reduced clutter and side lobe
   B. Improved temporal resolution
   C. Reduced mechanical index
   D. Increased FOV

B.98 Which type of Doppler provides the least amount of spatial information?
   A. Spectral
   B. Color
   C. Power
   D. Continuous

B.99 What type of Doppler is used to detect slow flow at a large Doppler angle?
   A. Spectral
   B. Color
   C. Power
   D. Continuous

B.100 What type of flow has the broadest spectral Doppler wave?
   A. Parabolic
   B. Plug
   C. Laminar
   D. Turbulent

PRACTICE EXAMINATION B:
Answers and Explanations

B.1 **A** (Atomic nuclei). X-rays are produced when energetic electrons are decelerated in the electric field of tungsten nuclei (bremsstrahlung).

B.2 **B** (30%). About 70% incident photon energy is absorbed within a patient, 30% scattered out of the patient, and less than 1% gets to the image receptor to generate an image.

B.3 **B** (24 keV). X-ray energies that are very low (5 keV), or just above the K-edge energy (26 and 32 keV) are strongly absorbed, so only 24 keV photons will be transmitted through an Ag filter.

B.4 **C** (Effective dose). Effective dose gives the whole-body equivalent dose that would give the same stochastic risk as the exam of interest. Since all effective doses are essentially whole-body doses, they can be directly compared and combined.

B.5 **B** (3 mm). Approximately 3 mm. It is actually a bit higher than 3 mm since adding 3 mm Al will harden the x-ray beam (knock out mainly low-energy photons) making the beam a bit more penetrating. However, the hardened beam will not require anywhere near 10 mm additional.

B.6 **B** (2). Tumor suppressor genes are recessive and require both copies to be impacted for loss of function.

B.7 **C** (>0%...). The threshold is the dose where there is a chance of the effect for the most radiosensitive people. Average people are very unlikely to see any effect at the threshold dose.

B.8 **C** (more transparent ribs). The higher energy decreases photoelectric interactions leading to more radiolucent ribs.

B.9 **C** (10 bits). Eight bits can code 256 shades of gray (2^8), and adding a bit doubles the shades of gray, so 9 bits give 512 shades and 10 bits are required to code for 1,024 shades of gray.

B.10 **A** (Low-pass filtering). A low-pass filter removes high spatial frequency components of the image and removes noise but also blurs the image.

B.11 **D** (Body part too small). A finger is smaller than the AEC cell meaning that most of the cell will be hit by the unattenuated beam. This will typically result in an acquisition that is too short and a poor image.

B.12 **C** (Low contrast). The presence of noise affects the detection of low-contrast lesions; for high-contrast lesions, the presence of noise is of little practical importance.

B.13 **D** (Spatial resolution). A bar phantom is imaged and the limiting spatial resolution is where you can no longer identify individual bars in the image due to system blur.

B.14 **A** (Image intensifier systems and digital systems increase). Both systems increase dose, image intensifier systems to maintain brightness and digital systems to mitigate the appearance of noise in the zoomed image.

B.15 **A** (Larger area under the curve is better.). The area under the curve (AUC) ranges from 0 to 1. A value of 0 implies no sensitivity and all false positives. A value of 1 implies perfect sensitivity with no false positives.

B.16 **C** (Maximizes iodine contrast). The K-edge of iodine is ~33 keV. Just above this, attenuation of iodine (and thus iodine subject contrast) is maximized while maintaining soft tissue penetration. Just below or much above 33 keV, attenuation is much lower. At very low energies, iodine attenuation is high, but so is soft tissue attenuation, resulting in too much image noise.

B.17 C (100 mGy). The American College of Obstetrics and Gynecology and American Association of Physicists in Medicine do no support discussion of therapeutic abortion below the threshold for fetal tissue effects (100 mGy). Even at this threshold, there is >94% chance of no fetal effects.

B.18 A (Colon). The colon has the highest tissue weighting factor (W_T) of 0.12, whereas the bladder, liver, and thyroid each have a lower tissue weighting factor (W_T) of 0.04.

B.19 C Moderate (1-10 mSv). A chest CT has an effective dose of ~5 mSv.

B.20 D (Fluoroscopic interventional procedures). Interventional fluoroscopy procedures are in the tens of mSv with the high end toward 90 mSv (spine embolization). CT perfusion is a few mSv. DEXA is <0.01 mSv. A VQ scan is also a few mSv.

B.21 B (4 Gy). The oxygen enhancement ratio is the ratio of dose for a certain level of cell kill in hypoxic cells divided by dose for the same cell kill in aerated cells.

B.22 C (10 Gy). GI Syndrome occurs for acute whole-body doses of about 10 Gy.

B.23 C (15 Gy). Moist desquamation is most likely observed as an early effect at peak skin doses approaching 15 Gy.

B.24 D (Bone cancer). Licking the paint brush with radium on it resulted in huge doses to the jaw and development of bone cancer.

B.25 B (Three). A young child likely is three times more sensitive than a 25 year old in terms of radiation induced carcinogenesis.

B.26 C (DICOM). DICOM is the standard in radiology and IHE is used to resolve conflicts communicating with the larger hospital which will primarily use HL7.

B.27 D (Too much attenuation). At such low energies the beam will not penetrate the patient resulting in high dose, long acquisition times and too much noise.

B.28 B (overestimate; underestimate). Dosimeters worn above the lead apron (grossly) overestimate operator effective doses, and those worn under the lead apron will underestimate doses.

B.29 D (150 mSv). The dose limit for the eye lens in the United States is 150 mSv/y for occupational exposure. Outside the United States, the International Commission on Radiological Protection in 2011 recommended a lower limit and is now a regulatory limit in some countries (e.g., UK) but not in the United States.

B.30 B (5 mSv). The annual dose limit is 5 mSv and should be evenly distributed throughout the gestation (i.e., ~<0.5 mSv/mo). The fetus is thus not a member of the public (1 mSv limit each year), which allows women of reproductive capacity to be radiation workers (e.g., NM technologists) who receive 2 to 3 mSv each year.

B.31 B (Never). For modern scanners, dose is low enough that major organizations no longer recommend shielding during CT, since it may cause artifacts or even increase patient dose if used incorrectly.

B.32 B (Rayleigh scatter). Rayleigh scatter (aka Thompson or coherent) redirects the photon but is elastic (i.e., does not transfer any energy).

B.33 D (1%). Most x-ray tubes convert about 1% of the deposited energy into x-rays. This improves as kV increases which is why radiation oncology has ~10% x-rays production.

B.34 B (FOV). Heel effect severity increases with increasing FOV because the change in the number of photons is highest between the two image edges and gets bigger as they move further apart.

B.35 D (250). EI = 250 (i.e., K_{air} is 2.5 µGy at the image receptor) typically gives acceptable noise levels without excess dose to the patient.

B.36 B (Flicker artifact). If the television screen refreshes too slowly (60 fps progressive or 30 fps interlaced), then the image will appear to flicker. This causes increased eyestrain that causes headaches and can reduce detectability in the image.

B.37 A (less attenuation). Glass has high-Z materials that drastically attenuate the low-energy mammography beam. The higher energies used in other modalities makes glass acceptable.

B.38 C (Decrease focal spot size). Magnification also magnifies the focal spot which would cause a loss of spatial resolution. To combat that, the focal spot size decreases from 0.3 to 0.1 mm.

B.39 C (Accordion). Out-of-slice structures are blurred and their intensity decreased due to the tomosynthesis reconstruction process. This blurring can cause the skin line to appear thickened, as blurry out-of-slice skin is superimposed on the in-plane skin line.

B.40 D (Increase filter K-edge energy). Increasing the filter K-edge energy by changing the filter material (i.e., atomic number) results in the highest increase in x-ray beam quality (e.g., Mo to Rh filter for a Mo target, or Rh to Ag for a W target), and much higher than only adjusting tube voltage.

B.41 C (Reduced). Techniques are generally reduced (e.g., 100-70 mAs) because the removal of a grid eliminates losses of primary photons in the grid.

B.42 B (Organ malformation). At high doses (>100 mGy), tissue effects can occur for a fetus. During the fourth week of gestation, the fetus is undergoing organogenesis, so organ malformation is the primary concern.

B.43 D (Increase light brightness). An image intensifier operated in normal mode has a brightness gain of about 5,000 which is due to the flux gain (e.g., X 50) and minification gain (e.g., X 100).

B.44 B (Urological). Urological examinations normally have an over-the-table x-ray tube to minimize geometric magnification of the kidneys. In all other examinations, this geometry is avoided to minimize operator doses, especially to the eye lens.

B.45 C (100%; 0%). Switching from the Normal to Mag 1 mode will most likely double the skin dose but not affect the Kerma-area product (increase in beam intensity (dose) is offset by an reduction in beam area).

B.46 D (~200 mGy/min). Current US regulations require the maximum entrance K_{air} rate incident on a patient undergoing HLC fluoroscopy to be 20 R/min is roughly 200 Gy/min (175 mGy/min).

B.47 C (500 mGy). Highest skin doses in fluoroscopy-guided GI/GU studies are about 500 mGy, which is well below the threshold dose for erythema.

B.48 C (lower than). For small fields of view, doses are lower for FPDs, because application of electronic magnification with image intensifiers *requires* increased doses for smaller areas (automatic brightness control active). Use of Mag 2 with an image intensifier would likely quadruple the incident intensity (K_{air}), but the corresponding FOV on a FPD would only double K_{air}.

B.49 B (1 day). Although an exact time is dependent on the radiochemical structure, recent simplified guidance by the NRC states breast-feeding should cease for 1 day for Tc-99m. Milk should be pumped and discarded during this time.

B.50 A (Effective dose…). Effective doses are essentially equivalent doses to the whole body. As a result, they are virtually hitting the same tissue and can be added. All the other combinations are to different pieces of tissue and so cannot be added.

B.51 A (Fluoroscopy). Last image hold will leave a processed version of the last frame (or combination of frames) up on the screen for inspection whenever the foot pedal is released.

B.52 C (65%). Wearing leaded glasses reduces eye lens doses only by about 60% to 70%, with the eye lens doses mainly due to "scatter" from radiation incident on skin around the glasses.

B.53 A (Improve radiation uniformity). The bow tie filter is designed to be thicker where the patient is thin (periphery) to give more uniform radiation across the patient and improve the image contrast. The correct size bow tie is necessary as is centering the patient in the bore.

B.54 C (Soft tissue contrast). HU values are not accurate in cone-beam CT and soft tissue image contrast is much worse due partially to the large amount of scatter received by the detector. Cone-beam CT has usually much lower dose and much worse temporal resolution.

B.55 A (Image noise). Statistical iterative reconstruction substantially reduces image noise.

B.56 D (Water). Hounsfield units are attenuation coefficients of tissues relative to water, with positive values attenuating more than water, and negative values attenuating less than water.

B.57 B (Does not affect). The HU of water (by definition) is always zero and is therefore not affected by x-ray tube voltage or photon energy.

B.58 B (VQ scan). The ventilation part of a VQ scan utilizes radioactive aerosols or gasses. The room is kept at negative pressure so that when the door is opened air rushes into the room and prevents the radioactive aerosol/gas to escape.

B.59 C (Pitch). CT pitch values are very low (e.g., 0.2) in retrospectively gated CT coronary angiography, which results in especially high effective doses.

B.60 D (decreased; decreased). Both CT voltage and tube output (mAs) need to be reduced when performing CT scans of infants.

B.61 A (DSA dose is larger.). The dose rate from DSA is much larger than HLC (e.g., boost mode). This is why low frame rates are utilized for DSA.

B.62 A (Next to the detector). The dose is much lower for the operator if they stand next to the detector during cross-table acquisitions. The beam is limited to the size of the detector and the patient attenuates almost all of the beam so that a much lower amount of scatter will hit the operator.

B.63 B (Reduce overfitting of the model). The training set is used to train new features for the model. The final metrics for model performance are reported based on the testing set. A validation set increases training time but mitigates tuning the model parameters to a specific training set and thus reduces overfitting.

B.64 D (60 mGy). Directly irradiated organs in routine head CT scans likely receive about 60 mGy.

B.65 A (metastable). The term metastable (m) means the lifetime of the excited nuclear energy level is relatively long (defined by physicists to be 10^{-9} seconds).

B.66 A (0.1%). After 10 half-lives, 0.1% of the initial activity remains $(1/2^{10})$; we typically hold radioactivity for 10 half-lives and then check its activity to confirm it is not above natural background before disposing of it.

B.67 D (daughter; daughter). Radionuclide equilibrium occurs after four daughter half-lives for both transient and secular equilibria. By convention, if the parent is long lived it is called secular equilibrium, and when the parent is short lived, it is called transient equilibrium, but it is exactly the same phenomenon and both obey exactly the same "rules."

B.68 A (Labeled sulfur colloids). Sulfur colloid is used to assess liver and spleen function is an example of phagocytosis, GI bleed studies is compartmental leakage, Bone uptake of pyrophosphates is physiochemical absorption, and labeled leukocytes is cell sequestration.

B.69 B (10%). Broadening of the photopeak, as measured by the full width at half maximum, is generally 10% for scintillators. The width of the ^{123}I peak on a gamma ray spectrum will be about 16 keV, which translates into a 10% broadening as the peak occurs at 160 keV.

B.70 B (constant; degraded). Parallel-hole collimator sensitivity is constant with increased distance from collimator, whereas the corresponding spatial resolution performance is degraded.

B.71 B (10 half-lives). After 10 half-lives, the emissions are typically at or below natural background. The material can be disposed of in normal trash or drains after surveying to confirm it is at background levels..

B.72 C (8 mm). A full width at half maximum of 8 mm would likely be obtained for a SPECT image of a line source, which is (just a bit) larger than a gamma camera's resolution.

B.73 B (They are about the same.). The dose for a dual-energy acquisition is about the same as a single because the high- and low-dose acquisitions are each acquired at doses lower than a single energy acquisition. If two phases (with and without contrast) are acquired, then dual energy may have a much lower dose if the noncontrast acquisition is removed and virtual noncontrast images utilized.

B.74 D (Chemical fat saturation). Fat sat is based on the Larmor frequency of fat. In the presence of an inhomogeneity, the Larmor frequency is altered and the RF pulse used during fat sat will not excite the fat protons (fat sat will fail).

B.75 B (PET). Highest attenuation correction factors are in PET because it is the total path length that is used, not just the distance from activity to the exit point used in SPECT. In PET, attenuation correction factors can easily be as high as a factor of 10.

B.76 C (PET). It is PET facilities that use the highest energies and handle the largest number of patients and would require shielding much more substantial than a CT facility (i.e., much more than ~2 mm Pb). ^{131}I has lower-energy gamma rays than 511 keV PET annihilation photons and has a very low patient throughput.

B.77 A (3 ppm). Only 3 per million protons contribute to the net tissue magnetization at a magnetic field of 1 T. Doubling the magnetic field generally doubles the number of protons contributing to net magnetization (i.e., why radiologists want higher fields).

B.78 C (T2*). Ferritin and hemosiderin cause a change in the local magnetic field, leading to dephasing of spins from T2* decay.

B.79 B (long; short). T1 times in all solids such as bone are extremely long (i.e., seconds), and T2 times are extremely short (i.e., microseconds); the latter fact explains why solids generally do not result in any signal (i.e., FID and echoes all disappear instantaneously).

B.80 A (Increased). Increasing the transmit RF bandwidth would likely increase the corresponding acquired image slice thickness.

B.81 A (Blurrier). The periphery of k-space contains high spatial frequencies that provide the edges and detail of images, and when these are missing, the image will be more blurred.

B.82 B (Zipper). Leaving a door open to the MR suite during image acquisition results in zipper artifacts. Each radio station frequency will produce a line along the PE gradient direction.

B.83 D (short; short). T1 weighting is obtained when TR is short, and TE is short.

B.84 C (Lower than). GRE sequences have echoes that are much weaker than echoes obtained during SE sequences (GRE is affected by T2*, whereas SE is not), so SNR in GRE is relatively low.

B.85 D (CSF). Fluids are suppressed by choosing a TI time of 1700 ms (i.e., FLAIR pulse sequence).

B.86 C (4; 2). Parallel imaging, in this case, will take one-fourth the time but reduces the SNR by a factor of sqrt(4) = 2, since some channels are dedicated to unwrapping the undersampled image.

B.87 D (T2). A long echo train length extends the effective echo time. A long echo time will introduce more T2 weighting into the image, and so large echo train lengths are typically only used for T2W images.

B.88 D (Using GRE instead of FSE). GRE imaging uses a <90° flip angle initially and eliminates the 180° pulse used in spin echo and fast spin echo sequences. Reducing the RF in this way substantially lowers the SAR due to less RF depositing energy in the patient.

B.89 B (Utilize compound imaging). Anisotropy occurs because the beam is specularly reflected from the tissue, but the echo misses the transducer. Using compound imaging alters the angle that the beam hits the surface and may allow the specular reflection to be received by the transducer. Altering the placement and angle of the probe will also help.

B.90 A (<1%). Tissue air interfaces transmit negligible amounts of the incident sound (<1%), as the acoustic impedance mismatch ensures it is all reflected (>99%). This is why ultrasound gel and good patient contact are so important.

B.91 C (Speckle is not random.). Speckle is an interference pattern caused by the many reflections in the patient. If the transducer and tissue are held still, then speckle will not move but noise will be different from frame to frame, since it is random.

B.92 C (Axial resolution). Adding a damping block to an ultrasound transducer shortens the pulse length (and duration), which improves axial resolution.

B.93 A (Small footprint gives a short near-field distance.). The near-field distance is strongly dependent on the size of the transducer footprint. As footprint gets smaller, the near-field distance gets shorter and divergence in the far field happens more quickly.

B.94 B (Alters where color Doppler is displayed). Color priority is used to determine when a pixel shows the color Doppler signal and when it shows B-mode gray level values. Generally it is set so anechoic structures and very hypoechoic structures display Doppler color, but other tissues display gray level.

B.95 A (PRF). The pulse repetition frequency is the product of the lines per image and the image frame rate (Hz).

B.96 D (16 mmHG). The pressure difference from the simplified Bernoulli principle is 4 × velocity squared.

B.97 A (Reduced clutter and side lobe). Clutter and side lobe are mitigated in harmonic imaging. Clutter is reduced because the harmonic beam does not form until deeper into the tissue and side lobes are reduced because they are too weak to form harmonics powerful enough to be detected.

B.98 D (Continuous). All pulsed Doppler systems provide excellent spatial information. Continuous Doppler (CW) uses two transducers that are always on and compares the frequency difference to estimate flow, and the absence of "echo timing" severely limits spatial information. CW Doppler accurately measures very fast flows (e.g., >2 m/s).

B.99 C (Power). It is power Doppler that is most sensitive to slow flow, and is (approximately) independent of Doppler angle.

B.100 D (Turbulent). Spectral waveform thickness is proportional to the number of different velocities measured. Turbulence causes the blood to move at many different speeds and many directions, giving it a very broad waveform.

Physics Equations

X-Rays

Energy utilized is Power × Time.

Power (P; watts) dissipated in an electrical circuit with a voltage (V) and current (I) is I (amps) × V (volts).

Velocity of any wave (v) is the product of the wave frequency (f) and wavelength (λ) (i.e., $\lambda \times f$).

The photon energy (E) the product of the photon frequency (f) and Planck constant (h) (i.e., $h \times f$).

Number of x-rays transmitted (N) through an absorber thickness (t) and linear attenuation coefficient (μ) is $N_o \times e^{-(\mu \times t)}$, where N_o is the number of incident x-rays.

When μ is a small number (<0.1), this represents the fraction of incident x-rays that are absorbed in unit distance (i.e., $\mu = 0.1$ cm^{-1} means 10% of the rays are lost traveling through 1 cm).

The mass attenuation coefficient of a material with a linear attenuation coefficient (μ) and a density (ρ) is μ/ρ.

The number of transmitted x-rays is $N = N_o \times e^{-([\mu/\rho] \times [\rho t])}$, where $\rho \times t$ is the areal thickness of the absorber.

An exposure of 1 Roentgen corresponds to a Kerma (K_{air}) of 8.76 mGy.

The inverse square law predicts the radiation intensity I_2 at distance d_2, when the radiation intensity at distance d_1 is I_1. I_2 is equal to $I_1 \times (d_1/d_2)^2$ so that doubling the distance from a source reduces the radiation intensity fourfold.

X-ray fractional transmission through an absorber that is N half-value layers thick is $1/2^N$.

Radiation Protection and Dosimetry

Absorbed dose (D) in Gray is E/M, where E is the energy absorbed (joules) by an absorber of mass M (kg).

Skin dose (D_{skin}) is the product of the entrance Kerma (K_{air}), backscatter factor (BSF), and tissue "f-factor" (f) (i.e., $K_{air} \times BSF \times f$).

When patient entrance dose is $D_{entrance}$, and the patient exit dose is D_{exit}, the midline dose is the geometrical mean (i.e., $(D_{entrance} \times D_{exit})^{0.5}$).

The equivalent dose (H) in mSv is the product of the absorbed dose (D) in mGy and radiation weighting factor (w_R) (i.e., $w_R \times D$).

The effective dose to an exposed individual, (E) in mSv, is obtained from organ equivalent doses (H) in mSv and the corresponding organ weighting factors (w_T) using $E = \Sigma_i [H_i \times (w_T)_i]$, where i refers to the ith organ, and the summation is overall exposed organs in the exposed individual.

Projection Imaging

Geometrical magnification is SID/SOD, where SID is the source-to-image receptor distance, and SOD is the source-to-object distance.

Exposure index (EI) is approximately 100 times the average radiation intensity (K_{air}) incident on the image receptor (μGy) after being transmitted through the patient.

For constant x-ray beam intensity with an average of N photons per pixel incident on a digital image receptor, the interpixel standard deviation is $N^{0.5}$, and the relative interpixel fluctuations are $100/N^{0.5}$ %.

Bucky factor (BF) is the radiation intensity incident on a grid ($I_{incident}$) divided by the radiation intensity transmitted through the grid ($I_{transmitted}$) (i.e., $[I_{incident}]/[I_{transmitted}]$).

Image intensifier minification gain is the exposed image intensifier area at the input divided by the area of the image intensifier output, where the latter is typically 2.54 cm in diameter (i.e., 1″).

Flat-panel detector limiting spatial resolution is $1/(2 \times d)$ cycles per mm, where d is the pixel size in mm.

Computed Tomography

Pitch = table travel per rotation/beam width.

Pixels with a linear attenuation coefficient μ_x have a Hounsfield unit (HU_x) of $1000 \times (\mu_x - \mu_{water})/\mu_{water}$, where μ_{water} is the attenuation of water at the same x-ray photon energy.

Weighted CD dose index ($CTDI_w$) is obtained from measurements made at the center ($CTDI_c$) and periphery ($CTDI_p$) in cylindrical phantoms. Formally, $CTDI_w$ is equal to $1/3 \times CTDI_c + 2/3 \times CTDI_p$.

Volume CTDI (i.e., $CTDI_{vol}$) is $CTDI_w$ divided by the CT pitch (p) in helical scanning, or the effective pitch in axial CT (i.e., $CTDI_w/p$).

Dose-length product (DLP) is $CTDI_{vol} \times$ Scan length.

In CT, the patient effective dose is DLP $\times$ k, where k is a conversion factor that accounts for the CT region, as well as patient age and size.

Nuclear Medicine

Effective half-life (T_e) is obtained from physical half-life (T_p) and biological half-life (T_b) using the formula $1/T_e = 1/T_p + 1/T_b$.

Energy resolution ($E_{resolution}$) of a scintillator with photopeak energy ($E_{photopeak}$), and measured energy photopeak (E_{FWHM}), is $100 \times E_{FWHM}/E_{photopeak}$ (%).

If the intrinsic gamma camera resolution is $R_{intrinsic}$, and the collimator resolution is $R_{collimator}$, the system resolution (R_{system}) is obtained using the formula $R_{system} = ([R_{intrinsic}]^2 + [R_{collimator}]^2)^{0.5}$.

The total number of nuclear transformation for A Bq of activity with a half-life of $T_{1/2}$ seconds is $1.44 \times A \times T_{1/2}$.

Organ doses are obtained from the product of the total number of nuclear transformation in a source organ and the corresponding target organ dose per unit transformation in the source organ.

Fractional activity remaining after ten half-lives is $1/2^{10}$, or ~0.1%.

SPECT or PET attenuation correction factor is $e^{(\mu \times t)}$, where t is the tissue thickness and μ is the corresponding tissue attenuation factor.

Magnetic Resonance

Larmor frequency for any magnetic nucleus is $\gamma \times B$, where γ is the gyromagnetic ratio for the nucleus and B is the magnetic field.

Local field in a material with susceptibility χ in an magnetic field B is $B(1 + \chi)$ so that positive values of χ increase the local field and negative values of χ decrease the local field.

Following a 90° RF pulse, the relative longitudinal magnetization in a tissue with a longitudinal relaxation time T1 is given by $(1 - e^{-t/T1})$.

Following a 90° RF pulse, the relative transverse magnetization in a tissue with a transverse relaxation time T2 is given by $e^{-t/T2}$.

Imaging time in spin echo sequences for a repetition time TR, and a phase encode matrix size of N, is given by Imaging time = $N \times TR$

Imaging time in fast spin echo (FSE) with echo train length of ETL is $[N \times TR]/ETL$.

Imaging with a number of excitations E and parallel acceleration factor A is $[N \times TR \times E]/A$.

The matrix size of k-space for N echoes in SE imaging, each of which is sampled (digitized) M times, is $N \times M$, where N is phase encode direction and M is frequency encode direction.

Ultrasound

Sound period of a wave with a frequency f is $1/f$.

The relative intensity (in decibels) of a sound wave with intensity I is given by $10 \times \log_{10}(I/I_o)$, where I is the sound intensity and I_o is the initial sound intensity.

The maximum reflected intensity at an interface between two materials with impedances of Z_1 and Z_2 is given by $[Z_1 - Z_2]^2/[Z_1 + Z_2]^2$, and the maximum reflections occur at normal incidence (i.e., 90°).

Reflected sound intensity (%) plus transmitted sound intensity (%) is 100%.

Attenuation of sound is [Attenuation coefficient] × [Distance traveled], and the attenuation coefficient is [Attenuation coefficient per MHz] × [Frequency].

Transducer thickness is equal to one half the wavelength.

The transducer near zone for an element of effective radius r, and wavelength λ, is given by Near zone = r^2/λ.

Pulse repetition frequency is the product of lines per frame and the corresponding frame rate (frames/second).

Distance traveled is the product of the sound velocity (m/s) and elapsed time (s).

Doppler frequency shift is $2 \times f \times v \times \cos(\theta)/c$, where f is the operating frequency, v is the speed of the reflector, θ is the Doppler angle, and c is the sound velocity in the medium.

The maximum Doppler frequency shift that can be measured with no aliasing is one half of the pulse repetition frequency (PRF/2).

Glossary

90° pulse - radio frequency pulse that rotates the equilibrium magnetization vector through 90°

180° pulse - radiofrequency pulse that rotates the equilibrium magnetization vector through 180°

A-mode ultrasound - displays echo strength versus time

absolute risk - model of cancer induction where radiation induces a given number of cancers

absorbed dose - radiation energy absorbed per unit mass of a medium measured in gray

absorption efficiency - fraction of incident photons that are absorbed

acoustic enhancement - hyperechoic area distal to object with low attenuation (e.g., fluid-filled cyst)

acoustic impedance - product of density and velocity of sound measured in rayl

acoustic shadowing - hypoechoic area distal to object due to high attenuation or reflection

activity - number of nuclear transformations per unit of time measured in becquerel or curie

air gap - gap between a patient and the imaging receptor used in magnification examinations

ALARA - as low as reasonably achievable is the principle for minimizing all radiation doses

air kerma - measure of the intensity of x-ray beams obtained from the energy transferred to electrons per unit mass of air

aliasing - artifact caused by undersampling in digital imaging

alpha decay - emission of an alpha particle by a radionuclide

alpha particle - nuclear particle consisting of two neutrons and two protons

analog-to-digital converter (ADC) - converts analog signals into digital values

angiography - imaging of the vasculature achieved by the administration of iodinated contrast material that absorbs many more x-rays than tissues or blood

anode - positive side of an electric circuit

area under the curve (AUC) - measure of imaging performance based on area under a receiver operating characteristic curve (sensitivity vs false-positive fraction)

artificial intelligence - programs capable of performing tasks typically requiring human intelligence.

atom - basic constituent of matter that has a positive nucleus surrounded by electrons

atomic number (Z) - number of protons in the nucleus of an atom

attenuation coefficient (μ) - measure of the x-ray–attenuating property of a material, in mm^{-1}

automatic brightness control (ABC) - regulates x-ray tube radiation to maintain a constant brightness at image intensifier output

average glandular dose (AGD) - the average dose to the glandular breast tissue in mGy

axial resolution - ability to separate two objects lying *along* the axis of an ultrasound beam

B-mode ultrasound - brightness mode that displays echo intensity as a pixel brightness

background radiation - radiation doses from naturally occurring radioactivity and extraterrestrial cosmic radiation

backscatter - x-ray photons scattered from the patient that will increase the patient skin dose

bandwidth - *range* of frequencies that can be transmitted or processed by a system

beam hardening - increase in mean energy of polychromatic x-ray beams when lower energy photons are preferentially absorbed by a filter or patient

beam quality - penetrating ability of an x-ray beam, usually expressed as an aluminum thickness that reduces beam intensity by 50%

Becquerel - SI unit of radioactivity (1 Bq = 1 disintegration per second)

BEIR - Committee on Biological Effects of Ionizing Radiation of the US National Academy of Sciences

beta minus decay - nuclear process in which a neutron is converted to a proton

beta particle - electron or positron emitted from a nucleus during beta decay

beta plus decay - nuclear process in which a proton is converted to a neutron

biological half-life - time required to biologically clear one-half of the amount of a stable material in an organ or tissue

bit - (binary digit) smallest unit of computer memory that holds one of two values, 0 or 1

blur - loss of image detail produced by an imaging system

bow tie filter - beam shaping filter used to equalize x-ray transmission through the patient

bremsstrahlung radiation - "braking radiation" x-rays produced when electrons lose energy

brightness gain - ratio of the image brightness at the image intensifier output to the brightness produced at the input phosphor

Bucky - device that shakes a grid, named after its inventor

Bucky factor - ratio of incident to transmitted radiation through a grid

byte - unit of computer memory equal to 8 bits

CAD - computer-aided detection or diagnosis

candela/m^2 - measure of luminance (brightness)

cataract - eye lens opacity that can be caused by ionizing radiation

cathode - negative side of an electrical circuit

characteristic curve - plot of detector response against x-ray intensity (K_{air})

characteristic radiation - x-ray photon of characteristic energy emitted from an atom when an inner shell vacancy is filled by an outer shell electron

charge-coupled device (CCD) - two-dimensional electronic array for converting light patterns into electrical signals

chemical shift artifacts - artifacts in MR due to small differences in resonance frequencies of different chemical compounds (e.g., water and fat)

coherent scatter - photon scattered by an atom without suffering any energy loss (aka Rayleigh or classical scatter)

collimation - restriction of an x-ray beam or gamma rays by use of attenuators

color Doppler - measures changes in ultrasound frequency which are displayed as colors ranging from blue to red

compression - in breast imaging, a device used to compress the breast to a nominally uniform thickness

Compton interaction - photon interaction with an outer shell electron resulting in a scattered electron and photon of lower energy

computed tomography (CT) - x-ray imaging modality showing cross-sectional anatomy as represented by x-ray attenuation coefficients

computed radiography (CR) - digital radiography that uses photostimulable phosphor plates

contrast - difference in signal intensity between a lesion and the surrounding background

contrast agent - material administered to the patient that increases (or reduces) x-ray absorption to visualize structures that take up the agent

contrast improvement factor - ratio of image contrast levels obtained with, and without, the use of a scatter-reducing grid

contrast-to-noise ratio (CNR) - a relative measure of image quality that compares the contrast of a lesion to the surrounding noise levels

controlled area - area with potentially high dose rates supervised by a radiation safety officer

converging collimator - a NM collimator used for small organs that results in magnified images

convolutional neural network - a type of deep learning that maintains the spatial relationships of image data.

coulomb (C) - unit of electric charge

count density - used in nuclear medicine to specify the number of counts per unit area

CTDI - computed tomography dose index (CTDI) used to quantify CT output using measurements made in phantoms

cumulative activity - a measure of the total number of radioactive disintegrations obtained by integrating a time-activity curve

curie (Ci) - the non-SI unit of activity (1 Ci = 3.7 x 10^{10} disintegrations per second)

current - rate of flow of electric charge, measured in ampere

cyclotron - charged particle accelerator used to make radioisotopes

decay constant (λ) - the rate of decay of radionuclides ($\lambda = 0.69/T_{1/2}$, where $T_{1/2}$ is the half-life)

deep learning - machine learning using neural networks with many layers

depth gain compensation (DGC) - used in ultrasound to correct for increased attenuation of sound with tissue depth

deterministic effect - biological effect of radiation (e.g., epilation) that has a threshold dose (harmful tissue reaction)

DICOM (Digital Imaging and Communications in Medicine) - a standard used for digital images in radiology

digital - quantity specified by discrete numbers, as opposed to analog (continuous)

digital fluoroscopy - fluoroscopic imaging with TV signal digitized, and processed, in real time

digital photospot imaging - acquisition of a digital diagnostic quality image of the output of fluoroscopic imaging system (image intensifier or flat-panel detector)

digital radiography - use of a flat-panel detector array system to acquire a digital x-ray image

digital subtraction angiography (DSA) - digital images made before and after the introduction of iodine contrast are subtracted from each other

directly ionizing radiations - charged particles, such as electrons, which directly ionize atoms

diverging collimator - collimators for large organs (e.g., lungs) resulting in minified image

Doppler shift - change in ultrasound frequency from moving objects

dose - absorbed energy per unit mass, expressed in gray

dose-area product - product of the entrance kerma and cross-sectional area of an x-ray beam incident on a patient (aka kerma-area product)

dose calibrator - ionization chamber used in nuclear medicine to measure the amount of radioactivity prior to injection into a patient

dose-length product (DLP) - in CT, the product of the scan length and CT radiation intensity (i.e., $CTDI_{vol}$)

dual-energy CT - CT images created using two sets of images acquired at different energies (tube voltages)

dual-source CT - CT imaging systems that uses two x-ray tubes offset at 90° relative to each other

diffusion-weighted imaging (DWI) - MR imaging modality that employs paired gradients to identify and quantify molecular diffusion in tissues

dynamic range - ratio of the largest to smallest signal intensity

echo-planar imaging (EPI) - fast MR imaging mode

edge enhancement - enhancement of tissue margins using digital processing techniques

edge packing - nuclear medicine artifact that occurs at the periphery of the scintillator camera

effective atomic number - average atomic number obtained from a weighted summation of the atomic constituents of a compound

effective dose - uniform whole-body dose that has the same detriment as a given dose distribution

effective half-life - half-life of a radioactive material in an organ that is also being cleared biologically

electricity - flow of electrical charge (i.e., electrons) in a circuit

electromagnetic radiation - transverse wave in which electric and magnetic fields oscillate perpendicular to wave motion

electron - small constituent of matter and a negative charge

electron binding energy - energy that must be supplied to extract a bound atomic electron

electron capture - nuclear process in which a proton is converted to a neutron by capturing an electron

electron density - number of electrons per unit volume (electrons per cm^3)

electron volt (eV) - unit of energy corresponding to the kinetic energy gained by an electron when accelerated through an electrical potential of 1 volt

electrostatic force - force that results from charges, which holds atoms together

elevational resolution - ultrasound resolution in the slice thickness direction

energy - ability to do work measured in joule (J)

entrance skin dose - absorbed radiation dose to skin where the x-ray beam enters the patient

equivalent dose - product of the absorbed dose and radiation weighting factor expressed in sievert (Sv)

excited state - any energy level above the lowest energy ground state in an atom or nucleus

extrinsic flood - scintillator camera image obtained of a uniform source of activity with the collimator in place

faraday cage - radiofrequency copper shielding sheets built into the wall around an MR scanner

fast spin echo (FSE) - MR technique that uses multiple spin echoes to reduce imaging times in comparison to spin-echo imaging

ferromagnetic - material (e.g., iron and nickel) with large intrinsic magnetic fields produced by a regular array of unpaired atomic electrons in a domain

field uniformity - a measure of the uniformity of a nuclear medicine scintillator camera

filament - wire on the cathode of an x-ray tube that is heated to emit electrons

file transfer protocol (FTP) - method for transferring files across a computer network

filter - aluminum, copper, or other absorber placed in an x-ray beam to preferentially absorb low-energy x-rays

filtered back projection - computed tomography image reconstruction technique

flat-panel detectors - digital x-ray detector consisting of an x-ray absorber (photoconductor or scintillator) and a two-dimensional readout array

flip angle - angle through which net magnetization vector is rotated by an RF pulse

flux gain - number of light photons at the output phosphor of an image intensifier per light photon produced at the input phosphor

focal spot - region in the x-ray tube anode where x-ray beam is produced

focused transducer - ultrasound transducer that focuses the beam with an acoustic lens or shaped transducer

force - directed energy that can change the motion of a mass

Fourier analysis - analysis of time signals that identifies the individual signal frequencies

Fraunhofer zone - the far zone of an ultrasound beam where it diverges

free induction decay (FID) - decreasing MR signal following a 90° pulse

frequency - number of oscillations per second (i.e., hertz)

frequency encode gradient - magnetic field gradient applied during the acquisition (readout) of a free induction decay signal

Fresnel zone - near zone of an ultrasound beam used for imaging

fringe field - magnetic field at a distance from a magnet

full width at half maximum (FWHM) - a measure equal to the width of any distribution at points where the intensity is reduced to one-half the maximum

functional imaging - MR imaging modality that measures changes in regional blood flow arising from mental activity

fusion imaging - combination of two images such as CT and PET

gadolinium - paramagnetic contrast material used in MR imaging

gamma camera - nuclear medicine imaging system that detects gamma rays (i.e., scintillation camera)

gamma decay - nuclear transformation that results in the emission of a gamma ray

gamma rays - high-frequency electromagnetic radiation produced by nuclear processes

Gaussian distribution - a bell-shaped statistical distribution that is symmetrical about the mean value and whose spread is characterized by the standard deviation σ

Geiger counter - ionization chamber with a high voltage that produces amplified signals (electron avalanche) following detection of any ionizing particle

generator (radionuclide) - produces radionuclides such as ^{99m}Tc in nuclear medicine

genetically significant dose (GSD) - an estimate of the genetic significance of gonad radiation doses, which accounts for the child expectancy of exposed individuals

geometric unsharpness - image blur resulting from the finite size of the x-ray focal spot

gradient coils - current-carrying coils in magnetic resonance that create small magnetic field gradients superimposed on the large stationary magnetic field

gradient-recalled echo (GRE) - magnetic resonance spin echo created using gradients rather than a 180° rephasing RF pulse

gray (Gy) - the SI unit of absorbed dose (1 Gy = 1 J/kg)

grid - strips of lead in a radiolucent matrix used to reduce scattered radiation

grid line density - the number of grid lines per unit length

grid ratio - ratio of height to separation gap of the attenuating strips in a grid

ground state - lowest energy level of an atom or nucleus

gyromagnetic ratio (γ) - determines the Larmor precession frequency of a magnetic nucleus

half-life (physical) ($T_{1/2}$) - time for the activity of a radioisotope to decrease by a factor of 2

half-value layer (HVL) - thickness of specified material (e.g., aluminum) needed to reduce the x-ray beam intensity by 50%

heel effect - x-ray intensity is greater at the cathode side and lower at the anode side

hereditary effects - radiation damage in the gametes that is passed onto the offspring of irradiated individuals

hertz (Hz) - frequency expressed in cycles per second

HL7 - Health Level 7 is a standard for the exchange of medical information

Hounsfield unit (HU) - the attenuation coefficient of a material relative to that of water as used in computed tomography

ICRP - International Commission on Radiological Protection is an international agency that issues recommendations regarding radiation safety

ICRU - International Commission on Radiological Units and Measurements is an international agency that defines radiation units

IHE (Integrating the Healthcare Enterprise) - electronic (digital) integration of medical enterprises, including digital images

image compression - reduction of the data required to store or transfer a digital image

image contrast - difference in intensity of a lesion and the adjacent background tissues

image intensifier - converts incident x-ray pattern to a light image

image quality - a term that includes the resolution, noise, and contrast properties of any medical image

indirectly ionizing radiation - uncharged radiation that produces ionization via charged particles (e.g., x-rays via photo-electrons or Compton electrons)

integral dose - a measure of the total amount of energy (joules) imparted to a patient during a radiological examination

internal conversion - electron emitted from a nucleus in lieu of a gamma ray

intrinsic flood - scintillator camera image of a uniform source obtained *without* a collimator

intrinsic resolution - spatial resolution of a scintillator camera *without* a collimator

inverse square law - air kerma decreases in proportion to the square of the distance from the source

inversion recovery (IR) - magnetic resonance pulse sequence designed to emphasize T1 differences

ionization - production of electrons and positive ions following the absorption of radiation energy

ionization chamber - gas chamber used to measure x-ray air kerma by measuring the charge liberated in a given mass of air

ionizing radiation - radiation that can eject electrons from atoms

isobars - nuclides with the same total number of neutrons and protons (mass number [A])

isomers - nuclides with an excited nuclear state

isometric state - metastable state that exists for more than 10^{-9} seconds

isotones - nuclides with the same number of neutrons

isotopes - nuclides with the same number of protons

joule (J) - SI unit of energy

K-edge - binding energy of K-shell electrons

kerma - *k*inetic *e*nergy *r*eleased to *ma*tter, which refers to the transfer of energy from uncharged to charged particles

kerma-area product (KAP) - product of the air kerma incident on a patient, and the corresponding x-ray beam cross-sectional area

kinetic energy - energy associated with motion

lag - afterglow of an image on a screen or television camera

Larmor frequency - precession frequency of a magnetic nucleus in an applied magnetic field

lateral resolution - ability to resolve two laterally adjacent objects

latitude - the range of air kerma values over which an image recording system can operate

LD$_{50}$ - radiation dose that kills 50% of the irradiated cells or people

leakage radiation - radiation emerging from an x-ray unit when the collimators are closed

limiting resolution - highest spatial frequency resolved by an imaging system

line focus principle - result of viewing an x-ray tube anode at an angle, thus reducing its apparent size

line density - in ultrasound, the number of lines used to generate an image

line spread function (LSF) - image of a narrow line

linear attenuation coefficient (μ) - the fraction of photons lost from an x-ray beam in traveling a unit of distance, measured in mm^{-1}

linear energy transfer (LET) - energy absorbed by the medium per unit of length traveled, measured in keV per μm

longitudinal magnetization - component of magnetization that is oriented parallel to the main magnetic field in a magnetic resonance scanner

lookup table - used to relate digital data into an image brightness

luminance - the brightness of a light-emitting source (e.g., view box or display monitor)

M-mode ultrasound - displays depth versus time and permits motion to be observed

Machine learning - an AI technique where a machine may learn to perform tasks directly from data without explicit task programming from human expertise

magnetic moment - strength of nuclear or electronic magnetism

magnetic susceptibility - the inherent property of a substance that modifies the local magnetic field when placed in a strong applied (external) field

mass - resistance to acceleration (inertia) of matter measured in kilograms (kg)

mass attenuation coefficient - linear attenuation coefficient divided by the physical density, measured in cm^2/g

mass number (A) - total number of nucleons (protons and neutrons) in the nucleus of an atom

matching layer - layer of material placed in front of an ultrasound transducer to improve the efficiency of energy transfer into a patient

matrix size - the number of pixels allocated to each linear dimension in a digital image

maximum intensity projection (MIP) - an image processing method used in CT and MR

mean - the average value of any distribution of values

median - value of a statistical distribution where half the distribution is higher and half is lower

metastable state (isomeric state) - transient energy state of an atom whose half-life is >10^{-9} seconds

minification gain - ratio of the area of the image intensifier input to area of the output phosphor

modulation transfer function (MTF) - ratio of output to input signal amplitude as a function of spatial frequency, used to quantify resolution imaging systems

monochromatic radiation - radiation where all photons have the same energy

motion blur - unsharpness resulting from motion that occurs during the image acquisition time

mottle - random fluctuations in image intensity for the same nominal input air kerma

MPR - multiplanar reformatting used in tomographic imaging to generate sagittal, coronal, and oblique views from axial sections

MQSA - Mammography Quality Standards Act passed into law in the United States in 1992 and requires all mammography facilities to be accredited

MRA (MR angiography) - techniques for imaging the flow of blood using MR

MRS (MR spectroscopy) - MR techniques that permit the identification of chemical compounds such as phosphorus or proton metabolites

multidetector CT (MDCT) - CT scanners that can acquire more than one slice per single rotation of the x-ray tube and detector array

National Council on Radiation Protection and Measurements (NCRP) - a US agency that advises on radiation protection issues

natural background radiation - radiation doses from cosmic radiation and naturally occurring radionuclides (~3 mSv / year in the United States)

negative predictive value - probability of not having a disease given a negative diagnostic test result

neural network - a type of machine learning where many regression models (nodes) are connected to each other and arranged into layers to create an output (the final layer)

neutrons - uncharged particles found in the atomic nucleus

noise - unwanted signals in images

nonspecular reflection - diffuse ultrasound reflections (scatter) at irregular (rough) surfaces and small structures

nuclear medicine - imaging modality that enables the visualization of radiopharmaceuticals in patients

Nuclear Regulatory Commission (NRC) - US federal agency responsible for regulating nuclear materials

nucleon - neutron or proton

nuclides - nuclei with differing numbers of protons or neutrons

Nyquist frequency - the highest spatial frequency that can be faithfully reproduced when digitally sampling data

occupational dose limit - regulatory dose limits applied to radiation workers (e.g., 50 mSv/yr)

organ dose - absorbed radiation dose to a specified organ or tissue

PACS - **p**icture **a**rchiving and **c**ommunication **s**ystems receive, store, transfer, and display medical images

paramagnetism - substance with a positive susceptibility enhances the local magnetic field due to the presence of unpaired atomic electrons (e.g., gadolinium)

parallel processing - performing several computer tasks *simultaneously*

partial volume artifact - artifact caused by tissues with different attenuations within a voxel

peak voltage (kV$_p$) - maximum voltage across the x-ray tube

phase encode gradient - magnetic resonance gradient applied perpendicular to the frequency encode gradient and the slice select gradient

photoconductor - solid-state device that converts absorbed x-ray energy into charge that can be collected by an applied voltage

photoelectric effect - a photon is absorbed by an atom and a photoelectron is emitted

photomultiplier tube - electronic device that converts light into an electric signal

phototimer - x-ray detector used to terminate a radiographic exposure

photon - bundle of electromagnetic radiation that behaves like a particle, with an energy proportional to frequency

photopeak - signal produced in a scintillator camera crystal from a photoelectric absorption

photospot image - image of the output of an image intensifier

photostimulable phosphor - barium fluorohalide material used to capture radiographic images

piezoelectric effect - conversion of electric energy into mechanical motion (and vice versa)

pin cushion distortion - image distortion associated with image intensifiers

pinhole collimator - collimator used in NM for imaging small structures (e.g., thyroid)

pitch - term used in helical CT, defined as the ratio of table advancement per 360° rotation of x-ray tube to the total x-ray beam width

pixel - **pi**cture **el**ement comprising the smallest component of a digital image

planar imaging - projection imaging such as a chest x-ray where all tissues are superimposed on each other

pocket dosimeter - small device that can be worn to assess radiation doses using an instant (real-time) readout mechanism

point spread function (PSF) - image of a point source quantifying the degradation caused by the imaging system

Poisson distribution - random distribution in which the variance is equal to the mean value

positive predictive value - probability of having a disease given a positive diagnostic test result

positron emission tomography (PET) - nuclear medicine imaging modality that detects the annihilation radiation (511 keV gamma rays) from positrons

positron - particle identical to an electron but with a positive electric charge

potential energy - energy associated with the location of a particle at a high-energy potential, such as an electron at a cathode

power - rate of doing work (i.e., energy divided by time) measured in watt (W)

power Doppler - way of displaying frequency shift information in Doppler ultrasound that uses the number of frequency shifts, not their average value

primary transmission - fraction of an x-ray beam passing unattenuated through a patient or grid

progressive scan mode - method of TV scanning where all the lines are scanned successively

projection data - attenuation data set acquired in CT at one x-ray tube angle

protons - positively charged particles found in the nucleus

pulse height analyzer (PHA) - used in a scintillator camera to select energies that correspond to the photopeak and used to generate an NM image

pulse repetition frequency (PRF) - the number of ultrasound pulses generated by the transducer each second

pulse sequence - sequence of RF pulses and magnetic gradients used to produce MR images

pulse wave Doppler - Doppler imaging that compares the frequency shifts between emitted and reflected pulses

quantum mottle - image noise resulting from the discrete nature of x-ray photons

radiation weighting factor (w_R) - used to convert absorbed dose into equivalent dose

radiobiology - study of the effects of ionizing radiations on biological systems

radiochemical purity - a measure of chemical impurity assessed by thin-layer chromatography

radiofrequency (RF) coils - coils used to transmit RF pulses in MR and detect RF signals from patients

radiographic mottle - random fluctuations (noise) in an image with a *uniform* air kerma

radioisotopes - atoms with unstable nuclei

radiomics - derivation of quantitative diagnostic information (a feature) from medical images.

radionuclide - an unstable nuclide that decays exponentially

radionuclide purity - a measure of radioactive contaminants (other radionuclides)

radiopharmaceutical - chemical or pharmaceutical that is labeled with a radionuclide

radon (^{222}Ra) - radioactive gas produced when naturally occurring radium (^{226}Ra) decays; found at high levels in some home basements

RAID (redundant array of inexpensive disks) - computer data storage medium with rapid access time

random access memory (RAM) - volatile computer memory that loses information when the computer power supply is switched off

range - distance traveled by a charged particle in losing its energy

read-only memory (ROM) - permanent memory in computers

real-time ultrasound imaging - cross-sectional image updated 20 to 40 times per second, allowing motion to be followed

receiver operating characteristic (ROC) curve - curve that plots the true-positive fraction versus false-positive fraction and used to measure imaging performance

reciprocating grid - a grid that moves during a radiographic exposure, "smearing" the Pb lines

rectification - changing an alternating voltage to one polarity (i.e., AC to DC)

refraction - change of direction of any wave when moving from one medium to another

relative risk - model of cancer induction in which radiation dose increases the natural incidence by a fixed percentage

repetition time (TR) - time period over which an MR pulse sequence is repeated

resolution (spatial) - ability to see small details (e.g., edges) in images

reverberation - artifact in ultrasound caused by multiple echoes from parallel tissue interfaces

ring artifact - artifact resembling rings produced in CT and SPECT

roentgen (R) - unit of exposure that measures charge liberated in air

scatter - radiation deflected from its initial direction

scintillator - material that emits light after absorption of radiation

secular equilibrium - occurs after four half-lives of the daughter with a *long lived parent* radionuclide

sensitivity - the ability of a test to detect disease

septal penetration - gamma rays that penetrate the collimator septa

shim coils - current-carrying coils used in MR to improve the magnetic field homogeneity

signal-to-noise ratio (SNR) - a measure image quality that depends on the diagnostic task

skin dose (peak) - the highest absorbed dose to any region of a patient's skin in interventional radiology

slice sensitivity profile - broadening of CT slice thickness along the patient axis

somatic effects - radiation effects such as cancer that occur in the exposed individual

spatial frequency - sinusoidal signal intensity expressed in line pairs or cycles per millimeter

spatial peak temporal average intensity (I_{SPTA}) - ultrasound intensity obtained at a single point and averaged over many pulses, which quantifies thermal effects

spatial resolution - ability to discriminate between two adjacent high-contrast objects

specificity - the ability to identify the absence of disease

SPECT - single-photon emission computed tomography, which is tomographic imaging technique where a scintillator camera is rotated around a patient

spectroscopy - magnetic resonance analysis of the chemical species (e.g., ^{31}P may be present as adenosine triphosphate, inorganic phosphorus, and so on)

spectrum - display of the number (photons, beta particles, etc.) that are present at each energy

specular reflection - ultrasound reflections from large smooth surfaces

spin echo (SE) - MR pulse sequence in which echoes are generated by rephasing spins in the transverse plane

spot film - radiographic image taken using a digital detector instead of the fluoroscopy imaging chain

standard deviation - a measure of the spread of a statistical distribution

stochastic effect - radiation effect such as carcinogenesis and genetic effects whose occurrence depends on the absorbed dose

streak artifacts - CT artifacts caused by patient motion or metallic implants

strong force - holds the nucleus of an atom together

subject contrast - difference in x-ray beam intensities emerging from a lesion and adjacent background tissues

superconductivity - property of zero electrical resistance when cooled to very low temperatures

superparamagnetism - magnetic property similar to ferromagnetism but occurring in small aggregates of atoms (single domains)

T1 - spin lattice or longitudinal relaxation time

T2 - spin-spin or transverse relaxation time

T2* - rapid reduction of free induction decay signals due to magnetic field inhomogeneities

TE (time to echo) - time from the initial 90° radiofrequency pulse to the echo signal in magnetic resonance spin-echo sequences

tenth-value layer (TVL) - thickness of material needed to reduce an x-ray beam intensity to 10% of its initial value

teratogenic - malformations of the embryo or fetus

thermoluminescent dosimeter (TLD) - solid-state dosimeter that, after exposure to x-rays, emits light when heated

threshold dose - dose below which deterministic radiation effects do not occur

TI - time to inversion or the time interval between the initial 180° pulse and subsequent 90° radiofrequency pulse in an inversion recovery pulse sequence

tissue magnetization - equilibrium magnetization in a tissue in the presence of a fixed external magnetic field

tomography - imaging that generates slices rather than projections

TR - repetition time in magnetic resonance pulse sequences

transducer - device that converts mechanical energy into electric current and vice versa

transformer - device used to increase or decrease voltages

transient equilibrium - equilibrium between the parent and daughter radionuclides in which the *parent half-life is short*

transverse magnetization - magnetization vector oriented in a plane perpendicular to the main external magnetic field in magnetic resonance

tungsten (W) - heavy atom with a high atomic number (74) that is used as a target material in x-ray tubes

ultrasound - sound waves with frequencies in excess of 20 kHz and used in medical imaging and therapy

UNSCEAR - United Nations Scientific Committee on the Effects of Atomic Radiation is a UN body that assesses radiation doses received by populations.

unsharp masking - image processing method used to enhance the visibility of edges

unstable nuclei - nuclei that will decay by emission of radiation in the form of varying forms of energy (alpha, beta, or gamma)

vignetting - peripheral reduction of light intensity in image intensifiers

veiling glare - loss of contrast due to light scattering

voxel - volume element obtained from the product of pixel size and the image section thickness

watt (W) - unit of power (1 W = 1 J/s)

waveform ripple - temporal variation in voltage across an x-ray tube

wavelength - the distance between two consecutive crests of a wave

weight - gravitational attractive force due to gravity

work - product of force and distance, measured in joule

x-rays - high-frequency (energetic) electromagnetic radiation produced using electrons

Bibliography

General Radiologic Imaging

Bushberg JT, Seibert JA, Leidholdt EM, Boone JM. *The Essential Physics of Medical Imaging.* 4th ed. Lippincott, Williams & Wilkins; 2020.

Bushong SC. *Radiologic Science for Technologists: Physical, Biology, and Protection.* 10th ed. CV Mosby; 2013.

Carlton RR, Adler AM. *Principles of Radiographic Imaging: An Art and a Science.* 6th ed. Cengage Learning (Clifton Park, NY); 2019.

Hall EJ, Giaccia A. *Radiobiology for the Radiologist.* 8th ed. Lippincott, Williams & Wilkins; 2018.

Klein J, Brant WE, Helms CA, Vinson EN. *Brant and Helms' Fundamentals of Diagnostic Radiology.* 5th ed. Lippincott Williams & Wilkins; 2018.

Orth D. *Essentials of Radiologic Science.* 2nd ed. Lippincott Williams & Wilkins; 2017.

Vosper M, England A, Major V, Graham DT. *Graham's Principles and Applications of Radiological Physics.* 7th ed. Elsiever; 2019.

Yucel-Finn A, McKiddie F, Prescott S, Bentley R. *Farr's Physics for Medical Imaging.* 3rd ed. Elsevier; 2023.

Breast Imaging

American College of Radiology (ACR). *Mammography Quality Control Manual.* ACR; 2018.

Andolina VF, Lillé SL. *Mammographic Imaging: A Practical Guide.* 3rd ed. Lippincott Williams & Wilkins; 2010.

Computed Tomography

Romans LE. *Computer Tomography for Technologists: Exam Review.* 2nd ed. Lippincott Williams & Wilkins; 2018.

Romans LE. *Computer Tomography for Technologists: A Comprehensive Text.* Lippincott Williams & Wilkins; 2018.

Seeram E. *Computed Tomography: Physical Principles, Clinical Applications, and Quality Control.* 3rd ed. WB Saunders; 2009.

Szczykutowicz TP. *The CT Handbook: Optimizing Protocols for Today's Feature-Rich Scanners.* American Association of Physicists in Medicine; 2020.

Nuclear Medicine

Chandra R, Rahmim A. *Nuclear Medicine Physics: The Basic.* 8th ed. Lippincott Williams & Wilkins; 2017.

Cherry SR, Sorensen JA, Phelps ME. *Physics in Nuclear Medicine.* 4th ed. Saunders; 2012.

Gibbons JP. *Khan's The Physics of Radiation Therapy.* 6th ed. Wolters Kluwer Health, Lippincott Williams & Wilkins; 2019.

Mettler FA, Guibertean MJ. *Essentials of Nuclear Medicine Imaging.* 7th ed. WB Saunders; 2018.

Powsner RA, Palmer MR, Powsner ER. *Essentials of Nuclear Medicine Physics, Instrumentation, and Radiobiology.* 4th ed. Wiley-Blackwell; 2021.

Ultrasound

de Jong MR. *Sonography Scanning: Principles and Protocols.* 5th ed. Elsevier; 2020.

Hoskins PR, Martin M, Thrush A. *Diagnostic Ultrasound: Physics and Equipment.* 2nd ed. Cambridge University Press; 2010.

Kremkau FW. *Sonography Principles and Instruments.* 10th ed. Saunders, Elsevier; 2019.

Odwin CS, Fleischer AC, Berdejo GL. *Lange Review: Ultrasonography Examination.* 5th ed. McGraw-Hill; 2021.

Penny SM, Fox TB. *Examination Review for Ultrasound: SPI—Sonographic Principles & Instrumentation.* 2nd ed. Wolters Kluwer Health, Lippincott Williams & Wilkins; 2017.

Pozniak MA, Allan PL. *Clinical Doppler Ultrasound.* 3rd ed. Churchill Livingstone, Elsevier; 2014.

Magnetic Resonance

Brown MA, Semelka RC. *MRI: Basic Principles and Applications.* 4th ed. Wiley-Blackwell; 2010.

Hashemi RH, Bradley WG, Lisanti CJ. *MRI: The Basics*. 4th ed. Wolters Kluwer Health; 2017.

McRobbie DW, Moore EA, Graves MJ. *MRI From Picture to Proton*. 3rd ed. Cambridge University Press; 2018.

Runge VM, Wolfgang RN, Schmeets SH. *The Physics of Clinical MR Taught Through Images*. 4th ed. Thieme; 2018.

Westbrook C, Talbot J. *MRI in Practice*. 5th ed. Wiley-Blackwell; 2018.

Appendices

Selected Radiologic Physics Websites

American Association of Physicists in Medicine (AAPM): www.aapm.org
American Board of Radiology (ABR): www.theabr.org
American College of Radiology (ACR): www.acr.org
American Institute of Ultrasound in Medicine (AIUM): www.aium.org
American Journal of Roentgenology (AJR): www.ajronline.org
American Society of Radiologic Technologists (ASRT): www.asrt.org
Conference of Radiation Control Program Directors (CRCPD): www.crcpd.org
Food and Drug Administration (FDA): www.fda.gov
Health Physics Society (HPS): www.hps.org
Image Gently: https://imagegently.org
Image Wisely: www.imagewisely.org
International Commission on Non-Ionizing Radiation Protection (ICNIRP): www.icnirp.de
International Commission on Radiation Units and Measurements (ICRU): www.icru.org
International Commission on Radiological Protection (ICRP): www.icrp.org
National Council on Radiation Protection and Measurements (NCRP): www.ncrponline.org
Radiation Research Society: www.radres.org
RadioGraphics and *Radiology* journals: https://pubs.rsna.org/
Radiological Society of North America (RSNA): www.rsna.org
Society for Imaging Informatics in Medicine (SIIM): www.siim.org
Society of Nuclear Medicine and Molecular Imaging (SNMMI): www.snm.org
The Joint Commission: www.jointcommission.org
U.S. National Institute of Standards and Technology (NIST): www.nist.gov
U.S. Nuclear Regulatory Commission (NRC): www.nrc.gov

TABLE I — Summary of SI and Non-SI Units for General Quantities

Quantity	SI Unit	Non-SI Unit
Length	meter (m)	foot (ft)
Mass	kilogram (kg)	—
Time	second (s)	—
Electrical current	ampere (A)	—
Amount of substance	mole (mol)	—
Frequency	hertz (Hz)	—
Force	newton (N)	dyne
Energy	joule (J)	erg
Power	watt (W)	erg/s
Electrical charge	coulomb (C)	ESU
Electrical potential	volt (V)	—
Magnetic field strength	tesla (T)	gauss (G)

Although commonly called Magnetic Field Strength in Medical Physics, this is more correctly called magnetic flux density.

331

TABLE II	Summary of Prefix Names and Magnitudes	
Prefix Name	Symbol	Magnitude
Exa	E	10^{18}
peta	P	10^{15}
tera	T	10^{12}
giga	G	10^9
mega	M	10^6
kilo	k	10^3
hecto	h	10^2
deca	da	10
deci	d	10^{-1}
centi	c	10^{-2}
milli	m	10^{-3}
micro	μ	10^{-6}
nano	n	10^{-9}
pico	p	10^{-12}
femto	f	10^{-15}
atto	a	10^{-18}

TABLE III	Summary of Units for Radiologic Quantities			
Quantity	SI Unit	Non-SI Unit	SI to Non-SI Conversions	Non-SI to SI Conversions
Air kerma	gray (J/kg)	roentgen	1 Gy = 114 R	1 R = 8.76 mGy
Absorbed dose	gray (J/kg)	rad (100 erg/g)	1 Gy = 100 rad	1 rad = 10 mGy
Equivalent dose	sievert	rem	1 Sv = 100 rem	1 rem = 10 mSv
Activity	becquerel	curie	1 MBq = 27 μCi	1 mCi = 37 MBq

TABLE IV	Summary of Units for Photometric[a] Quantities		
Quantity	SI Unit	Non-SI Unit	To Convert Non-SI Units to SI Units
Luminance[b] (light scattered or emitted by a surface)	cd/m² (nit)	foot-lamberts	foot-lamberts × 3.43 = cd/m²
Illuminance (light falling on a surface)	lumen/m² (lux)	foot-candles	foot-candles × 10.8 = lumen/m²

[a]Photometric units take into account the spectral sensitivity of the eye.
[b]One lux falling on a perfectly diffusing surface with no absorption produces a luminance of $1/\pi$ cd/m².

TABLE V	Approximate Illuminance Values
Illuminance (lux)	Conditions
5,000	Full daylight
500	Overcast day
250	Average office
20	Radiologist reading room
5	Twilight
0.1	Moonlight
0.001	Starlight

Index